The 2010 Year Book Series

Year Book of Anesthesiology and Pain Management™: Drs Chestnut, Abram, Black, Gravlee, Lien, Mathru and Roizen

Year Book of Cardiology®: Drs Gersh, Cheitlin, Elliott, Gold, Graham, and Suri

Year Book of Critical Care Medicine®: Drs Dellinger, Parrillo, Balk, Dorman, Dries, and Zanotti-Cavazzoni

Year Book of Dermatology and Dermatologic Surgery™: Dr Del Rosso

Year Book of Diagnostic Radiology®: Drs Osborn, Abbara, Birdwell, Elster, Manaster, Oestreich, Offiah, Rosado de Christenson, and Walker

Year Book of Emergency Medicine®: Drs Hamilton, Bruno, Handly, Mullin, Quintana, and Ramoska

Year Book of Endocrinology®: Drs Schott, Apovian, Clarke, Eugster, Ludlam, Meikle, Ovalle, Schinner, Schteingart, and Toth

Year Book of Gastroenterology™: Drs Talley, Ambikaipaker, Bollipo, DeVault, Harnois, Pearson, Picco, Rombeau, Scolapio, and Smith

Year Book of Hand and Upper Limb Surgery®: Drs Yao and Steinmann

Year Book of Medicine®: Drs Barker, Berney, Garrick, Gersh, Khardori, LeRoith, Talley, and Thigpen

Year Book of Neonatal and Perinatal Medicine®: Drs Fanaroff, Benitz, Donn, Neu, Papile, Polin, and van Marter

Year Book of Neurology and Neurosurgery®: Drs Klimo and Rabinstein

Year Book of Obstetrics, Gynecology, and Women's Health®: Drs Dungan and Shulman

Year Book of Oncology®: Drs Arceci, Bauer, Gordon, Lawton, and Thigpen

Year Book of Ophthalmology®: Drs Rapuano, Cohen, Flanders, Hammersmith, Milman, Myers, Nelson, Penne, Pyfer, Sergott, Shields, and Vander

Year Book of Orthopedics®: Drs Morrey, Beauchamp, Huddleston, Swiontkowski, and Trigg

Year Book of Otolaryngology-Head and Neck Surgery®: Drs Sindwani, Balough, Franco, Gapany, and Mitchell

Year Book of Pathology and Laboratory Medicine®: Drs Raab, Parwani, Bejarano, and Bissell

Year Book of Pediatrics®: Dr Stockman

2010 YEAR BOOK OF NEUROLOGY AND NEUROSURGERY®

Year Book of Plastic and Aesthetic Surgery™: Drs Miller, Gosain, Gurtner, Gutowski, Ruberg, Salisbury, and Smith

Year Book of Psychiatry and Applied Mental Health®: Drs Talbott, Ballenger, Buckley, Frances, Krupnick, and Mack

Year Book of Pulmonary Disease®: Drs Barker, Jones, Maurer, Raza, Tanoue, and Willsie

Year Book of Sports Medicine®: Drs Shephard, Cantu, Feldman, Jankowski, Khan, Lebrun, Nieman, Pierrynowski, and Rowland

Year Book of Surgery®: Drs Copeland, Behrns, Daly, Eberlein, Fahey, Huber, Jones, Mozingo, and Pruett

Year Book of Urology®: Drs Andriole and Coplen

Year Book of Vascular Surgery®: Drs Moneta, Gillespie, Starnes, and Watkins

2010
The Year Book of NEUROLOGY AND NEUROSURGERY®

"Published without interruption since 1902"

Neurology

Editor

Alejandro Rabinstein, MD

Associate Professor of Neurology, Department of Neurology, Mayo Clinic College of Medicine, Rochester, Minnesota

Neurosurgery

Editor

Paul Klimo, Jr, MD, MPH

Neurosurgeon, Semmes-Murphey Neurologic and Spine Institute, Memphis, Tennessee

ELSEVIER
MOSBY

ELSEVIER
MOSBY

Vice President, Continuity: Kimberly Murphy
Editor: Ruth Malwitz
Supervisor, Electronic Year Books: Donna M. Skelton
Electronic Article Manager: Jennifer C. Pitts
Illustrations and Permissions Coordinator: Dawn Vohsen

2010 EDITION

Composition by TnQ Books and Journals Pvt Ltd, India

Editorial Office:
Elsevier
1600 John F. Kennedy Blvd.
Suite 1800
Philadelphia, PA 19103-2899

International Standard Serial Number: 0513-5117
International Standard Book Number: 978-0-323-06835-2

Associate Editors

Adam S. Arthur, MD, MPH

Department of Neurosurgery, the University of Tennessee and Semmes-Murphey Clinic, Memphis, Tennessee

John P. Blass, MD, PhD

Professor of Neurology, Cornell University, Burke Rehabilitation Hospital, White Plains, New York

Galen N. Breningstall, MD

Pediatric Neurology, Gillette Children's Specialty Healthcare, St Paul, Minnesota

Martin J. Brodie, MD, FRCP

Director, Epilepsy Unit, Western Infirmary, Glasgow, Scotland

Brian A. Crum, MD

Assistant Professor of Neurology, Department of Neurology, Mayo Clinic, Rochester, Minnesota

Paul A. House, MD

Assistant Professor of Neurosurgery, Department of Neurosurgery, University of Utah, Hospitals and Clinics, Salt Lake City, Utah

Jacqueline Leavitt, MD

Associate Professor of Ophthalmology, Department of Ophthalmology, Mayo Clinic, Rochester, Minnesota

James K. Liu, MD

Assistant Professor of Neurosurgery and Director of Skull Base and Pituitary Surgery, Department of Neurological Surgery, UMDNJ-New Jersey Medical School, Neurological Institute of New Jersey, Newark, New Jersey

Alexander M. McKinney IV, MD

Associate Professor of Radiology, Department of Radiology, University of Minnesota School of Medicine, Minneapolis, Minnesota

Bruce Nolan, MD, FACP, FAASM

Associate Professor of Neurology and Psychiatry, Sleep Center Medical Director, UHealth Sleep Medicine Program, Leonard M. Miller School of Medicine/University of Miami, Miami, Florida

Ashok Panagariya, MD, DM

Professor and Head, Department of Neurology, SMS University Hospital and Medical College, Jaipur, India

Spyridon Papapetropoulos, MD, PhD

Voluntary Associate Professor, Department of Neurology, University of Miami Leonard M. Miller School of Medicine, Miami, Florida

Brian T. Ragel, MD

Assistant Professor of Neurosurgery, Oregon Health Sciences University, Portland, Oregon

Ganesh Rao, MD
Assistant Professor of Neurosurgery, the University of Texas MD Anderson Cancer Center, Houston, Texas

Ron Riesenburger, MD
Assistant Professor of Neurosurgery, Tufts Medical Center, Boston, Massachusetts

Ronald J. Tusa, MD, PhD
Professor of Neurology, Otolaryngology and Ophthalmology, Dizziness and Balance Center, Emory University, Atlanta, Georgia

Joon Uhm, MD
Assistant Professor of Neurology, Departments of Neurology and Oncology, Mayo Clinic, Rochester, Minnesota

Diederik van de Beek, MD, PhD
Neurologist, Academic Medical Center, University of Amsterdam, Amsterdam, The Netherlands

Ashok Verma, MD, DM, MBA
Professor of Neurology; Medical Director, Kessenich Family MDA-ALS Center, Leonard M. Miller School of Medicine/University of Miami; Attending Neurologist, Jackson Memorial Hospital, Miami, Florida

Table of Contents

Journals Represented

Journals represented in this YEAR BOOK are listed below.

Acta Ophthalmologica
AJNR American Journal of Neuroradiology
AJR American Journal of Roentgenology
American Journal of Hypertension
American Journal of Neuroradiology
American Journal of Obstetrics and Gynecology
Anesthesia & Analgesia
Annals of Epidemiology
Annals of Neurology
Archives of General Psychiatry
Archives of Neurology
Archives of Surgery
Biochemistry
Biomaterials
Brain
Brain Pathology
Brain Research Bulletin
Cancer Research
Circulation Cardiovascular Quality and Outcomes
Clinical Cancer Research
Clinical Infectious Diseases
Clinical Pediatrics
Diabetes
Epilepsia
European Journal of Heart Failure
European Journal of Paediatric Neurology
European Radiology
European Respiratory Journal
General Hospital Psychiatry
Headache
International Journal of Radiation Oncology Biology Physics
Journal of Antimicrobial Chemotherapy
Journal of Clinical Neuroscience
Journal of Clinical Oncology
Journal of Laryngology and Otology
Journal of Lipid Research
Journal of Nervous and Mental Disease
Journal of Neurology
Journal of Neurology Neurosurgery and Psychiatry
Journal of Neurosurgery
Journal of Neurosurgery Pediatrics
Journal of Neurosurgery Spine
Journal of Pharmacology and Experimental Therapeutics
Journal of the American College of Cardiology
Journal of the American Medical Association
Journal of the Neurological Sciences
Journal of Thoracic and Cardiovascular Surgery

Lancet
Lancet Neurology
Laryngoscope
Medicine and Science in Sports and Exercise
MMWR Morbidity and Mortality Weekly Report
Muscle & Nerve
Nature
Neurobiology of Aging
Neurology
Neuro-Oncology
Neurosurgery
New England Journal of Medicine
Nursing Research
Ophthalmology
Otolaryngology-Head and Neck Surgery
Otology & Neurotology
Pain
Pediatric Neurology
Pediatric Research
Pediatrics
Proceedings of the National Academy of Sciences of the United States of America
Radiology
Sleep
Spine
Stroke

Standard Abbreviations

The following terms are abbreviated in this edition: acquired immunodeficiency syndrome (AIDS), cardiopulmonary resuscitation (CPR), central nervous system (CNS), cerebrospinal fluid (CSF), computed tomography (CT), deoxyribonucleic acid (DNA), electrocardiography (ECG), health maintenance organization (HMO), human immunodeficiency virus (HIV), intensive care unit (ICU), intramuscular (IM), intravenous (IV), magnetic resonance (MR) imaging (MRI), ultrasound (US), and ribonucleic acid (RNA).

Note

The Year Book of Neurology and Neurosurgery is a literature survey service providing abstracts of articles published in the professional literature. Every effort is made to assure the accuracy of the information presented in these pages. Neither the editors nor the publisher of the Year Book of Neurology and Neurosurgery can be responsible for errors in the original materials. The editors' comments are their own opinions. Mention of specific products within this publication does not constitute endorsement.

To facilitate the use of the Year Book of Neurology and Neurosurgery as a reference tool, all illustrations and tables included in this publication are now identified as they appear in the original article. This change is meant to help the reader recognize that any illustration or table appearing in the Year Book of Neurology and Neurosurgery may be only one of many in the original article. For this reason, figure and table numbers will often appear to be out of sequence within the Year Book of Neurology and Neurosurgery.

NEUROLOGY

ALEJANDRO RABINSTEIN, MD

1 Alzheimer's Disease and Dementia

Alzheimer's disease phenotypes and genotypes associated with mutations in presenilin 2

Jayadev S, Leverenz JB, Steinbart E, et al (Univ of Washington, Seattle; et al)
Brain 133:1143-1154, 2010

Mutations in presenilin 2 are rare causes of early onset familial Alzheimer's disease. Eighteen presenilin 2 mutations have been reported, although not all have been confirmed pathogenic. Much remains to be learned about the range of phenotypes associated with these mutations. We have analysed our unique collection of 146 affected cases in 11 Volga German families, 101 who are likely to have the same N141I mutation in presenilin 2 (54 genotyped confirmed). We have also assessed the detailed neuropathologic findings in 18 autopsies from these families and reviewed the world's literature on other presenilin 2 mutations; presenting a novel mutation that is predicted to lead to a premature truncation codon. Seven presenilin 2 mutations reported in the literature have strong evidence for pathogenicity whereas others may be benign polymorphisms. One hundred and one affected persons, with sufficient historical information from the Volga German pedigrees (N141I mutation), had a mean onset age of 53.7 years ± 7.8 (range 39–75) and mean age at death of 64.2 years ± 9.8 (range 43–88). These figures overlap with and generally fall between the results from the subjects in our centre who have late onset familial Alzheimer's disease or mutations in presenilin 1. Seizures were noted in 20 (30) of 64 subjects with detailed medical records. Two mutation carriers lived beyond age 80 without developing dementia, representing uncommon examples of decreased penetrance. Two persons had severe amyloid angiopathy and haemorrhagic stroke. Eighteen cases had detailed histopathology available and analysed at our institution. Braak stage was five or six, amyloid angiopathy and neuritic plaques were common and more than 75 had Lewy bodies in the amygdala. TAR DNA-binding protein-43 inclusions were uncommon. In addition, a 58-year-old female with a 2 year course of cognitive decline and no family history of dementia has abnormal fludeoxyglucose-positron emission tomography imaging and a novel 2 base pair deletion in presenilin 2 at nucleotide 342/343, predicted to produce a frame-shift and premature termination. We conclude that mutations in presenilin 2 are rare with only seven being well documented in the literature. The best studied N141I mutation produces an Alzheimer's disease phenotype with a wide range of onset ages overlapping both early and late onset Alzheimer's disease, often associated with seizures, high penetrance and typical Alzheimer's disease neuropathology. A novel premature termination mutation supports loss of function or haploinsufficiency as pathogenic mechanisms in presenilin 2 associated Alzheimer's disease.

▶ This elegant scholarly review from Seattle points out the wide range of clinical phenotypes associated with mutations in presenilin 2. The range is disconcertingly wide even within the Volga German families, who presumably have the same mutation; some patients are clinically normal even though they are older than 80 years. The history of inborn errors illustrates that tight relationships between mutations in specific genes and specific clinical syndromes often reflect observer bias. Specific genes were closely associated with specific syndromes such as Tay Sachs disease when the genes (or earlier the gene product) were examined mainly or only in children with the syndrome. As genetic screening became technically more feasible and was more widely applied to unselected populations, the varieties of clinical presentation associated with mutations in the responsible genes have in general widened. It is not surprising to see such wide variation in clinical presentation of a gene predisposing to a disorder, which does not generally present clinically until later life.

J. P. Blass, MD, PhD

Association Between Acute Care and Critical Illness Hospitalization and Cognitive Function in Older Adults

Ehlenbach WJ, Hough CL, Crane PK, et al (Univ of Washington, Seattle; et al)
JAMA 303:763-770, 2010

Context.—Studies suggest that many survivors of critical illness experience long-term cognitive impairment but have not included premorbid measures of cognitive functioning and have not evaluated risk for dementia associated with critical illness.

Objectives.—To determine whether decline in cognitive function was greater among older individuals who experienced acute care or critical illness hospitalizations relative to those not hospitalized and to determine whether the risk for incident dementia differed by these exposures.

Design, Setting, and Participants.—Analysis of data from a prospective cohort study from 1994 through 2007 comprising 2929 individuals 65 years old and older without dementia at baseline residing in the community in the Seattle area and belonging to the Group Health Cooperative. Participants with 2 or more study visits were included, and those who had a hospitalization for a diagnosis of primary brain injury were censored at the time of hospitalization. Individuals were screened with the Cognitive Abilities Screening Instrument (CASI) (score range, 0-100) every 2 years at follow-up visits, and those with a score less than 86 underwent a clinical examination for dementia.

Main Outcome Measures.—Score on the CASI at follow-up study visits and incident dementia diagnosed in study participants, adjusted for baseline cognitive scores, age, and other risk factors.

Results.—During a mean (SD) follow-up of 6.1 (3.2) years, 1601 participants had no hospitalization, 1287 had 1 or more noncritical illness hospitalizations, and 41 had 1 or more critical illness hospitalizations. The CASI score was assessed more than 45 days after discharge for 94.3% of participants. Adjusted CASI scores averaged 1.01 points lower for visits following acute care illness hospitalization compared with follow-up visits not following any hospitalization (95% confidence interval [CI], −1.33 to −0.70; $P < .001$) and 2.14 points lower on average for visits following critical illness hospitalization (95% CI, −4.24 to −0.03; $P = .047$). There were 146 cases of dementia among those not hospitalized, 228 cases of dementia among those with 1 or more noncritical illness hospitalizations, and 5 cases of dementia among those with 1 or more critical illness hospitalizations. The adjusted hazard ratio for incident dementia was 1.4 following a noncritical illness hospitalization (95% CI, 1.1 to 1.7; $P = .001$) and 2.3 following a critical illness hospitalization (95% CI, 0.9 to 5.7; $P = .09$).

Conclusions.—Among a cohort of older adults without dementia at baseline, those who experienced acute care hospitalization and critical illness hospitalization had a greater likelihood of cognitive decline compared with those who had no hospitalization. Noncritical illness hospitalization was significantly associated with the development of dementia.

▶ The families of older patients who have gone through a severe medical illness often perceive the patients as not having come back all the way, mentally or spiritually. The patients themselves and their doctors often come to the same conclusion. This meticulous epidemiological study from the University of Washington in Seattle documents the accuracy of this impression. A major medical illness does not condemn an elderly patient to developing dementia but does significantly increase the risk.

J. P. Blass, MD, PhD

Association Between Lifetime Cigarette Smoking and Lewy Body Accumulation

Tsuang D, Larson EB, Li G, et al (Univ of Washington, Seattle)

Brain Pathol 20:412-418, 2010

Cigarette smoking has been associated repeatedly in observational studies with decreased risk of Parkinson's disease (PD), but its relationship to the risk of dementia or Alzheimer's disease (AD) is inconsistent. All of these studies have used clinical diagnoses of disease. We tested the hypothesis that lifetime cigarette use might be associated with reduced risk of neuropathologic changes of Lewy-related pathology (LRP) in multiple brain regions or with reduced risk of consensus neuropathologic changes of AD in a prospective community-based study of brain aging and dementia, the Adult Changes in Thought (ACT) study. We observed that heavy lifetime cigarette smoking (>50 pack years) was associated with significantly reduced relative risk (RR) for LRP, but not AD-type pathologic changes, after correcting for selection bias, and with significantly reduced frequency of LRP in the substantia nigra. These findings are the first of which we are aware to associate reduced LRP in human brain with any exposure, and substantiate observational studies that have associated cigarette smoking with reduced risk of PD. Although cigarette smoking is too toxic to suggest as a treatment, if confirmed, these findings may guide future therapeutic strategies that attempt to suppress LRP in human brain by other means.

▶ This population-based epidemiological study provides further documentation that smoking cigarettes protects against Parkinson disease (PD). Cigarette smoking is an unhealthy habit, and the authors do not recommend it. They do recommend research to find out what it is about cigarette smoking that appears to protect against PD. Unfortunately, one obvious candidate—nicotine—appears to have only minor clinical benefits in established PD.[1]

J. P. Blass, MD, PhD

Reference

1. Quik M, O'Leary K, Tanner CM. Nicotine and Parkinson's disease: implications for therapy. *Mov Disord.* 2008;23:1641-1652.

Brain tissue volumes in relation to cognitive function and risk of dementia

Ikram MA, Vrooman HA, Vernooij MW, et al (Erasmus MC Univ Med Ctr, Rotterdam, The Netherlands)

Neurobiol Aging 31:378-386, 2010

We investigated in a population-based cohort study the association of global and lobar brain tissue volumes with specific cognitive domains and risk of dementia. Participants ($n = 490$; 60–90 years) were non-demented at baseline (1995–1996). From baseline brain MRI-scans we obtained global and lobar volumes of CSF, GM, normal WM, white matter lesions and hippocampus. We performed neuropsychological testing at baseline to assess information processing speed, executive function, memory function and global cognitive function. Participants were followed for incident dementia until January 1, 2005. Larger volumes of CSF and WML were associated with worse performance on all neuropsychological tests, and an increased risk of dementia. Smaller WM volume was related to poorer information processing speed and executive function. In contrast, smaller GM volume was associated with worse memory function and increased risk of dementia. When investigating lobar GM volumes, we found that hippocampal volume and temporal GM volume were most strongly associated with risk of dementia, even in persons without objective and subjective cognitive deficits at baseline, followed by frontal and parietal GM volumes.

▶ This meticulous, prospective, epidemiological study provides evidence that losing brain substance is likely to impair mentation. The more brain one loses, the more prominent the impairment is likely to be. How much brain substance must be lost to cause clinically significant problems depends in part on how much—and what—the patient has to do. Those are points neurologists and psychiatrists will have little trouble in accepting. Losing gray matter is more likely to cause impairment than losing white matter, and losing gray matter in the areas of the brain associated with memory is particularly likely to impair mentation. Those areas include the mesial temporal cortex and specifically the hippocampus. On the other hand, losing white matter can also cause dementia, as in Binswanger disease.

J. P. Blass, MD, PhD

Cognitive deficits in chronic heart failure

Pressler SJ, Subramanian U, Kareken D, et al (Univ of Michigan, Ann Arbor)
Nurs Res 59:127-139, 2010

Background.—Patients with heart failure (HF) have been found to have cognitive deficits, but it remains unclear whether these deficits are associated with HF or with aging or comorbid conditions common in HF.

Objectives.—The purpose of this study was (a) to determine the types, the frequency, and the severity of cognitive deficits among patients with chronic HF compared with age- and education-matched healthy participants and participants with major medical conditions other than HF, and (b) to evaluate the relationships between HF severity, age, and comorbidities and cognitive deficits.

Methods.—A sample of 414 participants completed the study (249 HF patients, 63 healthy and 102 medical participants). The HF patients completed measures of HF severity, comorbidity (multiple comorbidity, depressive symptoms), and neuropsychological functioning. Blood pressure and oxygen saturation were assessed at interview; clinical variables were abstracted from records. Participants in the comparison groups completed the same measures as the HF patients except those specific to HF.

Results.—Compared with the healthy and medical participants, HF patients had poorer memory, psychomotor speed, and executive function. Significantly more HF patients (24%) had deficits in three or more domains. Higher (worse) HF severity was associated with more cognitive deficits; HF severity interacted with age to explain deficits in executive function. Surprisingly, men with HF had poorer memory, psychomotor speed, and visuospatial recall ability than women. Multiple comorbidity, hypertension, depressive symptoms, and medications were not associated with cognitive deficits in this sample.

Discussion.—HF results in losses in memory, psychomotor speed, and executive function in almost one fourth of patients. Patients with more severe HF are at risk for cognitive deficits. Older patients with more severe HF may have more problems in executive function, and men with HF may be at increased risk for cognitive deficits. Studies are urgently needed to identify the mechanisms for the cognitive deficits in HF and to test innovative interventions to prevent cognitive loss and decline.

▶ This article from the nursing literature documents that perhaps a quarter of patients with chronic heart failure have problems with cognition. Higher heart failure severity and advanced age increase the risk. This is a phenomenon with which nurses and physicians are familiar. Surprisingly, there are articles in the medical literature that deny the existence of this syndrome. They depend on drawing conclusions from mental testing in all patients with heart failure, that is, from the majority who do not have mental problems and the minority who do have mental problems. This is a classic error in statistical analysis—losing a significant subgroup by analyzing group data from a nonhomogeneous sample. (The cliché is: the correct statistical view of 9 virgins and a pregnant woman is not that each of the virgins are one-tenth pregnant and the pregnant woman is nine-tenths a virgin.) For the subgroup of patients with heart failure who have cardiac dementia and for those caring for them, the mental problems are significant.

J. P. Blass, MD, PhD

Does cognitive impairment predict poor self-care in patients with heart failure?

Cameron J, Worrall-Carter L, Page K, et al (Australian Catholic Univ, Melbourne, Australia; St Vincent's/ACU Centre for Nursing Res, Fitzroy, Melbourne, Australia; et al)

Eur J Heart Fail 12:508-515, 2010

Aims.—Cognitive impairment occurs often in patients with chronic heart failure (CHF) and may contribute to sub-optimal self-care. This study aimed to test the impact of cognitive impairment on self-care.

Methods and Results.—In 93 consecutive patients hospitalized with CHF, self-care (Self-Care of Heart Failure Index) was assessed. Multiple regression analysis was used to test a model of variables hypothesized to predict self-care maintenance, management, and confidence. Variables in the model were mild cognitive impairment (MCI; Mini-Mental State Exam and Montreal Cognitive Assessment), depressive symptoms (Cardiac Depression Scale), age, gender, social isolation, education level, new diagnosis, and co-morbid illnesses. Sixty-eight patients (75%) were coded as having MCI and had significantly lower self-care management ($\eta^2 = 0.07$, $P < 0.01$) and self-confidence scores ($\eta^2 = 0.05$, $P < 0.05$). In multivariate analysis, MCI, co-morbidity index, and NYHA class III or IV explained 20% of the variance in self-care management ($P < 0.01$); MCI made the largest contribution explaining 9% of the variance. Increasing age and symptoms of depression explained 13% of the variance in self-care confidence scores ($P < 0.01$).

Conclusion.—Cognitive impairment, a hidden co-morbidity, may impede patients' ability to make appropriate self-care decisions. Screening for MCI may alert health professionals to those at greater risk of failed self-care.

▶ This reasonably large Australian study concludes that people with chronic heart failure tend to take poorer care of themselves if they are older, depressed, or cognitively impaired. The effects are, however, surprisingly small. Increasing age and depression together account for only 13% of the variance; minimal cognitive impairment accounts for only 9%. Physicians should, of course, stay on the lookout for these interferences with self-care in their patients with heart failure, even if they interfere less often with self-care than many of us have thought we found in our own practices.

J. P. Blass, MD, PhD

Enrichment of cholesterol in microdissected Alzheimer's disease senile plaques as assessed by mass spectrometry

Panchal M, Loeper J, Cossec J-C, et al (Hôpital de la Salpêtrière, Paris, France; Centre de Génétique Moléculaire, Gif-sur-Yvette, France; Centre de Recherche de l'ICM [UPMC, INSERM UMR S 975, CNRS UMR 7225], Paris, France; et al)

J Lipid Res 51:598-605, 2010

Extensive knowledge of the protein components of the senile plaques, one of the hallmark lesions of Alzheimer's disease, has been acquired over the years, but their lipid composition remains poorly known. Evidence suggests that cholesterol contributes to the pathogenesis of Alzheimer's disease. However, its presence within senile plaques has never been ascertained with analytic methods. Senile plaques were microdissected from sections of the isocortex in three Braak VI Alzheimer's disease cases and compared with a similar number of samples from the adjoining neuropil, free of amyloid-β peptide (Aβ) deposit. Two cases were apoε4/apoε3, and one case was apoε3/apoε3. A known quantity of ^{13}C-labeled cholesterol was added to the samples as a standard. After hexane extraction, cholesterol content was analyzed by liquid chromatography coupled with electrospray ionization mass spectrometry. The mean concentration of free cholesterol was 4.25 ± 0.1 attomoles/μm^3 in the senile plaques and 2.2 ± 0.49 attomoles/μm^3 in the neuropil ($t = 4.41$, $P < 0.0009$). The quantity of free cholesterol per senile plaque (67 ± 16 femtomol) is similar to the published quantity of Aβ peptide. The highly significant increase in the cholesterol concentration, associated with the increased risk of Alzheimer's disease linked to the apoε4 allele, suggests new pathogenetic mechanisms.

▶ Current theories of the biology of Alzheimer disease have not led to significant improvements in therapy. That includes the still popular amyloid cascade hypothesis. New ideas are badly needed. This stimulating study from the Salpêtrière in Paris reports that free cholesterol is at as high a concentration in Alzheimer plaques as is amyloid protein. Variations in a lipoprotein gene, apolipoprotein E4 (*apoE4*), are a known risk factor for Alzheimer disease. That supports the possibility that cholesterol may play a role in Alzheimer pathophysiology. This is not a new idea; the literature contains more than 1000 articles on the subject of cholesterol and Alzheimer disease. Unfortunately, statins, which lower blood cholesterol levels, have not been found to benefit Alzheimer dementia. Nevertheless, the role of cholesterol in this disease deserves further study.

J. P. Blass, MD, PhD

Insight, cognition and quality of life in Alzheimer's disease

Hurt CS, on behalf of the AddNeuroMed Consortium (King's College London, UK; et al)

J Neurol Neurosurg Psychiatry 81:331-336, 2010

Background.—The detrimental impact of dementia upon patient health-related quality of life (HRQL) is well established, as is the importance of improving HRQL. However, relatively little is known about the natural history of HRQL in dementia and those factors influencing it. This limited knowledge potentially restricts the evaluation of the efficacy of interventions designed to improve HRQL. One such area concerns the relationship between HRQL and patient insight. It remains unclear what impact, if any, impaired insight has upon a patient's HRQL. The present study aimed to investigate the relationship between insight and HRQL in a sample of patients with Alzheimer's disease (AD) and their carers.

Methods.—256 patients with AD were recruited as part of AddNeuroMed, a multicentre European AD biomarkers study. Of these, 174 completed a quality-of-life measure in addition to a comprehensive battery of clinical and neuropsychological assessments.

Results.—Insight was found to be differentially related to patient perceptions of HRQL in mild and moderate dementia. Within moderate dementia, impaired insight was associated with better perceived HRQL. Conversely, cognition, but not insight, was associated with impaired HRQL in mild dementia. Insight was not found to be associated with carer perceptions of patient HRQL.

Conclusion.—Impairment of insight is associated with better HRQL in moderate dementia. This finding has implications for interventions which focus on increasing patient awareness and orientation, as impairment of insight appears to have a positive impact upon HRQL.

▶ Denial is a classic psychological defense mechanism. It sometimes interferes with patient care, for instance, the smoker who denies his or her cough has anything to do with their use of cigarettes. On the other hand, denial can be a major comfort to people with incurable diseases, particularly in the later stages of their illnesses. This article indicates that people in London with dementia feel better about themselves if they minimize the degree of their impairment. So long as that does not interfere with appropriate treatment or with protecting them from the consequences of their disability, why not let them fool themselves, if that makes them happier?

J. P. Blass, MD, PhD

Levels of reduced and oxidized coenzyme Q-10 and 8-hydroxy-2′-deoxyguanosine in the CSF of patients with Alzheimer's disease demonstrate that mitochondrial oxidative damage and/or oxidative DNA damage contributes to the neurodegenerative process

Isobe C, Abe T, Terayama Y (Iwate Med Univ, Morioka, Japan)

J Neurol 257:399-404, 2010

To investigate the possibility that mitochondrial oxidative damage, oxidative DNA damage or both contribute to the neurodegenerative process of Alzheimer's disease (AD), we employed highperformance liquid chromatography using an electrochemical detector to measure the concentrations of the reduced and oxidized forms of coenzyme Q-10 (CoQ-10) and 8-hydroxy-2'-deoxyguanosine (8-OHdG) in the cerebrospinal fluid (CSF) of 30 patients with AD and in 30 age-matched controls with no neurological disease. The percentage of oxidized/total CoQ-10 (%CoQ-10) in the CSF of the AD group (78.2 ± 18.8%) was significantly higher than in the control group (41.3 ± 10.4%) ($P < 0.0001$). The concentration of 8-OHdG in the CSF of AD patients was greater than in the CSF of controls ($P < 0.0001$) and was positively correlated with the duration of illness ($r_s = 0.95$, $P < 0.0001$). The %CoQ-10 was correlated with concentrations of 8-OHdG in the CSF of AD patients ($r_s = 0.66$, $P < 0.001$). The present study suggests that both mitochondrial oxidative damage and oxidative

DNA damage play important roles in the pathogenesis of early AD development.

▶ This article adds to the ever-growing mountain of evidence that free radical metabolism is abnormal in Alzheimer disease. The authors conclude with the suggestion that the alterations in free radicals contribute to the pathogenesis of Alzheimer disease. This suggestion is frequently made, but accepting it requires experimental proof. One can make an equally reasonable argument that alterations in free radicals are adaptations—perhaps healthy adaptations—to more fundamental disease process. There are many examples in biology of free radicals being beneficial and many examples of them being harmful.

J. P. Blass, MD, PhD

Mechanisms of enzymatic degradation of amyloid Beta microfibrils generating nanofilaments and nanospheres related to cytotoxicity

Numata K, Kaplan DL (Tufts Univ, Medford, MA)

Biochemistry 49:3254-3260, 2010

Amyloid beta (Abeta) fibrils are found in the brain tissue of persons with Alzheimer's disease (AD), where they accumulate as plaques. One way to reduce the level of accumulation of Abeta in the brain and potentially treat AD is with Abeta-degrading enzymes such as neprilysin (NEP) and insulin-degrading enzyme (IDE). However, enzymatic responses and degradation mechanisms of Abeta fibrils (crystalline-state Abeta) have not been investigated, particularly with respect to how to avoid cytotoxicity of the degradation products to neuronal cells. Thus, insight into mechanisms of enzymatic degradation of Abeta fibrils would be instructive as a route to elucidating different structural features related to degradation and to cytotoxicity. We report mechanisms of enzymatic degradation of Abeta with crossbeta structures and show the series of steps involved in the digestion of Abeta microfibrils to nanospheres or nanofilaments by protease XIV or alpha-chymotrypsin, respectively. These degradation products, which contained almost the same secondary structures, exhibited different cytotoxicities, indicating that relationships between nanoassembled structures and cytotoxicity of Abeta peptides are more significant than the beta-sheet content. In addition, the enzymatic digestion at the Lys28 loop region linking the two beta-sheets in Abeta fibrils is suggested as a key target related to cytotoxicity, a feature that can be selectively targeted on the basis of the choice of protease.

▶ Erudite studies of Alzheimer amyloid protein continue to appear, despite increasing evidence that brings into question the amyloid cascade hypothesis of this disease. That evidence includes the following: (1) amyloid, including diagnostic number of plaques and tangles, can occur without clinically significant cognitive impairment,[1] (2) removing amyloid (for instance by immunization against it) does not significantly alter the course of the disease,[2] and (3) most disappointing, the many excellent studies of these proteins have not led to notable improvements in the care of patients with this disorder.

J. P. Blass, MD, PhD

References

1. Schmitt FA, Davis DG, Wekstein DR, Smith CD, Ashford JW, Markesbery WR. "Preclinical" AD revisited: neuropathology of cognitively normal older adults. *Neurology.* 2000;55:370-376.
2. Holmes C, Boche D, Wilkinson D, et al. Long-term effects of Abeta42 immunisation in Alzheimer's disease: follow-up of a randomised, placebo-controlled phase I trial. *Lancet.* 2008;372:216-223.

Physical Activity, Cognitive Function, and Mortality in a US National Cohort

Gillum RF, Obisesan TO (Howard Univ College of Medicine, Washington, DC)
Ann Epidemiol 20:251-257, 2010

Purpose.—Increasing physical activity is postulated to slow cognitive decline associated with aging. Low levels of both physical activity and cognitive function are associated with increased risk of mortality. We test the hypothesis that the relative protective effect of high physical activity level as related to mortality is greater in persons with impaired cognitive function than in others.

Methods.—Data were analyzed from a longitudinal mortality follow-up study of 5903 American men and women aged 60 years and older examined in 1988 to 1994 who were followed an average of 8.5 years. Measurements at baseline included self-reported leisure-time physical activity (LTPA), a short index of cognitive function (SICF), sociodemographic data, health status, and physical and biochemical measurements.

Results.—Death during follow-up occurred in 2431 persons. In bivariate cross-sectional analyses, more frequent LTPA was associated with greater cognitive function. In proportional hazards regression analysis, no significant interaction of LTPA with cognitive function was found; however, there was a significant age- LTPA interaction. After adjusting for confounding by baseline sociodemographic data and health status at ages 60 to 74, the hazards ratio (95% confidence intervals) was for LTPA more than 8 times weekly compared with none (0.51; 0.38–0.76, $p < .001$) and for low SICF score compared with high 1.43 (1.36; 1.00–1.84, $p < .05$). After controlling for health behaviors, blood pressure, and body mass, C-reactive protein, and high-density lipoprotein cholesterol, the LTPA hazards ratio was 0.52 (0.35–0.78; $p = .002$), but cognitive function was no longer significant. At ages 75 and older, results were similar for LTPA, but cognitive function remained significant after adjustment.

Conclusions.—In a nationwide cohort of older Americans, analyses demonstrated a lower risk of death independent of confounders among those with frequent LTPA. Much of the effect of low cognitive function could be explained by other risk factors at ages 60 to 74 but not 75 years and older.

▶ This large study indicates that physical activities during leisure time were associated with a decreased risk of dementia in people who are 75 years and older. This is yet another addition to the large pile of evidence that older people who keep physically active tend to be healthier. An obvious question is whether healthier people stay more active or whether active people stay healthier. Also, one wonders what part of the life of most people who are 75 years or older does not consist of leisure time.

J. P. Blass, MD, PhD

Quality of end-of-life care for dementia patients during acute hospital admission: a retrospective study in Ireland

Afzal N, Buhagiar K, Flood J, et al (Beaumont Hosp, Dublin, Ireland; Royal Free and Univ College London Med School, UK)

Gen Hosp Psychiatry 32:141-146, 2010

Objectives.—To examine the quality of end-of-life care received by patients with and without dementia on acute medical wards during their final hospitalization.

Methods.—A retrospective clinical case note review of patients aged over 65 who had died on acute medical wards within a 6-month period in a general hospital in Dublin was conducted. Seventy-five multidisciplinary clinical notes were available for scrutiny in order to identify cognitive status, measure the frequency of invasive procedures undertaken and examine the quality of palliative care as benchmarked with the Liverpool Care Pathway for the Dying Patient (LCP) program. Comparison between patients with and without dementia was made.

Results.—Eighteen (24.0%) subjects had dementia, 32 (42.7%) subjects were described as "cognitively intact" and 25 subjects did not have reference to cognitive status. Of the 50 patients with known cognitive status, 27 (54.0%) had had a Mini Mental State Examination (MMSE) conducted (10 dementia vs. 17 nondementia). Patients were equally subjected to invasive interventions regardless of their cognitive status. However, dementia patients were significantly less likely to be referred to palliative care interventions (P=.007), to be prescribed palliative drugs (P=.017) and to have carers involved in decision making (P=.006).

Conclusion.—Individuals with dementia may be receiving different end-of-life care from those without. The effective delivery of robust multidisciplinary frameworks for the palliation of symptoms of hospitalized dementia patients remains an important clinical goal.

▶ This small study from Dublin claims that systematic differences in the type of care allotted to patients with dementia compared with those who are cognitively intact persists even in the well-regarded Irish health care system—ranked by the World Health Organization as 19 in the world. (The United States ranks 37.) However, is considering mental status inappropriate in designing care plans? Cognitive abilities are certainly not the only qualities that provide humans with full moral agency, but common sense and individualizing care remain key parts of medical practice. Dogmatic statements of moral absolutes are best left to ethicists. Their judgments are not clouded by having actually provided care to living human beings and their families.

J. P. Blass, MD, PhD

The inhibition of prions through blocking prion conversion by permanently charged branched polyamines of low cytotoxicity

Lim Y-B, Mays CE, Kim Y, et al (Yonsei Univ, Seoul, Republic of Korea; Univ of Kentucky, Lexington)

Biomaterials 31:2025-2033, 2010

Branched polyamines are effective in inhibiting prions in a cationic surface charge density dependent manner. However, toxicity associated with branched polyamines, in general, often hampers the successful application of the compounds to treat prion diseases. Here, we report that constitutively maintained cationic properties in branched polyamines reduced the intrinsic toxicity of the compounds while retaining the anti-prion activities. In prion-infected neuroblastoma cells, quaternization of amines in polyethyleneimine (PEI) and polyamidoamine (PAMAM) dendrimers markedly increased the nontoxic concentration ranges of the compounds and still supported, albeit reduced, an appreciable level of anti-prion activity in clearing prions from the infected cells. Furthermore, quaternized PEI was able to degrade prions at acidic pH conditions and inhibit the in vitro prion propagation facilitated by conversion of the normal prion protein isoform to its misfolded counterpart, although such activities were decreased by quaternization. Quaternized PAMAM was least effective in degrading prions but efficiently inhibited prion conversion with the same efficacy as unmodified PAMAM. Our results suggest that quaternization represents an effective strategy for developing nontoxic branched polyamines with potent anti-prion activity. This study highlights the importance of polyamine structural control for developing polyamine-based anti-prion agents and understanding of an action mechanism of quaternized branched polyamines.

▶ A major effort is underway in many laboratories to find potential treatments for prion diseases. These conditions are still rare, but they will become a major public health problem if fears about mad cow disease prove justified. This report from South Korea provides encouraging evidence that quarternary amines, which are already normal constituents of human cells, may prove useful. One hopes!

J. P. Blass, MD, PhD

Volume changes in Alzheimer's disease and mild cognitive impairment: cognitive associations

Evans MC, the Alzheimer's Disease Neuroimaging Initiative (Dementia Res Centre, Queen Square, London, UK)

Eur Radiol 20:674-682, 2010

Objective.—To assess the relationship between MRI-derived changes in whole-brain and ventricular volume with change in cognitive scores in Alzheimer's disease (AD), mild cognitive impairment (MCI) and control subjects.

Material and Methods.—In total 131 control, 231 MCI and 99 AD subjects from the Alzheimer's Disease Neuroimaging Initiative (ADNI) cohort with T1-weighted volumetric MRIs from baseline and 12-month follow-up were used to derive volume changes. Mini mental state examination (MMSE), Alzheimer's disease assessment scale (ADAS)-cog and trails test changes were calculated over the same period.

Results.—Brain atrophy rates and ventricular enlargement differed between subject groups ($p < 0.0005$) and in MCI and AD were associated with MMSE changes. Both measures were additionally associated with ADAS-cog and trails-B in MCI patients, and ventricular expansion was associated with ADAS-cog in AD patients. Brain atrophy ($p < 0.0005$) and ventricular expansion rates ($p = 0.001$) were higher in MCI subjects who progressed to AD within 12 months of follow-up compared with MCI subjects who remained stable. MCI subjects who progressed to AD within 12 months had similar atrophy rates to AD subjects.

Conclusion.—Whole-brain atrophy rates and ventricular enlargement differed between patient groups and healthy controls, and tracked disease progression and psychological decline, demonstrating their relevance as biomarkers.

▶ Brain scans for anatomy but not function—for example, MRI rather than functional MRI—have been known for decades to give primarily negative information in the differential diagnosis of dementia. They do identify such alternate diagnoses as brain tumors or previously undetected strokes, including small lesions in white matter. People with Alzheimer dementia can have brains well within the normal range of sizes, and people with walnut brain can have cognition well within the normal range for their age. Progressive atrophy has, however, been considered to be a better indication of the presence and the progress of dementia. This study from Queen Square of almost 500 individuals provides solid objective support for that view.

J. P. Blass, MD, PhD

2 Cerebrovascular Disease

Aspirin vs anticoagulation in carotid artery dissection: A study of 298 patients

Georgiadis D, Arnold M, von Buedingen HC, et al (Univ Hosp Zürich, Switzerland; Univ Hosp Bern, Switzerland; et al)

Neurology 72:1810-1815, 2009

Background.—No randomized study has yet compared efficacy and safety of aspirin and anticoagulants in patients with spontaneous dissection of the cervical carotid artery (sICAD).

Methods.—Prospectively collected data from 298 consecutive patients with sICAD (56% men; mean age 46 ± 10 years) treated with anticoagulants alone (n = 202) or aspirin alone (n = 96) were retrospectively analyzed. Admission diagnosis was ischemic stroke in 165, TIA in 37, retinal ischemia in 8, and local symptoms and signs (headache, neck pain, Horner syndrome, cranial nerve palsy) in 80 patients, while 8 patients were asymptomatic. Clinical follow-up was obtained after 3 months by neurologic examination (97% of patients) or structured telephone interview. Outcome measures were 1) new cerebral ischemic events, defined as ischemic stroke, TIA, or retinal ischemia, 2) symptomatic intracranial hemorrhage, and 3) major extracranial bleeding.

Results.—During follow-up, ischemic events were rare (ischemic stroke, 0.3%; TIA, 3.4%; retinal ischemia, 1%); their frequency did not significantly differ between patients treated with anticoagulants (5.9%) and those treated with aspirin (2.1%). The same was true for hemorrhagic adverse events (anticoagulants, 2%; aspirin, 1%). New ischemic events were significantly more frequent in patients with ischemic events at onset (6.2%) than in patients with local symptoms or asymptomatic patients (1.1%).

Conclusions.—Within the limitations of a nonrandomized study, our data suggest that frequency of new cerebral and retinal ischemic events in patients with spontaneous dissection of the cervical carotid artery is low and probably independent of the type of antithrombotic treatment (aspirin or anticoagulants).

▶ The main findings of this study are that cervical carotid artery dissections are associated with very low risk of recurrent ischemia (especially in patients without retinal or cerebral ischemia at presentation) and aspirin and warfarin confer similar protection. These results are mostly confirmatory but nonetheless reassuring and quite useful.

No controlled randomized trials have been conducted to define the best strategy to prevent cerebrovascular events after a carotid dissection. However, a meta-analysis of reported series found no significant difference between antiplatelet therapy and anticoagulation.[1] Given the low rate of cerebrovascular events in these patients, it is unlikely that a randomized controlled trial of adequate size will be conducted. Therefore, data such as that presented in this study will have to suffice to guide clinical decisions.

Warfarin is more cumbersome and perhaps more dangerous than aspirin. Hence, in the absence of any definite proof of superiority, warfarin cannot be generally recommended for patients with carotid dissections. Future studies should focus on determining whether there are any high-risk populations that could benefit from anticoagulation (such as patients presenting with cerebral or retinal ischemia who also have severe stenosis and frequent microembolic signals on emboli detection studies).

A. Rabinstein, MD

Reference

1. Lyrer P, Engelter S. Antithrombotic drugs for carotid artery dissection. *Cochrane Database Syst Rev.* 2003;3:CD000255.

Atraumatic convexal subarachnoid hemorrhage: Clinical presentation, imaging patterns, and etiologies

Kumar S, Goddeau RP Jr, Selim MH, et al (Beth Israel Deaconess Med Ctr, Boston, MA)

Neurology 74:893-899, 2010

Objective.—To identify patterns of clinical presentation, imaging findings, and etiologies in a cohort of hospitalized patients with localized nontraumatic convexal subarachnoid hemorrhage.

Methods.—Twenty-nine consecutive patients with atraumatic convexal subarachnoid hemorrhage were identified using International Classification of Diseases–9 code from 460 patients with subarachnoid hemorrhage evaluated at our institution over a course of 5 years. Retrospective review of patient medical records, neuroimaging studies, and follow-up data was performed.

Results.—There were 16 women and 13 men between the ages of 29 and 87 years. Two common patterns of presentations were observed. The most frequent presenting symptom in patients ≤60 years (n = 16) was a severe headache (n = 12; 75%) of abrupt onset (n = 9; 56%) with arterial narrowing on conventional angiograms in 4 patients; 10 ($p = 0.003$) were presumptively diagnosed with a primary vasoconstriction syndrome. Patients >60 years (n = 13) usually had temporary sensory or motor symptoms (n = 7; 54%); brain MRI scans in these patients showed evidence of leukoaraiosis and/or hemispheric microbleeds and superficial siderosis (n = 9; 69%), compatible with amyloid angiopathy (n = 10; $p < 0.0001$). In a small group of patients, the presentation was more varied and included lethargy, fever, and confusion. Four patients older than 60 years had recurrent intracerebral hemorrhages in the follow-up period with 2 fatalities.

Conclusion.—Convexal subarachnoid hemorrhage is an important subtype of nonaneurysmal subarachnoid bleeding with diverse etiologies, though a reversible vasoconstriction syndrome appears to be a common cause in patients 60 years or younger whereas amyloid angiopathy is frequent in patients over 60. These observations require confirmation in future studies.

▶ This case series presents a simple, clinically useful message that can be summarized as follows: when you encounter a patient with subarachnoid hemorrhage confined to the sulci in the brain hemispheric convexity, if the patient is younger than 60 years and presents with sudden headache, think of reversible cerebral vasoconstriction syndrome and benign prognosis with rare recurrences; if the patient is older than 60 years and presents with focal motor or sensory deficits (most often transient), think of cerebral amyloid angiopathy and the possibility of future parenchymal (lobar) hemorrhages. In younger patients, posterior reversible encephalopathy syndrome can be found on brain MRI, with or without documented vasoconstriction. Among older patients, brain MRI may show cortical microhemorrhages.

The reader of this article should be advised that the subarachnoid hemorrhages reported in this series were probably quite small or even subtle. The simple differential diagnosis presented should not be applied to patients with subarachnoid blood in the cisterns or fissures. When in doubt, it is always best to obtain a cerebral angiogram (the smaller the suspected vascular abnormality, the more important it is to favor a catheter study rather than noninvasive options). If the patient is febrile, infective endocarditis should always be kept in mind.

A. Rabinstein, MD

Characteristics, Performance Measures, and In-Hospital Outcomes of the First One Million Stroke and Transient Ischemic Attack Admissions in Get With The Guidelines-Stroke

Fonarow GC, on behalf of the GWTG-Stroke Steering Committee and Investigators (Univ of California, Los Angeles)

Circ Cardiovasc Qual Outcomes 3:291-302, 2010

Background.—Stroke results in substantial death and disability. To address this burden, Get With The Guideline (GWTG)-Stroke was developed to facilitate the measurement, tracking, and improvement in quality of care and outcomes for acute stroke and transient ischemic attack (TIA) patients in the United States.

Methods and Results.—We analyzed the characteristics, performance measures, and in-hospital outcomes in the first 1 000 000 acute ischemic stroke, intracerebral hemorrhage, subarachnoid hemorrhage, and TIA admissions from 1392 hospitals that participated in the GWTG-Stroke Program 2003 to 2009. Patients were 53.5% women, 73.3% white, and with mean age of 70.1 ± 14.9 years. There were 601 599 (60.2%) ischemic strokes, 108 671 (10.9%) intracerebral hemorrhages, 34 945 (3.5%) subarachnoid hemorrhages, 26 977 (2.7%) strokes not classified, and 227 788 (22.8%) TIAs. Performance measures showed small to moderate differences by cerebrovascular event type. In-hospital mortality rate was highest among intracerebral hemorrhage (25.0%) and subarachnoid hemorrhage (20.4%), and intermediate in ischemic stroke (5.5%) patients and lowest among TIA patients (0.3%). Significant improvements over time from 2003 to 2009 in quality of care were observed: all-or-none measure, 44.0% versus 84.3% (+40.3%, $P<0.0001$). After adjustment for patient and hospital variables, the cumulative adjusted odds ratio for the all-or-none measure over the 6 years was 9.4 (95% confidence interval, 8.3 to 10.6, $P<0.0001$). Temporal improvements in length of stay and risk-adjusted in-hospital mortality rate (for ischemic stroke and TIA) were also observed.

Conclusions.—With more than 1 million patients enrolled, GWTG-Stroke represents an integrated stroke and TIA registry that supports national surveillance, innovative research, and sustained quality improvement efforts facilitating evidence-based stroke/TIA care.

▶ This is a remarkable milestone that merits attention and compliment for those directing the efforts of hospital participation in Get with the Guidelines Stroke Program. Designed as a voluntary registry focused on performance improvement and application of evidence-based interventions, the program has been a great success in acute stroke as it had been previously in acute coronary syndromes. The number of participating hospitals has grown steadily since the inception of the program in 2003. Strong temporal improvements in all measures were collected to monitor the quality of stroke care. Adherence to these quality measures has already resulted in meaningful improvements in clinical outcomes.

The metrics may change in the future, but the principle of the importance of monitoring the quality of care delivered to our patients will not. There is a very good reason to be optimistic about the continuous growth of this valuable enterprise and also about its enormous potential to serve as a source of creative and solid clinical research.

A. Rabinstein, MD

Clinical-Diffusion Mismatch and Benefit From Thrombolysis 3 to 6 Hours After Acute Stroke

Ebinger M, Iwanaga T, Prosser JF, et al (The Royal Melbourne Hosp, Parkville, Australia; Austin Hosp, Melbourne, Australia; et al)

Stroke 40:2572-2574, 2009

Background and Purpose.—The clinical-diffusion mismatch (CDM) model has been proposed as a simpler tool than perfusion-diffusion mismatch (PDM) to select acute ischemic stroke patients for thrombolytic therapy. We hypothesized that in the 3- to 6-hour time window, the effect of tPA was significantly greater in patients with CDM than in patients without CDM.

Methods.—This is a substudy of EPITHET, a double-blind multi-center study of 100 patients randomized to tPA or placebo 3 to 6 hours after stroke onset. MRI was obtained before treatment, and at 3 to 5 days and 90 days after treatment. Presence of PDM (perfusion deficit/DWI_{volume} >1.2 and perfusion deficit at least 10 mL>DWI_{volume}) and CDM (NIHSS ≥8 and DWI_{volume} ≤25 mL) was determined for each patient. We assessed lesion growth and neurological improvement (decrease in NIHSS ≥8 points between baseline and 90 days, or a 90-day NIHSS ≤1).

Results.—86% of the patients had PDM, but only 41% had CDM. CDM detected PDM with a sensitivity of 46% and a specificity of 86%. We found statistically significant effects of reperfusion on the rate of neurological improvement (OR 9.92, 95% CI 1.91 to 51.64; $P < 0.01$) and on absolute growth (difference: −59.60 mL, 95% CI −95.40 mL to −23.81 mL; $P < 0.01$). Neither treatment with tPA nor reperfusion had a significantly different impact on lesion growth or clinical course in CDM patients compared to patients without CDM.

Conclusions.—There was no increased benefit from tPA in patients with CDM. The beneficial effects of reperfusion were similar in patients with and without CDM.

▶ Echoplanar Imaging Thrombolytic Evaluation Trial (EPITHET) was an observational study, which was aimed at examining the predictive value of perfusion-diffusion mismatch on MRI done before intravenous thrombolysis on the effects of thrombolytic therapy using an extended therapeutic time window. The main results of the study indicated that patients with mismatch who recanalized had less infarct growth and better chances of good recovery.[1] Most patients in this study (86%) had radiological penumbra at baseline (defined as a mismatch between perfusion and diffusion abnormalities greater than 20%).

This article is a useful subanalysis of EPITHET comparing clinical-diffusion mismatch versus perfusion-diffusion mismatch. In essence the question is whether acute reperfusion treatments can be best guided by detailed radiological information. Most acute stroke patients are currently treated without guidance from penumbral imaging. When patients are treated very early, avoiding any delays takes precedence because there is solid evidence that treatment with intravenous thrombolysis is safe and effective within the first 4.5 hours after stroke onset when administered simply based on clinical findings and the results of an unenhanced head CT scan. However, penumbral imaging may be essential to identify patients who might benefit from reperfusion therapy initiated later and to optimize the selection of candidates for endovascular interventions.

The results of this analysis of the EPITHET data clearly indicate that clinical-diffusion mismatch (ie, patients with severe deficits and relatively small areas of restricted diffusion) often fail to recognize persistent penumbra as defined by perfusion-diffusion mismatch. The specificity of clinical-diffusion mismatch was found to be quite good in this study and others.[2,3] Thus, patients with this presentation are very likely to have substantial perfusion-diffusion mismatch and, consequently, they can achieve favorable recovery if treatment results in recanalization of the occluded vessel. However, deciding not to pursue reperfusion attempts in patients without clinical-diffusion mismatch may be unwise because some of those patients might still have salvageable tissue. In fact, 79% of patients without clinical-diffusion mismatch who reperfused in this study exhibited neurological improvement.

A. Rabinstein, MD

References

1. Davis SM, Donnan GA, Parsons MW, et al. EPITHET investigators. Effects of alteplase beyond 3 h after stroke in the Echoplanar Imaging Thrombolytic Evaluation Trial (EPITHET): a placebo-controlled randomised trial. *Lancet Neurol.* 2008;7: 299-309.
2. Dávalos A, Blanco M, Pedraza S, et al. The clinical-DWI mismatch: a new diagnostic approach to the brain tissue at risk of infarction. *Neurology.* 2004;62: 2187-2192.
3. Prosser J, Butcher K, Allport L, et al. Clinical-diffusion mismatch predicts the putative penumbra with high specificity. *Stroke.* 2005;36:1700-1704.

Dabigatran versus Warfarin in Patients with Atrial Fibrillation

Connolly SJ, the RE-LY Steering Committee and Investigators (McMaster Univ, Hamilton, Ontario, Canada; et al)

N Engl J Med 361:1139-1151, 2009

Background.—Warfarin reduces the risk of stroke in patients with atrial fibrillation but increases the risk of hemorrhage and is difficult to use. Dabigatran is a new oral direct thrombin inhibitor.

Methods.—In this noninferiority trial, we randomly assigned 18,113 patients who had atrial fibrillation and a risk of stroke to receive, in a blinded fashion, fixed doses of dabigatran — 110 mg or 150 mg twice daily — or, in an unblinded fashion, adjusted-dose warfarin. The median duration of the follow-up period was 2.0 years. The primary outcome was stroke or systemic embolism.

Results.—Rates of the primary outcome were 1.69% per year in the warfarin group, as compared with 1.53% per year in the group that received 110 mg of dabigatran (relative risk with dabigatran, 0.91; 95% confidence interval [CI], 0.74 to 1.11; $P<0.001$ for noninferiority) and

1.11% per year in the group that received 150 mg of dabigatran (relative risk, 0.66; 95% CI, 0.53 to 0.82; P<0.001 for superiority). The rate of major bleeding was 3.36% per year in the warfarin group, as compared with 2.71% per year in the group receiving 110 mg of dabigatran (P = 0.003) and 3.11% per year in the group receiving 150 mg of dabigatran (P = 0.31). The rate of hemorrhagic stroke was 0.38% per year in the warfarin group, as compared with 0.12% per year with 110 mg of dabigatran (P<0.001) and 0.10% per year with 150 mg of dabigatran (P<0.001). The mortality rate was 4.13% per year in the warfarin group, as compared with 3.75% per year with 110 mg of dabigatran (P = 0.13) and 3.64% per year with 150 mg of dabigatran (P = 0.051).

Conclusions.—In patients with atrial fibrillation, dabigatran given at a dose of 110 mg was associated with rates of stroke and systemic embolism that were similar to those associated with warfarin, as well as lower rates of major hemorrhage. Dabigatran administered at a dose of 150 mg, as compared with warfarin, was associated with lower rates of stroke and systemic embolism but similar rates of major hemorrhage. (ClinicalTrials.gov number, NCT00262600.)

▶ Direct thrombin inhibitors have been studied for some time as potential alternatives to warfarin for chronic oral anticoagulation. Previously, agents such as ximelagatran were limited by toxicity. In this remarkable trial, known as Randomized Evaluation of Long-Term Anticoagulation Therapy (RE-LY), dabigatran compared favorably against warfarin for the prevention of cardiac embolism.

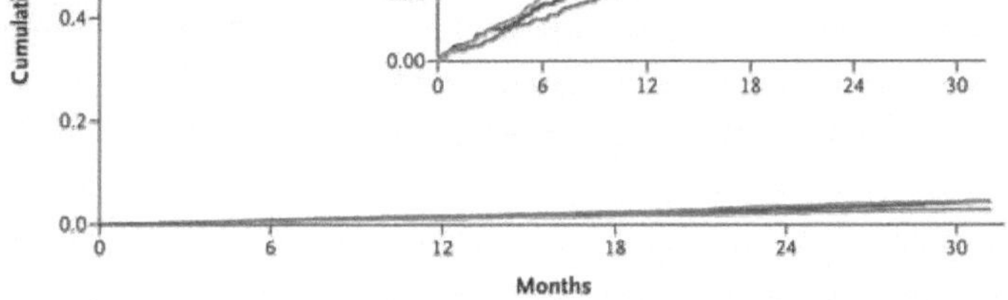

No. at Risk

Warfarin	6022	5862	5718	4593	2890	1322
Dabigatran, 110 mg	6015	5862	5710	4593	2945	1385
Dabigatran, 150 mg	6076	5939	5779	4682	3044	1429

FIGURE 1.—Cumulative Hazard Rates for the Primary Outcome of Stroke or Systemic Embolism, According to Treatment Group. (Reprinted from Connolly SJ, the RE-LY Steering Committee and Investigators. Dabigatran versus warfarin in patients with atrial fibrillation. *N Engl J Med.* 2009;361: 1139-1151. Copyright 2009 Massachusetts Medical Society. All rights reserved.)

The trial enrolled over 18 000 patients, of whom more than half had been on warfarin before enrollment into the study. Warfarin use was unblinded (the 2 doses of dabigatran were blinded), and patients on warfarin had therapeutic international normalized ratios (INRs) 64% of the time, which is comparable with prior trials involving oral anticoagulation. Dabigatran at a fixed dose of 150 mg twice daily outperformed not only the lower dose of this agent but also adjusted doses of warfarin (Fig 1).

The reductions in the risk of ischemic and hemorrhagic strokes, both disabling or fatal and nondisabling, were quite convincing. The consistent benefit across multiple subgroups and the stronger benefit in patients at higher risk of embolism (as predicted by higher $CHADS_2$ scores) are particularly promising. The lack of liver toxicity, seen with previous thrombin inhibitors, was reassuring, but not all findings were positive. Patients on dabigatran had greater risk of gastrointestinal bleeding (perhaps related to the acidic content of the pellets required to enhance the absorption of the drug) and myocardial infarction (without any clear reasons), and higher rates of discontinuation of the medication (also unexplained) compared with the warfarin group.

Overall, this trial offers great hope that we will have an option to replace warfarin in the near future. Having an agent that provides consistent anticoagulation without requiring frequent INR monitoring or close attention to diet or other medications would be a major advantage, even if it has to be taken twice daily. Yet, more randomized studies or, if regulatory approval is conceded, close postmarketing surveillance will be necessary to monitor the risks of gastrointestinal bleeding and myocardial ischemia on dabigatran.

A. Rabinstein, MD

Differing Risk Factor Profiles of Ischemic Stroke Subtypes: Evidence for a Distinct Lacunar Arteriopathy?

Jackson CA, Hutchison A, Dennis MS, et al (Univ of Edinburgh, UK; et al)
Stroke 41:624-629, 2010

Background and Purpose.—Differences in risk factor profiles between lacunar and other ischemic stroke subtypes may provide evidence for a distinct lacunar arteriopathy, but existing studies have limitations. We overcame these by pooling individual data on 2875 patients with first-ever ischemic stroke from 5 collaborating prospective stroke registers that used similar, unbiased methods to define risk factors and classify stroke subtypes.

Methods.—We compared risk factors between lacunar and nonlacunar ischemic strokes, altering the comparison groups in sensitivity analyses, and incorporated these data into a meta-analysis of published studies.

Results.—Unadjusted and adjusted analyses gave similar results. We found a lower prevalence of cardioembolic source (adjusted odds ratio, 0.33; 95% CI, 0.24 to 0.46), ipsilateral carotid stenosis (odds ratio, 0.21; 95% CI, 0.14 to 0.30), and ischemic heart disease (odds ratio, 0.75; 95% CI, 0.58 to 0.97) in lacunar compared with nonlacunar patients but no difference for hypertension, diabetes, or any other risk factor studied. Results were robust to sensitivity analyses and largely confirmed in our meta-analysis.

Conclusions.—Hypertension and diabetes appear equally common in lacunar and nonlacunar ischemic stroke, but lacunar stroke is less likely to be caused by embolism from the heart or proximal arteries, and the lower prevalence of ischemic heart disease in lacunar stroke provides additional support for a nonatherosclerotic arteriopathy causing many lacunar ischemic strokes. Our findings have implications for how clinicians classify ischemic stroke subtypes and highlight the need for additional research into the specific causes of and treatments for lacunar stroke.

▶ This study provides convincing confirmatory evidence that risk factors differ between lacunar and nonlacunar infarctions. Cardiac and arterial sources of embolism are much less common among cases of lacunar infarction. Furthermore, patients with lacunar strokes have a much lower prevalence of large artery atherosclerosis in the carotid and coronary vessels. Hence, these differential associations also suggest that lacunar infarctions are probably not simply caused by atherothrombosis of small vessels (although hypertension and to a lesser degree diabetes are very common in patients with lacunes, they were not more common than in other stroke patients in this study).

In my opinion, small vessel disease is the least understood mechanism of brain infarction. It was originally attributed to small vessel occlusion from lipohyalinosis, but more recent data indicate that cerebral lipohyalinosis is rather infrequent at present because of better control of blood pressure. Instead, other more complex mechanisms may play major roles in the development of subcortical brain ischemia by affecting the function of terminal penetrating arteries. Initial stuttering of deficits (arguing against a sudden occlusion of flow), frequent silent areas of ischemia, and the variety of clinical-radiological presentations (single symptomatic lacunes, multiple silent lacunes, coalescing white matter hyperintensities with progressive cognitive decline, and small subcortical infarctions combined with deep microhemorrhages) speak of the complexity of this disorder or perhaps spectrum of disorders.

Loss of vascular integrity leading to alterations in blood-brain barrier permeability, extravasation of fluid, and compromise of blood flow and nutrient supply to the perivascular parenchyma may lie at the core of the pathophysiology of this condition.[1,2] If that mechanism were to be confirmed by future research, we will need to rethink our approach to the prevention and treatment of subcortical ischemia.

A. Rabinstein, MD

References

1. Young VG, Halliday GM, Kril JJ. Neuropathologic correlates of white matter hyperintensities. *Neurology.* 2008;71:804-811.
2. Wardlaw JM, Doubal F, Armitage P, et al. Lacunar stroke is associated with diffuse blood-brain barrier dysfunction. *Ann Neurol.* 2009;65:194-202.

Effects of Intensive Medical Therapy on Microemboli and Cardiovascular Risk in Asymptomatic Carotid Stenosis

Spence JD, Coates V, Li H, et al (Stroke Prevention and Atherosclerosis Res Centre, London, Ontario, Canada; Univ of Western Ontario, London, Canada)

Arch Neurol 67:180-186, 2010

Objective.—To assess the effect of more intensive medical therapy on the rate of transcranial Doppler (TCD) microemboli and cardiovascular events in patients with asymptomatic carotid stenosis (ACS).

Design.—A prospective study.

Setting.—A teaching hospital.

Patients.—Four hundred sixty-eight patients with ACS greater than 60% by Doppler peak velocity.

Main Outcome Measures.—We compared (1) the proportion of ACS patients who had microemboli on TCD, (2) cardiovascular events, (3) rate of carotid plaque progression, and (4) baseline medical therapy, before and since 2003.

Results.—Among 468 ACS patients, 199 were enrolled between January 1, 2000, and December 31, 2002; and 269 were enrolled between January 1, 2003, and July 30, 2007. Microemboli were present in 12.6% before 2003 and 3.7% since 2003 ($P < .001$). The decline in microemboli coincided with better control of plasma lipids and slower progression of carotid total plaque area. Since 2003, there have been significantly fewer cardiovascular events among patients with ACS: 17.6% had stroke, death, myocardial infarction, or carotid endarterectomy for symptoms before 2003, vs 5.6% since 2003 ($P < .001$). The rate of carotid plaque progression in the first year of follow-up has declined from 69 mm^2 (SD, 96 mm^2) to 23 mm^2 (SD, 86 mm^2) ($P < .001$).

Conclusions.—Cardiovascular events and microemboli on TCD have markedly declined with more intensive medical therapy. Less than 5% of patients with ACS now stand to benefit from revascularization; patients with ACS should receive intensive medical therapy and should only be considered for revascularization if they have microemboli on TCD.

▶ This study from London, Ontario, presents further argument that intensive medical treatment of vascular risk factors in patients with asymptomatic carotid stenosis may confer greater benefit than that observed with carotid endarterectomy or stenting in available trials. The authors propose a particularly aggressive management strategy aimed at stopping progression of carotid atherosclerosis or even achieving regression of the plaque (which they quantify measuring the total plaque area described in their previous work).[1] They also check for the presence of microembolic signals (MESs) on transcranial Doppler to quantify stroke risk. Using this approach, they confirmed their previous findings that MESs are associated with a markedly increased risk of stroke, myocardial infarction, and death. In fact, the risk of stroke within the first year after documentation of the carotid stenosis was 10.3% among patients with MES but only 1.4% among those without MES (even lower in the later years of the study when intensive medical therapy had become standard in their practice). Hence, patients receiving intensive medical therapy and without MES at baseline have a very low risk of stroke, and carotid revascularization procedures would not be advisable in these patients.

The other important message of this study is reminding us that carotid plaques are an expression of severe arterial disease. Despite aggressive medical treatment, at least 5% of patients had died, suffered a major vascular event, or required revascularization over 2 years. Perhaps this is the main argument to focus on the treatment of vascular risk factors. The objective should be to control the atherosclerotic disease and not just one but all of its consequences.

A. Rabinstein, MD

Reference

1. Spence JD, Eliasziw M, DiCicco M, Hackam DG, Galil R, Lohmann T. Carotid plaque area: a tool for targeting and evaluating vascular preventive therapy. *Stroke*. 2002;33:2916-2922.

Low Risk of Ipsilateral Stroke in Patients With Asymptomatic Carotid Stenosis on Best Medical Treatment: A Prospective, Population-Based Study

Marquardt L, Geraghty OC, Mehta Z, et al (Univ of Oxford, UK)

Stroke 41:e11-e17, 2010

Background and Purpose.—The annual risk of ischemic stroke distal to ≥50% asymptomatic carotid stenoses was ≈2% to 3% in early cohort studies and subsequent randomized trials of endarterectomy. This risk might have fallen in recent years owing to improvements in medical treatment, but there are no published prognostic data from studies initiated within the last 10 years.

Methods.—In a population-based study of all patients with transient ischemic attack (TIA) or stroke in the Oxford Vascular Study, we studied the risk of TIA and stroke in patients with ≥50% contralateral asymptomatic carotid stenoses recruited consecutively from 2002 to 2009 and given intensive contemporary medical treatment.

Results.—Of 1153 consecutively imaged patients presenting with stroke or TIA, 101 (8.8%) had ≥50% asymptomatic carotid stenoses (mean age, 75 years; 39% women; 40% age ≥80 years). During 301 patient-years of follow-up (mean, 3 years), there were 6 ischemic events in the territory of an asymptomatic stenosis, 1 minor stroke (initially 50% to 69% stenosis), and 5 TIAs (2 initially 50% to 69% stenosis; 3 to 70% to 99% stenosis), 3 of which led to subsequent endarterectomy. The average annual event rates on medical treatment were 0.34% (95% CI, 0.01 to 1.87) for any ipsilateral ischemic stroke, 0% (95% CI, 0.00 to 0.99) for disabling ipsilateral stroke, and 1.78% (95% CI, 0.58 to 4.16) for ipsilateral TIA.

Conclusions.—In the first study of the prognosis of ≥50% asymptomatic carotid stenosis to be initiated in the last 10 years, the risk of stroke on intensive contemporary medical treatment was low. Larger studies are required to determine whether this apparent improvement in prognosis is generalizable.

▶ This population-based study prospectively assessed the risk of stroke in patients with asymptomatic carotid artery stenosis ≥50% maintained on medical therapy, the usual practice in the United Kingdom. Patients were identified after having a transient ischemic attack or minor stroke in another arterial territory at baseline (including 36/101 patients with contralateral carotid disease); thus, these were high-risk patients for additional vascular events. Still, the annual rate of cerebrovascular events was very low, and no patients had a disabling stroke during the time of follow-up (mean of 3 years). Although the asymptomatic carotid stenosis was severe at baseline in only one-third of the patients, the degree of stenosis did not appear to predict the risk of ipsilateral ischemia, as noted in previous endarterectomy trials such as ACAS and ACST.[1,2] When symptomatic patients were reimaged, no progression of the carotid stenosis was observed.

The investigators propose that the low rate of ipsilateral strokes observed in this population can be explained by the increasing use of medications, such as statins, that may reduce or abort the progression of atherosclerotic plaques. Still, these patients with asymptomatic carotid plaques had a fairly substantial risk of strokes in other vascular territories (annual risk of 8%), myocardial infarction (annual risk of 4.7%), and vascular death (annual risk of 7.7%). Therefore, the focus of care for these patients should not be carotid revascularization but rather the institution of intensive medical therapy for vascular risk factors to avoid the complications from atherosclerosis in various arterial beds.

A. Rabinstein, MD

References

1. Endarterectomy for asymptomatic carotid artery stenosis. Executive Committee for the Asymptomatic Carotid Atherosclerosis Study. *JAMA.* 1995;273: 1421-1428.
2. Halliday A, Mansfield A, Marro J, et al. Prevention of disabling and fatal strokes by successful carotid endarterectomy in patients without recent neurological symptoms: randomised controlled trial. *Lancet.* 2004;363:1491-1502.

Percutaneous closure of the left atrial appendage versus warfarin therapy for prevention of stroke in patients with atrial fibrillation: a randomised non-inferiority trial

Holmes DR, for the PROTECT AF Investigators (Mayo Clinic College of Medicine, Rochester, MN, et al)
Lancet 374:534-542, 2009

Background.—In patients with non-valvular atrial fibrillation, embolic stroke is thought to be associated with left atrial appendage (LAA) thrombi. We assessed the efficacy and safety of percutaneous closure of the LAA for prevention of stroke compared with warfarin treatment in patients with atrial fibrillation.

Methods.—Adult patients with non-valvular atrial fibrillation were eligible for inclusion in this multicentre, randomised non-inferiority trial if they had at least one of the following: previous stroke or transient ischaemic attack, congestive heart failure, diabetes, hypertension, or were 75 years or older. 707 eligible patients were randomly assigned in a 2:1 ratio by computer-generated randomisation sequence to percutaneous closure of the LAA and subsequent discontinuation of warfarin (intervention; n=463) or to warfarin treatment with a target international normalised ratio between 2·0 and 3·0 (control; n=244). Efficacy was assessed by a primary composite endpoint of stroke, cardiovascular death, and systemic embolism. We selected a one-sided probability criterion of non-inferiority for the intervention of at least 97·5%, by use of a two-fold non-inferiority margin. Serious adverse events that constituted the primary endpoint for safety included major bleeding, pericardial effusion, and device embolisation. Analysis was by intention to treat. This study is registered with Clinicaltrials.gov, number NCT00129545.

Findings.—At 1065 patient-years of follow-up, the primary efficacy event rate was 3·0 per 100 patient-years (95% credible interval [CrI] 1·9–4·5) in the intervention group and 4·9 per 100 patient-years (2·8–7·1) in the control group (rate ratio [RR] 0·62, 95% CrI 0·35–1·25). The probability of non-inferiority of the intervention was more than 99·9%. Primary safety events were more frequent in the intervention group than in the control group (7·4 per 100 patient-years, 95% CrI 5·5–9·7, *vs* 4·4 per 100 patient-years, 95% CrI 2·5–6·7; RR 1·69, 1·01–3·19).

Interpretation.—The efficacy of percutaneous closure of the LAA with this device was non-inferior to that of warfarin therapy. Although there was a higher rate of adverse safety events in the intervention group than in the control group, events in the intervention group were mainly a result of periprocedural complications. Closure of the LAA might provide an alternative strategy to chronic warfarin therapy for stroke prophylaxis in patients with non-valvular atrial fibrillation.

► Oral anticoagulation is associated with substantial risk of hemorrhage. In addition, warfarin has a narrow therapeutic range and frequent drug and food interactions. International normalized ratios need to be checked frequently, and they are too often nontherapeutic. Still, oral anticoagulation with warfarin is highly effective in reducing the risk of cardioembolic stroke in patients with atrial fibrillation.

The results of the PROTECT AF (WATCHMAN Left Atrial Appendage System for Embolic Protection in Patients with Atrial Fibrillation) trial suggest that percutaneous closure of the atrial appendage (left atrial appendage [LAA]) might become a reasonable alternative to warfarin for some patients with atrial fibrillation. In this study, the frequency of embolic events was comparable in patients treated with warfarin and those who underwent LAA

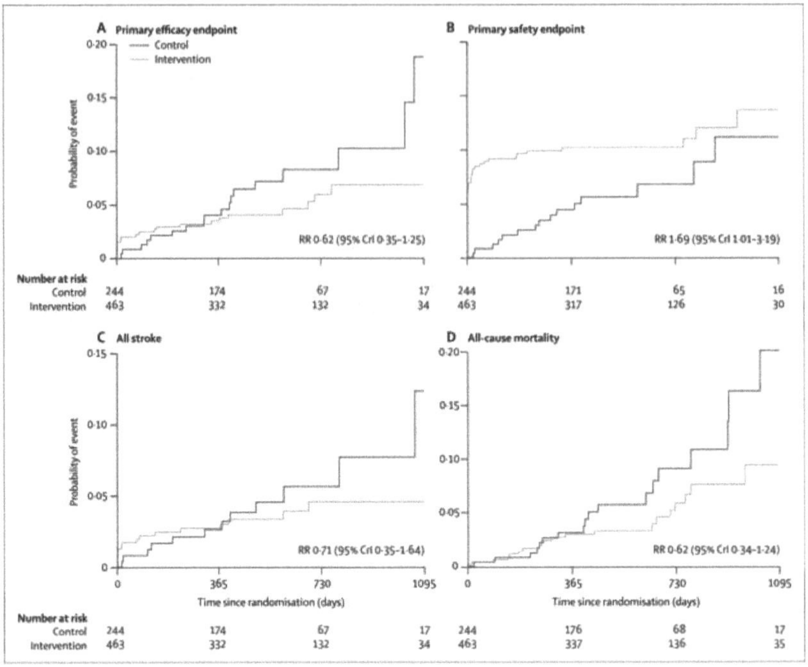

FIGURE 2.—Kaplan-Meier curves of incidence of study endpoints in intervention and control groups. RR=rate ratio. Incidence probabilities for the intention-to-treat analysis are shown with time calculated as the days since randomisation for the primary efficacy endpoint (A), the primary safety endpoint (B), all stroke (C), and all-cause mortality (D). (Reprinted from Holmes DR, for the PROTECT AF Investigators. Percutaneous closure of the left atrial appendage versus warfarin therapy for prevention of stroke in patients with atrial fibrillation: a randomised non-inferiority trial. *Lancet.* 2009;374:534-542, with permission from Elsevier.)

closure. The periprocedural risks of the percutaneous intervention were far from negligible (including 5 cases of air embolism with 2 deaths, 3 cases of device embolization, and a rate of pericardial effusion of 4.8%, necessitating pericardiocentesis in 15 cases and surgery in 7), but they were offset by greater risk of hemorrhage and embolism over the time of follow-up (Fig 2). The end point of noninferiority was reached in the intention-to-treat analysis, despite implantation failure in 9% of patients randomized to the intervention group and a relatively low incidence rate of stroke (1.6% per year) in the warfarin group. Protection from embolism was consistent across multiple subgroups. Of note, 92% of patients with successfully implanted devices had stopped taking warfarin 6 months after the intervention.

Still, some caveats apply to the interpretation of these promising results: (1) outcome assessment was unblinded; (2) maximal follow-up did not exceed 2 years; and (3) confidence intervals for all comparisons were quite wide. But most important of all, the patients enrolled in this study were not those who would be most strongly considered for LAA closure in practice (ie, patients with high stroke risk and high bleeding risk or poor compliance with the medication). These patients are most likely to have the greatest benefit from the intervention, and they should be the focus of future studies.

A. Rabinstein, MD

Population-based study of risk and predictors of stroke in the first few hours after a TIA

Chandratheva A, On behalf of the Oxford Vascular Study (Oxford Univ Dept of Clinical Neurology, UK)

Neurology 72:1941-1947, 2009

Background.—Several recent guidelines recommend assessment of patients with TIA within 24 hours, but it is uncertain how many recurrent strokes occur within 24 hours. It is also unclear whether the $ABCD^2$ risk score reliably identifies recurrences in the first few hours.

Methods.—In a prospective, population-based incidence study of TIA and stroke with complete follow-up (Oxford Vascular Study), we determined the 6-, 12-, and 24-hour risks of recurrent stroke, defined as new neurologic symptoms of sudden onset after initial recovery.

Results.—Of 1,247 first TIA or strokes, 35 had recurrent strokes within 24 hours, all in the same arterial territory. The initial event had recovered prior to the recurrent stroke (i.e., was a TIA) in 25 cases. The 6-, 12-, and 24-hour stroke risks after 488 first TIAs were 1.2% (95% confidence interval [CI]: 0.2–2.2), 2.1% (0.8–3.2), and 5.1% (3.1–7.1), with 42% of all strokes during the 30 days after a first TIA occurring within the first 24 hours. The 12- and 24-hour risks were strongly related to $ABCD^2$ score ($p = 0.02$ and $p = 0.0003$). Sixteen (64%) of the 25 cases sought urgent medical attention prior to the recurrent stroke, but none received antiplatelet treatment acutely.

Conclusion.—That about half of all recurrent strokes during the 7 days after a TIA occur in the first 24 hours highlights the need for emergency assessment. That the $ABCD^2$ score is reliable in the hyperacute phase shows that appropriately triaged emergency assessment and treatment are feasible.

▶ This study confirms the relatively high risk of stroke (approximately 5%) within the first 24 hours after a transient ischemic attack (TIA), even among patients who seek medical attention for the TIA symptoms. While applying the new definition of TIA requiring absence of brain infarction on neuroimaging[1] could reduce this numeric risk, it is clear that there are patients with true TIAs who suffer a stroke within hours of the initial transient symptoms. Those strokes can be disabling and even fatal, as shown in this study. Early initiation of adequate preventive measures has therefore enormous potential to avert brain damage.

An additional point of the study is to highlight the very good predictive performance of the $ABCD^2$ score, a simple measure to assess the risk of stroke after a TIA in the emergency department.[2] Yet, while useful, this score is not infallible, as it may be low in patients who have strokes within 1 week of the TIA.[3] High ABCD^2 scores reliably identify those patients at the greatest risk of stroke, but patients with lower ABCD^2 scores should also receive close attention.

The results of this study emphasize the undeniable importance of emergency evaluation of patients with TIA. Yet, being evaluated may not be enough. We still need to define the best way to treat these patients. This information reinforces the value of upcoming trials evaluating different early prevention strategies in this high-risk population.

A. Rabinstein, MD

References

1. Easton JD, Saver JL, Albers GW, et al. Definition and evaluation of transient ischemic attack: a scientific statement for healthcare professionals from the American Heart Association/American Stroke Association Stroke Council; Council on Cardiovascular Surgery and Anesthesia; Council on Cardiovascular Radiology and Intervention; Council on Cardiovascular Nursing; and the Interdisciplinary Council on Peripheral Vascular Disease. The American Academy of Neurology affirms the value of this statement as an educational tool for neurologists. *Stroke*. 2009;40:2276-2293.
2. Johnston SC, Rothwell PM, Nguyen-Huynh MN, et al. Validation and refinement of scores to predict very early stroke risk after transient ischemic attack. *Lancet*. 2007;369:283-292.
3. Fothergill A, Christianson TJ, Brown RD Jr, Rabinstein AA. Validation and refinement of the ABCD2 score: a population-based analysis. *Stroke*. 2009;40: 2669-2673.

Risk of recurrent subarachnoid hemorrhage, death, or dependence and standardised mortality ratios after clipping or coiling of an intracranial aneurysm in the International Subarachnoid Aneurysm Trial (ISAT): long-term follow-up

Molyneux AJ, Kerr RSC, Birks J, et al (Univ of Oxford and Oxford Radcliff Hosps NHS Trust, UK; Centre for Statistics in Medicine, Oxford, UK)

Lancet Neurol 8:427-433, 2009

Background.—Our aim was to assess the long-term risks of death, disability, and rebleeding in patients randomly assigned to clipping or endovascular coiling after rupture of an intracranial aneurysm in the follow-up of the International Subarachnoid Aneurysm Trial (ISAT).

Methods.—2143 patients with ruptured intracranial aneurysms were enrolled between 1994 and 2002 at 43 neurosurgical centres and randomly assigned to clipping or coiling. Clinical outcomes at 1 year have been previously reported. All UK and some non-UK centres continued long-term follow-up of 2004 patients enrolled in the original cohort. Annual follow-up has been done for a minimum of 6 years and a maximum of 14 years (mean follow-up 9 years). All deaths and rebleeding events were recorded. Analysis of rebleeding was by allocation and by treatment received. ISAT is registered, number ISRCTN49866681.

Findings.—24 rebleeds had occurred more than 1 year after treatment. Of these, 13 were from the treated aneurysm (ten in the coiling group and three in the clipping group; log rank p=0·06 by intention-to-treat analysis). There were 8447 person-years of follow-up in the coiling group and 8177 person-years of follow-up in the clipping group. Four rebleeds occurred from a pre-existing aneurysm and six from new aneurysms. At 5 years, 11% (112 of 1046) of the patients in the endovascular group and 14% (144 of 1041) of the patients in the neurosurgical group had died (log-rank p=0·03). The risk of death at 5 years was significantly lower in the coiling group than in the clipping group (relative risk 0·77, 95% CI 0·61–0·98; p=0·03), but the proportion of survivors at 5 years who were independent did not diff er between the two groups: endovascular 83% (626 of 755) and neurosurgical 82% (584 of 713). The standardised mortality rate, conditional on survival at 1 year, was increased for patients treated for ruptured aneurysms compared with the general population (1·57, 95% CI 1·32–1·82; p<0·0001).

Interpretation.—There was an increased risk of recurrent bleeding from a coiled aneurysm compared with a clipped aneurysm, but the risks were small. The risk of death at 5 years was signifi cantly lower in the coiled group than it was in the clipped group. The standardised mortality rate for patients treated for ruptured aneurysms was increased compared with the general population.

▶ The results of the long-term follow-up of the International Subarachnoid Aneurysm Trial (ISAT) patients are mostly confirmatory.[1] ISAT remains the most influential trial comparing clipping versus coiling of ruptured aneurysms. Only cases that fulfilled the condition of clinical equipoise were enrolled. In other words, only patients who were considered adequate candidates for clipping and for coiling were randomized. The initial report of the results of the study indicated that coiling was associated with a relative reduction in the risk of death and dependency at 1 year of 23.9% compared with clipping (absolute risk reduction 7.4%).[2] During the first year after treatment coiled patients had a slightly higher incidence of rebleeding from the treated aneurysm and required retreatment (typically additional coiling) 6.9 times more often than clipped patients.[2,3] However, there were concerns about the durability of coiling in patients who are often quite young at the time of their subarachnoid hemorrhage.

During a mean follow-up of 9 years (range 6-14 years) the risk of rebleeding from the treated aneurysm remained low in both groups, although it was higher in the coiling group (the difference was actually significant in the per protocol analysis which accounted for a patient assigned to the clipping group who requested to be coiled instead and later rebled). It is possible that current risk of aneurysm rebleeding after coiling could be lower than those seen in ISAT because technological improvement now allows higher rates of complete aneurysm obliteration, but this possibility remains to be proven. There were no differences in fatal cases of rebleeding between the 2 groups. Clipping did not eliminate the risk of late rebleeding from the treated aneurysm. Bleeding could also occur from another previously known but untreated aneurysm or from aneurysms that formed de novo after enrollment in the trial.

The risk of death at 5 years was significantly lower in the coiled group (relative risk 0.77). Yet, the chances of independent survival for those patients surviving 5 years were similar in both groups. This apparent discrepancy is probably explained by functional improvement of patients with initial moderate disability in both groups and the demise of some patients with severe disability, which had contributed to the difference in functional outcome among survivors at 1 year. Notably, the mortality rate of trial patients surviving more than 1 year was higher than the mortality expected for the general population (standardized mortality rate 1.57).

There are several important lessons to be learned from this follow-up data. All patients with subarachnoid hemorrhage should have follow-up angiograms, especially if they are smokers or have hypertension (unfortunately these 2 risk factors for aneurysm rupture and de novo aneurysm formation were not collected as part of ISAT). The timing of repeat angiograms, duration of angiographic monitoring, and relative value of noninvasive versus catheter angiograms in clipped and coiled patients need to be defined by future studies. The cost effectiveness of angiographic monitoring should also be analyzed. As correctly pointed out by the study investigators and the accompanying editorial,[4] coiling has benefits over clipping in patients who are adequate candidates for both treatments, but multiple factors (eg, anatomical features of the aneurysm, local expertise in each of the treatment options, age, and comorbid conditions of the patient), need to be weighed in the decision of which treatment modality should be chosen to secure the aneurysm.

A. Rabinstein, MD

References

1. Molyneux AJ, Kerr RS, Birks J; ISAT collaborators. Risk of recurrent subarachnoid haemorrhage, death, or dependence and standardised mortality ratios after clipping or coiling of an intracranial aneurysm in the International Subarachnoid Aneurysm Trial (ISAT): long-term follow-up. *Lancet Neurol.* 2009;8:427-433.
2. Molyneux AJ, Kerr RS, Yu LM, et al. International subarachnoid aneurysm trial (ISAT) of neurosurgical clipping versus endovascular coiling in 2143 patients with ruptured intracranial aneurysms: a randomised comparison of effects on survival, dependency, seizures, rebleeding, subgroups, and aneurysm occlusion. *Lancet.* 2005;366:809-817.
3. Campi A, Ramzi N, Molyneux AJ, et al. Retreatment of ruptured cerebral aneurysms in patients randomized by coiling or clipping in the International Subarachnoid Aneurysm Trial (ISAT). *Stroke.* 2007;38:1538-1544.
4. Broderick J. Clipping or coiling: the first step for ruptured aneurysms. *Lancet Neurol.* 2009;8:414-415.

Stroke treatment with alteplase given 3·0–4·5 h after onset of acute ischaemic stroke (ECASS III): additional outcomes and subgroup analysis of a randomised controlled trial

Bluhmki E, Chamorro Á, Dávalos A, et al (Boehringer Ingelheim, Biberach, Germany; Hosp Clinic, Barcelona, Spain; Hospital Universitari Germans Trias i Pujol, Barcelona, Spain; et al)

Lancet Neurol 8:1095-1102, 2009

Background.—In the European Cooperative Acute Stroke Study III (ECASS III), alteplase administered 3·0–4·5 h after the onset of stroke symptoms resulted in a significant benefit in the primary endpoint (modified Rankin scale [mRS] score 0–1) versus placebo, with no difference in mortality between the treatment groups. Compared with the 0–3 h window, there was no excess risk of symptomatic intracranial haemorrhage. We assessed the usefulness of additional endpoints and did subgroup and sensitivity analyses to further investigate the benefit of alteplase.

Methods.—In a double-blind, multicentre study in Europe, patients with acute ischaemic stroke were randomly assigned to intravenous alteplase (0·9 mg/kg bodyweight) or placebo. Additional outcome analyses included functional endpoints at day 90 or day 30 (mRS 0–1 [day 30], mRS 0–2, Barthel index ≥85, and global outcome statistic [day 30]) and treatment response (8-point improvement from baseline or 0–1 score on the National Institutes of Health stroke scale [NIHSS], and a stratified responder analysis by baseline NIHSS score). The subgroup analyses were based on the mRS 0–1 at day 90, symptomatic intracranial haemorrhage, and death. Analyses were by intention to treat and per protocol. This study is registered with ClinicalTrials.gov, number NCT00153036.

Findings.—418 patients were assigned to alteplase and 403 to placebo. Although not significant in every case, all additional endpoints showed at least a clear trend in favour of alteplase. Alteplase was effective in various subgroups, including older patients (<65 years: odds ratio 1·61, 95% CI 1·05–2·48; ≥65 years: 1·15, 0·80–1·64; p=0·230), and the effectiveness was independent of the severity of stroke at baseline (NIHSS 0–9: 1·28, 0·84–1·96; NIHSS 10–19: 1·16, 0·73–1·84; NIHSS ≥20: 2·32, 0·61–8·90; p=0·631). The incidence of symptomatic intracranial haemorrhage seemed to be independent of previous antiplatelet drug use (no: 2·41, 1·09–5·33; yes: 2·33, 0·79–6·90; p=0·962) and time from onset of symptoms to treatment (181–210 min: 1·62, 0·26–10·25; 211–240 min: 1·97, 0·82–4·76; 241–270 min: 3·15, 1·01–9·79; p=0·761), but not of age dichotomised at 65 years (<65 years: 0·74, 0·28–1·96; ≥65 years: 5·79, 2·18–15·39; p=0·004).

Interpretation.—Our results support the use of alteplase up to 4·5 h after the onset of stroke symptoms across a broad range of subgroups of patients who meet the requirements of the European product label but miss the approved treatment window of 0–3 h.

▶ It is reassuring to read this analysis indicating that the benefit from alteplase administered between 3 and 4.5 hours after acute stroke symptom onset in the European Cooperative Acute Stroke Study III trial was consistently maintained across multiple subgroups of patients. In other words, patients benefited from thrombolysis regardless of sex, comorbid conditions, stroke severity at baseline, and time to treatment (within the 90-minute window of this trial) (Fig 5). There were no statistically significant differences in the odds of favorable outcome

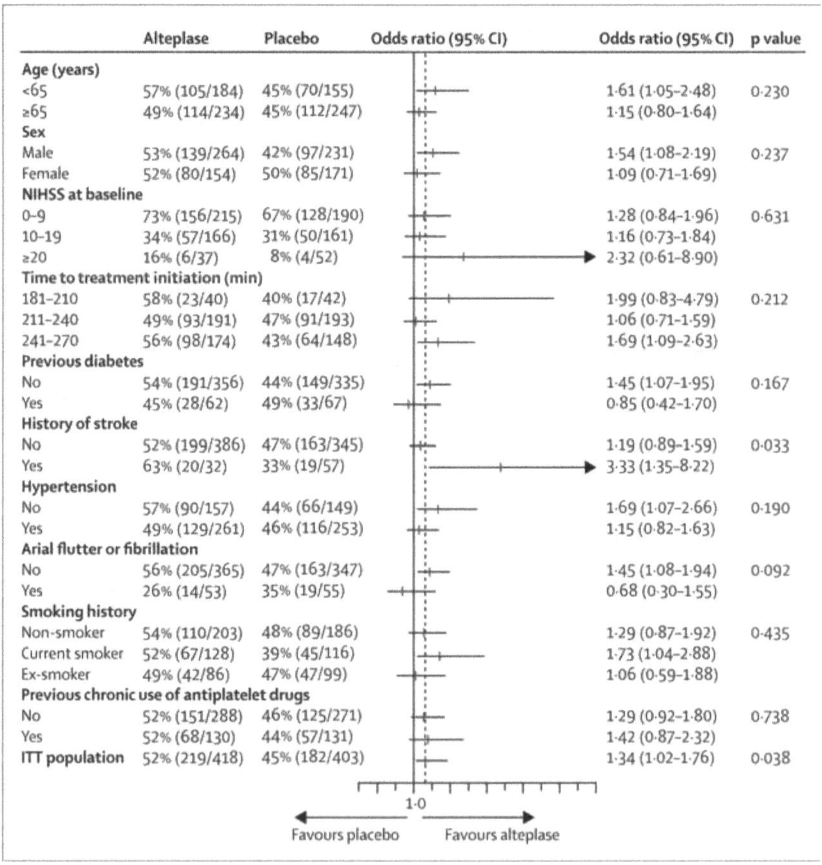

FIGURE 5.—Subgroup analysis of favourable outcome (modified Rankin scale 0–1) at day 90 according to demographic characteristics, baseline clinical data, and past medical history. Dashed vertical line represents the odds ratio for the whole intention-to-treat (ITT) population. Data are % (n/N), unless otherwise indicated. p values are for interaction based on logistic regression model with treatment, subgroup, and interaction term. NIHSS=National Institutes of Health stroke scale. (Reprinted from Bluhmki E, Chamorro Á, Dávalos A, et al. Stroke treatment with alteplase given 3·0–4·5 h after onset of acute ischaemic stroke (ECASS III): additional outcomes and subgroup analysis of a randomised controlled trial. *Lancet Neurol.* 2009;8:1095-1102, with permission from Elsevier.)

	Alteplase	Placebo	Odds ratio (95% CI)	p value
Age (years)				
<65	4% (8/184)	6% (9/155)	0·74 (0·28–1·96)	0·004
≥65	11% (25/234)	2% (5/247)	5·79 (2·18–15·39)	
Sex				
Male	9% (25/264)	3% (8/231)	2·92 (1·29–6·60)	0·340
Female	5% (8/154)	4% (6/171)	1·51 (0·51–4·44)	
NIHSS at baseline				
0–9	5% (10/215)	2% (3/190)	3·04 (0·82–11·22)	0·889
10–19	11% (19/166)	6% (9/161)	2·18 (0·96–4·98)	
≥20	11% (4/37)	4% (2/52)	3·03 (0·52–17·50)	
Time to treatment initiation (min)				
181–210	8% (3/40)	5% (2/42)	1·62 (0·26–10·25)	0·761
211–240	8% (15/191)	4% (8/193)	1·97 (0·82–4·76)	
241–270	8% (14/174)	3% (4/148)	3·15 (1·01–9·79)	
Previous diabetes				
No	8% (28/356)	3% (11/335)	2·51 (1·23–5·14)	0·724
Yes	8% (5/62)	4% (3/67)	1·87 (0·43–8·18)	
History of stroke				
No	9% (33/386)	3% (11/345)	2·84 (1·41–5·71)	0·966
Yes	0% (0/32)	5% (3/57)	..	
Hypertension				
No	8% (12/157)	5% (8/149)	1·46 (0·58–3·68)	0·175
Yes	8% (21/261)	2% (6/253)	3·60 (1·43–9·08)	
Arial flutter or fibrillation				
No	7% (24/365)	3% (10/347)	2·37 (1·12–5·04)	0·898
Yes	17% (9/53)	7% (4/55)	2·61 (0·75–9·06)	
Smoking history				
Non-smoker	10% (21/203)	3% (5/186)	4·18 (1·54–11·32)	0·250
Current smoker	5% (6/128)	3% (3/116)	1·85 (0·45–7·58)	
Ex-smoker	7% (6/86)	6% (6/99)	1·16 (0·36–3·75)	
Previous chronic use of antiplatelet drugs				
No	7% (22/288)	3% (9/271)	2·41 (1·09–5·33)	0·962
Yes	8% (11/130)	4% (5/131)	2·33 (0·79–6·90)	
ITT population	8% (33/418)	3% (14/403)	2·38 (1·25–4·52)	0·006

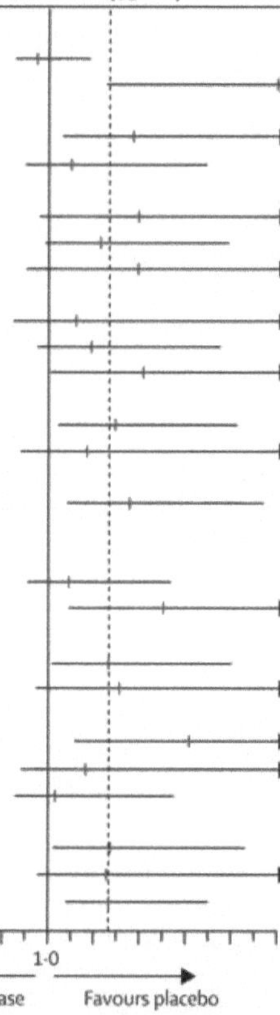

FIGURE7.—Subgroup analysis of symptomatic intracranial haemorrhage according to demographic characteristics, baseline clinical data, and past medical history. Dashed vertical line represents the odds ratio for the whole intention-to-treat (ITT) population. Data are % (n/N), unless otherwise indicated. p values are for interaction based on logistic regression model with treatment, subgroup, and interaction term. NIHSS=National Institutes of Health stroke scale. (Reprinted from Bluhmki E, Chamorro Á, Dávalos A, et al. Stroke treatment with alteplase given 3·0–4·5 h after onset of acute ischaemic stroke (ECASS III): additional outcomes and subgroup analysis of a randomised controlled trial. *Lancet Neurol.* 2009;8:1095-1102, with permission from Elsevier.)

between patients younger than 65 years and those between 65 and 80 years (patients older than 80 years were not enrolled in this trial), but careful review of the raw numbers reveals that the benefit from alteplase was much more robust and convincing in younger patients.

The subgroup analysis regarding the risk of symptomatic intracranial hemorrhage provided in this article is even more interesting and gave me a reason to pause (Fig 7). Patients ≥65 years had a significantly higher risk of hemorrhage (odds ratio 5.79 vs 0.74 in patients younger than 65 years). The rate of symptomatic intracranial hemorrhage in this group was 11%. Although these older patients still benefited from alteplase between 3 and 4.5 hours, the benefit was modest (odds ratio 1.15 for recovery with minimal or no deficits). Therefore, the risk-benefit ratio in older patients must be studied further for the extended time window. What to do at this point? Multiple studies have shown that older patients have worse outcomes after a stroke. Negating a potentially beneficial treatment precisely to these patients with worse prognosis is probably not the best course of action. Instead, I would favor discussing what is known about the risk and benefit of treatment in patients between 65 and 80 years by quoting a 15% increase in the likelihood of very favorable recovery and an 11% increase in the chance of symptomatic intracranial hemorrhage. For patients over age 80, I would abstain from offering intravenous thrombolysis after 3 hours because of the lack of safety and efficacy data.

A. Rabinstein, MD

The independent predictive utility of computed tomography angiographic collateral status in acute ischaemic stroke

Miteff F, Levi CR, Bateman GA, et al (John Hunter Hosp, New South Wales, Australia; et al)

Brain 132:2231-2238, 2009

It is unknown whether collateral vessel status, as seen on computed tomography angiography, can predict the fate of penumbral tissue identified on perfusion computed tomography and thereby influence clinical outcome. We tested this hypothesis in consecutive patients who underwent perfusion computed tomography/computed tomography angiography within 6 h of anterior circulation stroke, who also had repeat perfusion/infarct volume imaging at 24 h, and modified Rankin Scale at 3 months. Collateral status was graded as good or reduced depending on the extent of contrast visualized distal to the occlusion on computed tomography angiography. 'Perfusion computed tomography mismatch' ratio was calculated from the ratio of the mean transit time lesion/cerebral blood volume lesion. Of 92 patients with proximal intracranial vessel occlusion, good collateral status (51/92) was significantly associated with reduced infarct expansion and more favourable functional outcomes (modified Rankin Scale 0–2). Significant univariate predictors of favourable outcome were good collateral status, major reperfusion at 24 h, presence of perfusion computed tomography mismatch (for a range of ratios: ≥ 1.2, ≥ 2, ≥ 3, ≥ 3.5) and baseline National Institutes of Health Stroke Scale score. Notably, none of the 37 patients with a perfusion computed tomography mismatch ratio <3.0 had a favourable outcome. In patients with perfusion computed tomography mismatch, significant independent predictors of favourable outcome were good collateral status, major reperfusion and baseline National Institutes of Health Stroke Scale score. There was also a strong interaction between major reperfusion and good collateral status in the regression models. In patients with proximal vessel occlusion, perfusion computed tomography mismatch is a prerequisite for a favourable clinical response, but good collateral status appears a critical determinant of ultimate outcome, particularly if major reperfusion occurs.

▶ This study provides convincing evidence that the strength of the collateral flow is a major determinant of outcome in patients with acute ischemic stroke due to proximal large vessel occlusion. Good collateral flow was associated with less severe deficits upon presentation, smaller infarct cores, larger areas of ischemic penumbra (defined by the CT perfusion mismatch ratio calculated from mean transit time/cerebral blood volume lesion volume), and lower rates of infarct expansion. In order to be considered good, collateral flow from leptomeningeal vessels had to produce retrograde filling of the middle cerebral artery nearly up to the point of occlusion. This strong pattern of collateral flow was observed in 56% of the patients included in the analysis.

In patients with substantial mismatch on CT perfusion, the presence of good collateral flow and major reperfusion after thrombolytic treatment predicted better chances of favorable functional recovery. Conversely, patients with CT perfusion mismatch ratio <3 had uniformly unfavorable outcomes, regardless of treatment. Hence, these results highlight the value of CT perfusion not only to select good candidates for reperfusion therapy but also to select out those patients who do not have chances of recovery. Interestingly, in this study population, time from symptom onset (up to 6 hours) correlated very poorly with collateral status or the presence of ischemic penumbra.

The message of the study is clear. Adequate use of multimodal CT assessment (unenhanced CT, CT perfusion, and CT angiography) can be very useful to adopt the right course of action in patients with acute ischemic stroke due to anterior circulation large vessel occlusion. Furthermore, as the authors performed their analysis using an older version of CT perfusion with limited spatial resolution, the results may have been even more solid if the study were to be repeated using newer technology.

A. Rabinstein, MD

Unsuspected coagulopathy rarely prevents IV thrombolysis in acute ischemic stroke

Rost NS, Masrur S, Pervez MA, et al (Massachusetts General Hosp, Boston)
Neurology 73:1957-1962, 2009

Background.—American Heart Association/American Stroke Association guidelines recommend initiating treatment with IV tissue plasminogen activator (tPA) in acute ischemic stroke patients without suspected coagulopathy prior to availability of clotting results; however, little or no data support this practice. We sought to identify how often blood clotting abnormalities were responsible for withholding IV tPA at our institution.

Methods.—We conducted a retrospective review of our prospectively acquired Get With the Guidelines Stroke database from January 2003 to April 2008. All patients underwent clinical evaluation by a neurologist, diagnostic neuroimaging, and laboratory testing on admission. We classified patients with absolute contraindications to IV tPA as ineligible, and those with warnings/relative contraindications or potentially treatable factors as potentially eligible.

Results.—Of 2,335 considered for analysis, 470 (20.1%) patients presented to our emergency department (ED) within 3 hours. Among these, 147 (31.3%) received IV tPA in our ED, 102 (21.7%) had an absolute contraindication, and 221 (47%) had a reason to consider withholding tPA. Only 30/470 (6.4%) of potential thrombolysis patients were discovered to have international normalized ratio ≥ 1.7 or platelets $\leq 100{,}000/\mu L$, and of these, 28 were suspected a priori due to known coagulopathy from medication or illness. Only 2/470 (0.4%) patients had an unsuspected coagulopathy that ultimately prevented thrombolysis.

Conclusions.—Based on the experience of a large thrombolysis referral center, stroke patients without suspected clotting abnormality can safely begin thrombolytic therapy before clotting results are available. These data support the current practice guidelines, and may reassure clinicians that the benefits of early administration greatly outweigh the risks due to an unsuspected bleeding diathesis.

▶ The message of this study is simple and clinically valuable: intravenous thrombolysis should not be delayed until the results of the platelet count and INR become available unless the patient has a history of bleeding diathesis, liver disease, end-stage renal disease, or recent use of warfarin. The results from this analysis support the current recommendation in the American Heart Association guidelines for the treatment of acute ischemic stroke.[1] Time is precious in patients with acute stroke who are candidates for intravenous thrombolysis. Avoiding all but the most indispensable delays in these patients is of paramount importance.

As noted by the authors of this article, coagulation measures may be soon instantaneously available by using point-of-care fingerstick devices. Until then, the delay of waiting for clotting results from the laboratory should not be considered justifiable.

A. Rabinstein, MD

Reference

1. Adams HP Jr, del Zoppo G, Alberts MJ, et al. Guidelines for the early management of adults with ischemic stroke: a guideline from the American Heart Association/ American Stroke Association Stroke Council, Clinical Cardiology Council, Cardiovascular Radiology and Intervention Council, and the Atherosclerotic Peripheral Vascular Disease and Quality of Care Outcomes in Research Interdisciplinary Working Groups: the American Academy of Neurology affirms the value of this guideline as an educational tool for neurologists. *Stroke*. 2007;38: 1655-1711.

3 Epilepsy and Other Seizure Disorders

Adverse antiepileptic drug effects: toward a clinically and neurobiologically relevant taxonomy

Perucca P, Carter J, Vahle V, et al (Columbia Univ, NY)

Neurology 72:1223-1229, 2009

Background.—Adverse effects (AEs) of antiepileptic drugs (AEDs) are a major impediment to optimal dosing for seizure control. Better understanding of clinical properties of AEs is a prerequisite for systematic research of their neurobiological underpinnings. This study aimed to define specific patterns of AE occurrence and determine their clinical relevance based on their association with subjective health status.

Methods.—Two hundred subjects with epilepsy completed validated self-report health assessments, including the Adverse Event Profile (AEP) and Quality of Life in Epilepsy Inventory (QOLIE)-89. Factor analysis was performed on the 19 AEP items to identify distinct classes of AEs. Correlations between AE class scores and QOLIE-89 scores were evaluated. Multivariate analysis was used to assess contributions of AE class scores to QOLIE-89 scores after controlling for depression and seizure frequency. Relationships between changes in AE class scores and changes in QOLIE-89 scores were also investigated in a subgroup of 62 subjects enrolled in a randomized trial.

Results.—The mean number of AEs per subject was 6.5. AEs were segregated into five classes: Cognition/Coordination, Mood/Emotion, Sleep, Weight/Cephalgia, and Tegument/Mucosa. Higher scores in each AE class were associated with lower QOLIE-89 scores. Cognition/Coordination scores were the strongest predictor of QOLIE-89 scores. Improvements in Cognition/Coordination, Mood/Emotion, and Tegument/Mucosa scores were associated with improvements in QOLIE-89 scores. Improved Cognition/Coordination was the only predictor of improved QOLIE-89.

Conclusion.—Adverse effects (AEs) of antiepileptic drugs can be classified in five biologically plausible factors. When specific classes of AEs are identified and attempts are made to reduce them, quality of life is significantly improved.

▶ When a patient has a seizure, it is bad luck. When he or she suffers a side effect to the latest prescribed antiepileptic drug, it is the doctor's fault! Around 14 novel antiepileptic drugs have been licensed around the world over the last 20 years. All of these have a range of side effects, some of which are generic for the group and others peculiar to that individual drug. As pharmacotherapy for epilepsy often requires to be taken lifelong, new clinical problems can arise over the years, which may or may not be relevant to the treatment regimen. Clinicians, therefore, need to know what are the common, acute, and unusual chronic side effects for all of the "antiepileptic" drugs that their patients are likely to take.

Quality of life in people with epilepsy does not correlate with seizure numbers. Only seizure freedom produces a measurable improvement. However, the development of side effects to antiepileptic drug therapy has been consistently shown to predict worsening quality of life. Not surprisingly, therefore, relieving the patient of these additional burdens can be demonstrated to significantly improve their well-being. Systems that make drug-related side effects easier to recognize and remember will be helpful in optimizing the safe use of this ubiquitous group of therapeutic agents. This study classifies the adverse effects into 5 biologically plausible systems, thus helping neurologists to treat epilepsy successfully by recognizing drug-related problems, thereby reducing the burden of toxicity.

M. J. Brodie, MD, FRCP

Early-Onset Absence Epilepsy Caused by Mutations in the Glucose Transporter GLUT1

Suls A, Mullen SA, Weber YG, et al (VIB Department of Molecular Genetics; Univ of Melbourne; Univ of Ulm; et al)
Ann Neurol 66:415-419, 2009

Absence epilepsies of childhood are heterogeneous with most cases following complex inheritance. Those cases with onset before 4 years of age represent a poorly studied subset. We screened 34 patients with early-onset absence epilepsy for mutations in *SLC2A1*, the gene encoding the GLUT1 glucose transporter. Mutations leading to reduced protein function were found in 12% (4/34) of patients. Two mutations arose de novo, and two were familial. These findings suggest GLUT1 deficiency underlies a significant proportion of early-onset absence epilepsy, which has both genetic counseling and treatment implications because the ketogenic diet is effective in GLUT1 deficiency.

▶ The genetics of epilepsy is the currently most popular research avenue for understanding better this most heterogeneous group of common neurological disorders. Mutations in at least 25 different genes have been described over the past decade, although the strength of the evidence that these genes have a pathogenic role varies widely. Rather than throwing light on the neurobiology of common seizure disorders and rare pediatric syndromes, the epilepsy research community is slowly becoming aware of the ever increasing complexity governing their genetic basis. So far, most of the focus has been made on the most obvious targets for single gene mutations, such as voltage-gated (Na+, K+, Ca^2, Cl, and HCN) and ligand-gated channels (nicotinic acetylcholine and GABA receptors). Substantial phenotypic variation among affected family members substantially complicates our understanding of the genetic associations. The identification of new genes underpinning epilepsy syndromes may uncover promising areas for future research. This article includes data from children with onset of absence epilepsy before 4 years of age living in Belgium, Germany, Italy, and Australia, some of whom demonstrated a novel mutation in the glucose transporter GLUT1 gene. Although only present in 4 out of 34 (12%) patients, this observation points up new avenues for exploration. These patients, interestingly, may respond to treatment with the ketogenic diet. The complexity of epilepsy genetics is providing more questions than answers, but must represent the best way forward in identifying novel treatments for people with refractory epilepsy.

M. J. Brodie, MD, FRCP

Effects of Antiepileptic Drugs on Lipids, Homocysteine, and C-Reactive Protein

Mintzer S, Skidmore CT, Abidin CJ, et al (Thomas Jefferson Univ, Philadelphia, PA)

Ann Neurol 65:448-456, 2009

Objective.—The widely prescribed anticonvulsants phenytoin and carbamazepine are potent inducers of cytochrome P450 enzymes, which are involved in cholesterol synthesis. We sought to determine whether these drugs have an effect on cholesterol and other serological markers of vascular risk.

Methods.—We recruited 34 epilepsy patients taking carbamazepine or phenytoin in monotherapy whose physicians had elected to change treatment to one of the noninducing anticonvulsants lamotrigine or levetiracetam. Fasting blood samples were obtained both before and 6 weeks after the switch to measure serum lipid fractions, lipoprotein(a), C-reactive protein, and homocysteine. A comparator group of 16 healthy subjects underwent the same serial studies.

Results.—In the epilepsy patients, switch from either phenytoin or carbamazepine produced significant declines in total cholesterol (−24.8 mg/dl), atherogenic (non–high-density lipoprotein) cholesterol (−19.9 mg/dl), triglycerides (−47.1 mg/dl) (all $p < 0.0001$), and C-reactive protein (−31.4%; $p = 0.027$). Patients who stopped taking carbamazepine also had a 31.2% decline in lipoprotein(a) level ($p = 0.0004$), whereas those taken off phenytoin had a decrease in homocysteine level (−1.7 μmol/L;

$p = 0.005$). All of these changes were significant when compared with those seen in healthy subjects ($p < 0.05$). Results were similar whether patients were switched to lamotrigine or levetiracetam.

Interpretation.—Switching epilepsy patients from the enzyme-inducers carbamazepine or phenytoin to the noninducing drugs levetiracetam or lamotrigine produces rapid and clinically significant amelioration in several serological markers of vascular risk. These findings suggest that phenytoin and carbamazepine may substantially increase the risk for cardiovascular and cerebrovascular disease.

▶ Enzyme inducers stimulate the de novo synthesis of metabolic enzymes in the liver and elsewhere in the body with the potential to reduce the duration and intensity of the action of a wide range of lipid soluble drugs. This is a particular problem with broad spectrum inducers, such as phenobarbital, primidone (metabolized to phenobarbital), carbamazepine, and phenytoin. Target enzyme groups are monooxygenases (cytochrome P450 superfamily), glucuronyl transferases, and epoxide hydrolases. Substrates for these enzymes include oral contraceptives, anticoagulants, cytotoxic drugs, opioid analgesics, antiretrovirals, statins, antihypertensives, cardiac antiarrhythmias, and immunosuppressants. Enzyme induction will accelerate the clearance of these drugs by as much as 100%, thereby doubling the amount of drug (and its cost) required to achieve the same therapeutic response as in an uninduced patient. Conversely, withdrawal of an inducer will reverse the process over a month or 2, substantially increasing the circulating concentrations of the target agent risking severe toxicity unless the dose of the induced drug is appropriately reduced. There are also a number of endogenous substrates for this process, including steroid vitamins and hormones. In the above article substitution of inducing antiepileptic drugs, phenytoin, and carbamazepine by the noninducing lamotrigine or levetiracetam reduced total cholesterol, triglycerides, and C-reactive protein by 11%, 33%, and 31%, respectively. This observation supports epidemiological data that the prescription of enzyme inducing antiepileptic drugs may increase the risk of cardiovascular and cerebrovascular disease in later life. Given the wide range of antiepileptic drugs now available, do we now need to subject patients to the risks of lifelong enzyme induction? It is certainly not a cost-effective approach to treating the common epilepsies.

M. J. Brodie, MD, FRCP

Febrile Seizures and Primary Human Herpesvirus 6 Infection

Laina I, Syriopoulou VP, Daikos GL, et al (Athens Univ, Greece)

Pediatr Neurol 42:28-31, 2010

Primary human herpesvirus 6 infection is acquired mainly during the first two years of life and is often associated with febrile seizures. The aim of the present study was to investigate in Greece the frequency and clinical characteristics of primary human herpesvirus 6 (HHV-6) infection in hospitalized children with febrile seizures. Children aged from 6 months to 5 years without known neurologic disease were examined for primary HHV-6 infection, by real-time polymerase chain reaction in acute-phase plasma and by indirect immunofluorescent assay for antibody titers in acute and convalescent serum. Of 65 children included in the analysis, 55 experienced the first febrile episode of seizures and 10 the second. Primary HHV-6 infection was verified in 10 of 55 children with a first febrile episode (18%), whereas none of the 10 children with a second episode of seizures had primary HHV-6 infection. Eight children were infected with HHV-6 type B and two with type A. None of the 85 control subjects had primary HHV-6 infection, but 49% had immunoglobulin G antibodies against the virus. These findings suggest that primary HHV-6 infection is frequently associated with febrile seizures in children in this geographic region and should be considered, especially for a first episode of febrile seizures.

▶ There is increasing interest in the association of viral infection in infancy and the subsequent development of refractory epilepsy. Whether ongoing inflammation contributes to pharmacoresistance is a moot question. One of the prime targets implicated in this sequence of events is herpesvirus. After primary infection, the virus can remain latent within the central nervous system. As infection with this group of viruses is nearly ubiquitous in childhood, this is an important area of scientific inquiry. Herpesviruses have been identified as possible etiological factors in multiple sclerosis, myocarditis, and encephalitis, as well as causing febrile status epilepticus leading to the subsequent development of mesial temporal sclerosis. This scenario can result in the production of refractory epilepsy after a seizure-free interval of 10 to 20 years.

It has been suggested that infection with herpesvirus can interfere with excitatory amino acid transport, thereby contributing to chronic inflammatory damage. This work has led to increasing interest in the role of inflammation in epileptogenesis. Both human and animal data suggest that proinflammatory mediators, such as cytokines and interleukins, are upregulated after seizures and may contribute to increased cortical excitability. Similar mechanisms may also be implicated in the development of Rasmussen's encephalitis. These potentially important findings may help identify new therapeutic targets for the prevention and treatment of refractory epilepsy. In particular, if this relationship with herpesvirus infection is confirmed, specific antiviral interventions or anti-inflammatory medications may play a role in impeding epileptogenesis or in developing vaccines that prevent mesial temporal lobe epilepsy.

M. J. Brodie, MD, FRCP

Juvenile myoclonic epilepsy 25 years after seizure onset: A population-based study

Camfield CS, Camfield PR (IWK Health Centre and Dalhousie Univ, Halifax, Nova Scotia, Canada)

Neurology 73:1041-1045, 2009

Objective.—To document the long-term evolution of juvenile myoclonic epilepsy (JME) in a population-based cohort.

Methods.—All patients developing JME by 16 years of age in Nova Scotia between 1977 and 1985 were contacted in 2006-2008.

Results.—Twenty-four patients (17 women) had JME, 3.5% of all childhood-onset epilepsy. Age at first seizure was 10.4 ± 4.3 years. We contacted 23 of 24 (96%) at a mean age of 36 ± 4.8 years. All were initially treated with antiepileptic drugs (AEDs). At the end of a 25.8 ± 2.4-year follow-up, 11 (48%) had discontinued treatment: 6 were seizure-free (without AEDs for 5-23 years), 3 had myoclonic seizures only (without AEDs for >18 years), and 2 continued with rare seizures. Convulsive status epilepticus occurred in 8 (36%) and 3 had intractable epilepsy. About 70% reported good satisfaction with their health, work, friendships, and social life (Likert scales). Despite 87% high school graduation, 31% were unemployed. Sixteen live with a partner, 7 alone. Nine received antidepressant medications. Ten women had ≥1 pregnancy and 4 men fathered a child. Eleven pregnancies (80%) were unplanned, outside of a stable relationship. At least 1 major unfavorable social outcome was noted in 76%.

Conclusions.—Our sample size is modest but the long follow-up and population-based sampling is unique. All seizure types in juvenile myoclonic epilepsy (JME) resolved in 17% and for 13%, only myoclonus persisted. Therefore, one-third of people with JME have troublesome seizures vanish and antiepileptic drug treatment is no longer needed. Depression, social isolation, unemployment, and social impulsiveness complicate the lives of many patients.

▶ There is a general notion that juvenile myoclonic epilepsy (JME) requires lifelong pharmacotherapy. There is, as well, a tendency in epilepsy management to focus attention on seizure control and to overlook the psychological and social consequences of epilepsy. This review of the long-term status of patients with JME addresses both of these. This article shows that almost half of the JME patients were no longer receiving antiepileptic medication upon long-term follow-up. While half of these did still have seizures, these were either myoclonic only or rare convulsive seizures. Accordingly, the burden of taking medication in some instances may be greater than the burden of having seizures, another point to ponder. Despite the majority reporting themselves as very satisfied with their life situation and having educational success, a third were unemployed, the majority had received mood-altering medication, and pregnancies for the most part were unplanned. Three quarters had at least one unfavorable social outcome. As the authors indicate, further attention to unemployment, depression, social isolation, and inadvertent pregnancy is indicated.

G. N. Breningstall, MD

Juvenile myoclonic epilepsy 25 years after seizure onset: A population-based study

Camfield CS, Camfield PR (IWK Health Centre and Dalhousie Univ, Halifax, Nova Scotia, Canada)

Neurology 73:1041-1045, 2009

Objective.—To document the long-term evolution of juvenile myoclonic epilepsy (JME) in a population-based cohort.

Methods.—All patients developing JME by 16 years of age in Nova Scotia between 1977 and 1985 were contacted in 2006-2008.

Results.—Twenty-four patients (17 women) had JME, 3.5% of all childhood-onset epilepsy. Age at first seizure was 10.4 ± 4.3 years. We contacted 23 of 24 (96%) at a mean age of 36 ± 4.8 years. All were initially treated with antiepileptic drugs (AEDs). At the end of a 25.8 ± 2.4-year follow-up, 11 (48%) had discontinued treatment: 6 were seizure-free (without AEDs for 5-23 years), 3 had myoclonic seizures only (without AEDs for >18 years), and 2 continued with rare seizures. Convulsive status epilepticus occurred in 8 (36%) and 3 had intractable epilepsy. About 70% reported good satisfaction with their health, work, friendships, and social life (Likert scales). Despite 87% high school graduation, 31% were unemployed. Sixteen live with a partner, 7 alone. Nine received antidepressant medications. Ten women had ≥1 pregnancy and 4 men fathered a child. Eleven pregnancies (80%) were unplanned, outside of a stable relationship. At least 1 major unfavorable social outcome was noted in 76%.

Conclusions.—Our sample size is modest but the long follow-up and population-based sampling is unique. All seizure types in juvenile myoclonic epilepsy (JME) resolved in 17% and for 13%, only myoclonus persisted. Therefore, one-third of people with JME have troublesome seizures vanish and antiepileptic drug treatment is no longer needed. Depression, social isolation, unemployment, and social impulsiveness complicate the lives of many patients.

▶ Juvenile myoclonic epilepsy (JME) is a common form of idiopathic generalized epilepsy presenting usually in the teenage years. The diagnosis is often straightforward with patients complaining of early morning myoclonic jerks accompanied by tonic-clonic seizures and occasionally generalized absences. JME is regarded by most neurologists as a benign disorder that responds well to antiepileptic drug therapy. Relapse is likely in around 75% of patients if medication is withdrawn after a number of years of seizure freedom, although in some the epilepsy can remit. Over recent years, there have been a number of developments suggesting that this relatively reassuring situation may not be as clear-cut as previously thought. Firstly, the semiology and response to treatment differs substantially among this young patient population. Genetic studies support a range of epilepsies rather than a single JME syndrome. Functional brain imaging is often abnormal, possibly complementing the clinical observation that some patients display unreliable and impulsive behavior. This points up the possibility of frontal lobe dysfunction.

There are surprisingly few long-term studies of outcome in patients with JME. The Camfields followed up a relatively modest number of patients diagnosed in childhood. However, their results clearly demonstrate the substantial variation in prognosis. Seizure freedom with or without medication occurred in just less than half of their patients. Convulsive status epilepticus presented in just over a third, and around 13% of their population subsequently developed refractory epilepsy. Perhaps more importantly, depression, social isolation, and impulsiveness complicated the lives of many patients, around a third of whom remained unemployed. Thus, the good news message when JME is diagnosed must now be tempered with caution when discussing the prognosis with affected teenagers and their families. What can be done about the behavioral and psychiatric accompaniments to the diagnosis is not clear, but these problems clearly need to be identified at an early stage.

M. J. Brodie, MD, FRCP

Lorazepam versus diazepam–phenytoin combination in the treatment of convulsive status epilepticus in children: A randomized controlled trial

Sreenath TG, Gupta P, Sharma KK, et al (Univ College of Med Sciences and Guru Tegh Bahadur Hosp, Delhi, India)

Eur J Paediatr Neurol 14:162-168, 2010

Background.—Convulsive status epilepticus demands urgent and appropriate management with anticonvulsants. Intravenous diazepam is an established drug in the management of convulsive status epilepticus in adults as well as in children. The efficacy of intravenous lorazepam has not been well established in children.

Objective.—To determine whether intravenous lorazepam is as efficacious as diazepam–phenytoin combination in the treatment of convulsive status epilepticus in children.

Study Design.—Randomized controlled trial.

Methods.—A total of 178 children were enrolled in the study; 90 in the lorazepam group and 88 in the diazepam–phenytoin combination group. Enrolled subjects were between 1 and 12 years with a clinical diagnosis of convulsive status epilepticus, presenting in pediatric emergency of a tertiary care hospital. They were randomized to receive either intravenous lorazepam (0.1 mg/kg) or intravenous diazepam (0.2 mg/kg)–phenytoin (18 mg/kg) combination at admission and were followed up for subsequent 18 h.

Results.—The overall success rate of therapy was 100% in both the groups. There was no statistically significant difference in the two groups (lorazepam versus diazepam–phenytoin combination) in the median time taken to stop the seizure [20 s in both groups], the number of subjects requiring more than one dose of the study drug to stop the presenting seizure [lorazepam 6(6.7%) versus diazepam–phenytoin combination: 14 (15.9%); adjusted RR (95% CI) = 0.377 (0.377, 1.046); $P = 0.061$] and the number (%) of patients having respiratory depression [lorazepam 4(4.4%) versus diazepam–phenytoin combination 5 (5.6%)]. None of the patients in the two groups required additional anticonvulsant drug to stop the presenting seizure. No patient required mechanical ventilation and none of the patients in the two groups required cross-over to the alternative regimen.

Conclusion.—Lorazepam is as efficacious and safe as diazepam–phenytoin combination. We recommend use of lorazepam as a single drug to replace the two drug combination of diazepam–phenytoin combination to control the initial seizure in pediatric convulsive status epilepticus.

▶ The treatment of status epilepticus is old-fashioned and underresearched. We are still using benzodiazepines and phenytoin as first line drugs because little else is licensed or likely to be licensed soon. Prolonged epileptic seizures or status epilepticus can present at any time in life. The mortality rate has not changed over the last 25 years. No new treatments have been developed for status over a similar time period. The reason for this is that the complexity of the process required to obtain a license costs more than the likely financial rewards that could be recouped by the sponsor before the proprietary formulation was overtaken by a raft of generics. I am only aware of 2 major double-blind randomized controlled trials in the hospitalized patients, the last one being published in 1998.[1] One major reason for this is the complexity of the process needed to obtain consent from seizing patients' next of kin within a fairly short time window. What is needed is a regulatory compromise that would allow appropriate studies toward a license for status epilepticus to be undertaken expeditiously and cost-effectively. Sodium valproate, levetiracetam, and lacosamide are all available in parenteral formulations. All have some literature-suggesting efficacy in status epilepticus, but none will ever be granted a license for this indication.

What we are left with is a range of unblinded studies similar to one undertaken by Sreenath and colleagues in Delhi, which, although randomized, by necessity, lacks the rigor and the patient numbers needed to confirm superiority or equivalence sufficiently robustly to satisfy regulators. Nevertheless, this study does suggest that a simple regimen with intravenous lorazepam is as effective as the often-used "standard of care" combining diazepam with subsequent phenytoin. Timing was confined to the first 18 hours after treatment, and the article gives no data on long-term outcome. Considering all of the above, it is not surprising that the Cochrane systematic review undertaken in 2008 lamented that, "Significant gaps remain in the evidence base for the treatment of acute tonic-clonic convulsions and convulsive status epilepticus in childhood." This will remain the case for the foreseeable future.

M. J. Brodie, MD, FRCP

Reference

1. Treiman DM, Meyers PD, Walton NY, et al. A comparison of four treatments for generalized convulsive status epilepticus: Veterans Affairs Status Epilepticus Cooperative Study Group. *N Engl J Med.* 1998;339:792-798.

Relationship Between Antiepileptic Drugs and Suicide Attempts in Patients With Bipolar Disorder

Gibbons RD, Hur K, Brown CH, et al (Univ of Illinois at Chicago; et al)
Arch Gen Psychiatry 66:1354-1360, 2009

Context.—On January 31, 2008, the Food and Drug Administration issued an alert regarding increased risk of suicidal thoughts and behavior related to use of antiepileptic drugs (AEDs). On July 10, 2008, a Food and Drug Administration scientific advisory committee voted that, yes, there was a significant positive association between AEDs and suicidality but voted against placing a black box warning on AEDs for suicidality.

Objective.—To determine if AEDs increase the risk of suicide attempt in patients with bipolar disorder.

Design.—A pharmacoepidemiologic study in which suicide attempt rates were compared before and after treatment and with a medication-free control group. Analyses were restricted to AED and lithium monotherapy.

Setting.—We used the PharMetrics medical claims database to study the relationship between the 11 AEDs identified in the FDA alert, and lithium, to suicide attempts.

Main Outcome Measure.—Suicide attempts.

Patients.—A cohort of 47 918 patients with bipolar disorder with a minimum 1-year window of information before and after the index date of their illness.

Results.—Overall, there was no significant difference in suicide attempt rates for patients treated with an AED (13 per 1000 person-years [PY]) vs patients not treated with an AED or lithium (13 per 1000 PY). In AED-treated subjects, the rate of suicide attempts was significantly higher before treatment (72 per 1000 PY) than after (13 per 1000 PY). In patients receiving no concomitant treatment with an antidepressant, other AED, or antipsychotic, AEDs were significantly protective relative to no pharmacologic treatment (3 per 1000 vs 15 per 1000 PY).

Conclusions.—Despite Food and Drug Administration reports regarding increased risk of suicidality associated with AED treatment, the current study reveals that, as a class, AEDs do not increase risk of suicide attempts in patients with bipolar disorder relative to patients not treated with an AED or lithium. Use of AEDs reduces suicide attempt rates both relative to patients not receiving any psychotropic medication and relative to their pretreatment levels.

▶ Antiepileptic drugs (AEDs) are extensively used for other indications, including trigeminal neuralgia, prophylaxis of migraine, general anxiety, and mood disorders. In March 2005, the Food and Drug Administration (FDA) sent a letter to the sponsors of 11 AEDs requesting submission of their suicidality data from randomized clinical trials. They then conducted a meta-analysis of 199 placebo-controlled trials that included more than 40 000 patients. A total of 0.43% of 27 863 patients in drug-treatment groups reported suicidal behavior or ideation versus 0.22% of 16 029 patients randomized to placebo. Compared with placebo controls, 2.1 per 1000 more treated patients (95% confidence intervals 0.7-4.2) reported suicidal behavior or ideation. The resultant alert has caused much discussion, debate, and controversy.

This issue is now raised routinely in patients taking part in randomized trials but not necessarily in everyday clinical practice when a patient is commenced on a new AED. Because this is a group effect, all AEDs have been tarred with the same brush, although some, such as carbamazepine and lamotrigine, possess antidepressant properties. We are also, of course, now aware that around 30% of the patients with refractory epilepsy have depression as part of their pattern of brain dysfunction. Indeed, providing them with antidepressants has been shown to improve their quality of life. This debate has drawn attention to the importance of psychiatric comorbidities in people with epilepsy.

Nevertheless, do AEDs really increase suicidality or is the original observation, as many experts believe, flawed because all patients randomized to placebo were already receiving treatment with 1, or (more likely) 2, or 3 AEDs. Indeed, many of these patients were already receiving treatment with one or more of the drugs included in the active arm of previous randomized controlled trials. One alternative explanation could be that actively treated patients taking a fixed dose of a new drug were more likely to suffer side effects, feel miserable, and contemplate ending it all. The above study supports a number of others in finding no relationship between AED use and suicidality in patients this time with bipolar disorder.

M. J. Brodie, MD, FRCP

Seizure frequency and lateralization affect progression of atrophy in temporal lobe epilepsy

Coan AC, Appenzeller S, Bonilha L, et al (Univ of Campinas–UNICAMP, SP, Brazil)

Neurology 73:834-842, 2009

Background.—It is unclear which factors lead to progressive neuronal damage in mesial temporal lobe epilepsy (MTLE). The objective of this study was to evaluate whether progressive hippocampal and extrahippocampal atrophy occur in patients with MTLE and whether this atrophy is related to seizures.

Method.—We performed 2 MRI scans in 33 patients with clinical and electroencephalographic diagnosis of MTLE and in 24 healthy controls. MRI was performed in a 2-T scanner, and a T1-weighted gradient-echo sequence with 1 mm thickness was used for voxel-based morphometry analysis. Follow-up images were obtained at least 7 months after the first baseline MRI. Comparisons between the patient's follow-up and baseline MRIs, and between patients and controls, were performed. A corrected p value of 0.05 was set as the threshold for the statistical analysis.

Results.—Follow-up MRI was performed after a median interval of 39 months (range 7–85 months). Three patients were seizure-free between the first and second MRIs. We observed progressive white and gray matter atrophy ($p < 0.05$) in patients with MTLE. This progression was more intense in patients with left MTLE compared with right MTLE. A higher frequency of seizures and a longer duration of epilepsy were associated with progression of gray and white matter atrophy in patients with MTLE.

Conclusion.—The progression of white and gray matter atrophy in patients with mesial temporal lobe epilepsy (MTLE) was more intense in patients with left MTLE and was associated with poorer seizure control and a longer duration of epilepsy.

▶ Mesial temporal lobe epilepsy (MTLE) with hippocampal sclerosis is the commonest anatomical substrate for successful epilepsy surgery. Many patients will have had previous febrile convulsions with or without a family history of epilepsy. However, not all patients with MTLE and hippocampal sclerosis will develop refractory epilepsy. Some will go a number of years seizure free on antiepileptic drug therapy before relapsing and subsequently becoming pharmacoresistant. Others will remain controlled on antiepileptic medication. The pharmacotherapy of epilepsy prevents seizures, but none of the available agents have been shown to influence the neurobiologic processes causing them. A method of reviewing these patients to facilitate prediction of subsequent poor prognosis could be of clinical value.

In the above study, the size of the hippocampus was monitored over a number of years in a cohort of such patients. Progression of hippocampal atrophy was, perhaps not surprisingly, associated with longer duration of epilepsy and poorer seizure control. Less easy to explain was the observation that this process was more intense in patients with left compared with right MTLE. The International League against Epilepsy has just published in *Epilepsia*, a consensus definition of drug-resistant epilepsy that centers around failure of an adequate trial of 2 tolerated, appropriately dosed, and used antiepileptic drug schedules to achieve sustained seizure freedom. One of the major reasons for this initiative was to help reduce the delay in patients with MTLE associated with hippocampal atrophy being referred to an epilepsy surgery centre for work-up toward "curative" temporal lobectomy. Monitoring the size of the hippocampus could contribute to optimal management of these surgically treatable patients.

M. J. Brodie, MD, FRCP

Seizure Relapse and Development of Drug Resistance Following Long-term Seizure Remission

Schiller Y (Rambam Med Ctr, and Technion Med School, Haifa, Israel)
Arch Neurol 66:1233-1239, 2009

Objective.—To quantify and identify predictive risk factors for seizure relapse and development of drug resistance in patients who achieved long-term (>1 year) antiepileptic drug–induced seizure remission.

Design.—Prospective cohort study.

Setting.—Epilepsy Center, Rambam Medical Center.

Patients.—Two hundred fifty-six consecutive patients who entered long-term (>1 year) antiepileptic drug–induced seizure remission were followed up prospectively for 2 years or more.

Main Outcome Measures.—Seizure relapse and development of drug-resistant epilepsy.

Results.—Five years after entering seizure remission, 40.2% of patients experienced seizure relapse and 25.3% of patients developed drug-resistant epilepsy. The Kaplan-Meier curves could be fitted by monoexponential functions, with a maximal seizure relapse rate of 43.6%, maximal drug-resistance rate of 27.4%, and half-decay constant of 21.5 months for both curves. Treatment history served as a significant independent prognostic risk factor for both seizure relapse and development of drug resistance. The preremission seizure frequency and duration of epilepsy were also identified as significant prognostic risk factors in the univariant analysis but failed to reach statistical significance in the multivariate analysis.

Conclusion.—Seizure relapse commonly occurs in patients following long-term seizure remission. Treatment history and duration of epilepsy are predictive risk factors for both seizure relapse and development of drug resistance.

▶ There is increasing interest in the natural history of treated epilepsy. Many studies have been performed over the past 20 years in children, who can be regarded as a sort of captive population and whose prognosis tends to be better overall than in adults for idiopathic generalized and partial seizures. Around a decade ago, it became apparent that at either ends of the response spectrum there were 2 easily recognizable patient groups. Around 50% of adults with newly diagnosed epilepsy become seizure-free on their first antiepileptic drug. Randomized head-to-head trials suggest that for these individuals any appropriate choice will do the job. Indeed, two-thirds of this group will never have another seizure after taking the first drug dose. At the other end of the spectrum 25% to 33% of newly diagnosed adults never respond with a useful period of seizure freedom despite receiving different drugs with differing mechanisms of action used singly or in combination. There is some evidence that this group has shrunk a little with the recent introduction of a range of newer drugs with novel modes of action. It is now, however, increasingly being recognized that there is a third group of patients who do well initially with a sustained period of seizure freedom and then relapse and remit with some going on to develop refractory epilepsy and others continuing to experience a variable course. The neurobiological mechanisms underpinning these patterns are unknown, but are clearly important in identifying potentially successful treatment strategies for these individuals, who are constantly being disappointed when their seizures keep recurring. Optimal management of epilepsy depends on categorizing each patient into the appropriate outcome group and so making the best strategic plan for their management.

M. J. Brodie, MD, FRCP

Targeting Prostaglandin E_2 EP1 Receptors Prevents Seizure-Associated P-glycoprotein Up-Regulation

Pekcec A, Unkrüer B, Schlichtiger J, et al (Ludwig-Maximilians-Univ, Munich, Germany; et al)

J Pharmacol Exp Ther 330:939-947, 2009

Up-regulation of the blood-brain barrier efflux transporter P-glycoprotein in central nervous system disorders results in restricted brain access and limited efficacy of therapeutic drugs. In epilepsies, seizure activity strongly triggers expression of P-glycoprotein. Here, we identified the prostaglandin E2 receptor, EP1, as a key factor in the signaling pathway that mediates seizure-induced up-regulation of P-glycoprotein at the blood-brain barrier. In the rat pilocarpine model, status epilepticus significantly increased P-glycoprotein expression by 92 to 197% in the hippocampal hilus and granule cell layer as well as the piriform cortex. The EP1 receptor antagonist 8-chlorodibenz[*b*,*f*][1,4]oxazepine-10(11*H*)-carboxylic acid, 2-[1-oxo-3-(4- pyridinyl)propyl]hydrazide hydrochloride (SC-51089) abolished seizure-induced P-glycoprotein up-regulation and retained its expression at the control level. The control of P-glycoprotein expression despite prolonged seizure activity suggests that EP1 receptor antagonism will also improve antiepileptic drug efficacy. Preliminary evidence for this concept has been obtained using a massive kindling paradigm during which animals received a subchronic SC-51089 treatment. After withdrawal of the EP1 receptor antagonist, a low dose of the P-glycoprotein substrate phenobarbital resulted in an anticonvulsant effect in this pretreated group, whereas the same dosage of phenobarbital did not exert a significant effect in the respective control group. In conclusion, our data demonstrate that EP1 is a key signaling factor in the regulatory pathway that drives P-glycoprotein up-regulation during seizures. These findings suggest new intriguing possibilities to prevent and interrupt P-glycoprotein overexpression in epilepsy. Future studies are necessary to further evaluate the appropriateness of the strategy to enhance the efficacy of antiepileptic drugs.

▶ Despite the availability of an increasing number of antiepileptic drugs (AEDs) with different mechanisms of action, around 30% of the adult population have refractory epilepsy. The majority of these will be refractory de-novo, ie, never have a substantial period of seizure freedom despite being treated with a range of AEDs used singly and in combination. Although there is some evidence of a modest improvement in the overall prognosis in adult epilepsy over the past decade, there is a dearth of robust studies exploring this issue. Thus we are left with the conundrum of what is the problem in the brains of epilepsy patients who do not respond to AED pharmacotherapy. One of the main reasons to seek answers to this question is the hope that we can identify unique ways of treating pharmacoresistant epilepsy.

There are a number of hypotheses that have attracted the attention of the scientific community to explain the neurobiology of AED resistance. The 2 foremost ideas are the target hypothesis, which assumes that seizure-related changes in the properties of pharmacological targets in the brain result in reduced AED sensitivity. The other major idea is the transporter hypothesis, which requires overexpression of transporter proteins in brain capillary endothelium and glial cells that actively extrude AEDs from their intended sites of action. The best studied of these transporter proteins is P-glycoprotein. Attempts are underway to find novel ways of interfering with these processes that will have therapeutic potential. This article uniquely focuses on the prostaglandin E2 receptor, EP1, as a key factor in the signaling pathway that mediates seizure-induced up-regulation of P-glycoprotein at the blood brain barrier in the rat pilocarpine model of status epilepticus. Pharmacological interference with this process has the potential to point the way toward novel and safe treatments for people with refractory epilepsy that differ substantially from traditional AEDs.

M. J. Brodie, MD, FRCP

4 Headache

Cluster headache in children – Experience from a specialist headache clinic

Majumdar A, Ahmed MAS, Benton S (Bristol Royal Hosp for Children, UK; Queen's Hosp, Romford, UK; Hosp for Sick Children, London, UK)

Eur J Paediatr Neurol 13:524-529, 2009

Background.—Cluster headache is a primary headache disorder with the distinct clinical features: unilaterality, extreme pain, cranial autonomic features and periodicity. The prevalence of the disorder is 0.1% in adults and with a male predominance. The age of onset is usually in the second and third decade of life but the onset in the first decade is recognised. We describe our experience of cluster headache in children and review the literature. We have attempted to define the clinical features of cluster headache in children as compared to adults, the role of clinical investigations, reliability of clinical diagnosis, effective treatment and management options.

Methods.—A retrospective casenotes review was conducted on all children with suspected cluster headache seen in our centre from 2000 to 2005. Case ascertainment was conducted using International Headache Society guidelines, and by telephone interviews with the parents.

Results.—Eleven children were identified, (seven male and four female). The median age of onset was 8.5 years (range 2–14). The median age at diagnosis was 11.5 years (range 7–17). Eight children had episodic and 3 children had chronic cluster headaches. The average attack duration was 72 min. The commonest reported bout frequency was one per day. Several children had circadian and circumannual periodicity and most displayed the other features of the disorder, such as agitated movement and cranial autonomic activation. Oxygen, methysergide, verapamil, zolmitriptan and dihydroergotamine were the drugs which were effective in terminating the headache. Paracetamol, ibuprofen and paracetamol/codeine combinations were not.

Conclusion.—We describe our experience with cluster headache in eleven children who all presented before the age of 16.

▶ Pediatric headaches are not as well classified as in adults and more and more systematic data need to be gathered to identify headache patterns in children. Cluster headache (CH) is classically described in adults. Only anecdotal reports of CH in children are available in literature. The authors have presented a series of 11 children with episodic/chronic varieties of CH. They have not found any remarkable differences in the clinical characteristics in these cases as compared with adults, except that children exhibit a thrashing behavior or excessive crying as part of the agitation typically associated with CHs. The strict unilaterality, periodicity, and association with autonomic phenomena are the same as in adults, and a slight male preponderance has also been noted even in this small series of cases. It is therefore implied that the basic pathophysiology must be similar with underlying permissive and triggering role of hypothalamus in generation of pain. Just like adult patients, response of the acute attacks to analgesics and narcotics was poor, and preventive medications like valproate, topiramate, methysergide, and verapamil were found beneficial when given in doses adjusted according to age and weight. The authors have not used lithium in their cases, which is commonly used in adults and has usually been found to be quite effective.

Even though not very often seen in clinical practice, the challenge seems to lie in suspecting this rare disorder in children. Most often, children presenting with such severe unilateral headaches arouse a lot of concern in the parents as well as the physicians and even in the absence of localizing neurologic deficits, one is inclined to rule out any structural lesion by appropriate neuroimaging, which seems justified. If the clinical picture is suggestive, one should not refrain from considering the possibility of CH in children as well (despite its rarity in this age group) because the line of management is entirely different for this trigeminal autonomic cephalalgia and appropriate drugs might prove to be very effective.

A. Panagariya, MD, DM

Comprehensive Inpatient Treatment of Refractory Chronic Daily Headache

Lake AE III, Saper JR, Hamel RL (The Michigan Head-Pain and Neurological Inst, Ann Arbor)

Headache 49:555-562, 2009

Objective.—(1) To assess outcome at discharge for a consecutive series of admissions to a comprehensive, multidisciplinary inpatient headache unit; (2) To identify outcome predictors.

Background.—An evidence-based assessment (2004) concluded that many refractory headache patients appear to benefit from inpatient treatment, underscoring the need for more research, including outcome predictors.

Methods.—The authors completed a retrospective chart review of 283 consecutive admissions over 6 months. The inpatient program (mean length of stay = 13.0 days) included intravenous and oral medication protocols, drug withdrawal when indicated, cognitive-behavior therapy, and other services when needed, including anesthesiological intervention. Patient-reported pain levels and consensus of medical staff determined outcome status.

Results.—The 267 completers (94%) included 212 women and 55 men (mean age = 40.3 years, range = 13-74) from 43 states and Canada. The modal diagnosis was intractable, chronic daily headache (85%), predominantly migraine. Most (59%) had medication overuse headache (MOH), involving opioids (48%), triptans (16%), or butalbital- containing analgesics (10%). Psychiatric diagnoses included stress-related headache (82%), mood disorders (70%), anxiety disorders (49%), and personality disorders (PD, 26%). More patients with a PD (62%) had opioid-related MOH than those with no PD (38%), $P < .005$. Of the completers, 78% had moderate to significant pain reduction, with comparable improvement in mood, function, and behavior. Clinical factors predicting moderate-significant headache improvement were limited to MOH (84% vs 69%, $P < .007$) and presence of a PD (68% vs 81%, $P < .03$).

Conclusions.—Most patients (78%) improved following aggressive, comprehensive inpatient treatment. Maintenance of improvement is likely to depend on multiple post-discharge factors, including continuity of care, compliance, and home or work environment.

▶ Patients of chronic daily headache constitute the bulk of the neurology outpatients and indeed present a therapeutic challenge to physicians. Once an adequate diagnosis is made and appropriate treatment initiated, the treating doctors tend to keep on changing and adjusting the recommended drugs, many times without satisfactory results. Contrary to the patients presenting with acute severe headache who receive urgent attention, seldom are this group of patients considered for admission as inpatient services are already overwhelmed.

This article has highlighted the use of inpatient care in patients with refractory chronic daily headache.

A comprehensive approach to the management of refractory headache, as emphasized in the article, seems mandatory. Admitting patients and adminstering some intravenous medications for immediate relief would not suffice. An adequate counseling before admission regarding the whole approach, withdrawal of all medications temporarily in cases of medication overuse headache, psychotherapy, physiotherapy, opinions of experts from other disciplines like dentistry, ophthalmology, otolaryngorhinology, incorporation of aspects derived from alternative medicine during admission, are all important components of the attempt to reboot the chronically stressed neurochemistry. Hospital admission itself might provide some psychological benefit to these chronically disabled patients. It does offer a hope of being cured after years of not so fruitful outpatient care and might add to the improvement as a placebo.

The authors have concluded that in-hospital care may be the first step in transition from intractability to mild improvement by halting the vicious cycle of chronic pain. It can be inferred that comprehensive care in well designed and well equipped headache clinics on a regular basis might provide even more benefits in the long run. Therefore good centers must focus on the development of headache clinics with readily available multidisciplinary care with individualized treatment plans for patients.

A. Panagariya, MD, DM

Dizziness, migrainous vertigo and psychiatric disorders

Teggi R, Caldirola D, Colombo B, et al (Vita-Salute Univ, Milan, Italy)
J Laryngol Otol 124:285-290, 2010

Objectives.—This study sought to establish the prevalence of vestibular disorders, migraine and definite migrainous vertigo in patients with psychiatric disorders who were referred for treatment of dizziness, without a lifetime history of vertigo.

Study Design.—Retrospective study.

Setting.—Out-patients in a university hospital.

Materials and Methods.—Fifty-two dizzy patients with panic disorders and agoraphobia, 30 with panic disorders without agoraphobia, and 20 with depressive disorders underwent otoneurological screening with bithermal caloric stimulation. The prevalence of migraine and migrainous vertigo was assessed. The level of dizziness was evaluated using the Dizziness Handicap Inventory.

Results.—Dizzy patients with panic disorders and agoraphobia had a significantly $p = 0.05$ regarding the prevalence of peripheral vestibular abnormalities in the group of subjects with PD and agoraphobia and in those with depressive disorders. Migraine was equally represented in the three groups, but panic disorder patients had a higher prevalence of migrainous vertigo definite migrainous vertigo. Almost all patients with a peripheral vestibular disorder had a final diagnosis of definite migrainous vertigo according to Neuhauser criteria. These patients had higher Dizziness Handicap Inventory scores. The Dizziness Handicap Inventory total score was higher in the subgroup of patients with panic disorders with agoraphobia also presenting unilateral reduced caloric responses or definite migrainous vertigo, compared with the subgroup of remaining subjects with panic disorders with agoraphobia ($p < 0.001$).

Conclusions.—Our data support the hypothesis that, in patients with panic disorders (and especially those with additional agoraphobia), dizziness may be linked to malfunction of the vestibular system. However, the data are not inconsistent with the hypothesis that migrainous vertigo is the most common pathophysiological mechanism for vestibular disorders.

▶ A dizzy patient with a diverse constellation of symptoms with or without headache is a regular visitor in medical outpatient departments. Such patients make doctors feel helpless because they never seem to completely respond to any drug. This article linking dizziness, migrainous vertigo, depression, and other psychiatric diseases brings forth a few interesting facts. Migraine-associated vertigo, phobic disorders, and vestibular dysfunction may very well represent a continuum of a similar phenomenon.

The authors have found vestibular dysfunction in their patients with panic disorders, and many of these patients also fulfilled the criteria for migrainous vertigo, which implied that the same mechanisms were responsible for dizziness. Migraine-associated vertigo has been hypothesized to be due to both central and peripheral vestibular defects.

Panic, anxiety, and phobic disorders associated with vestibular dysfunction produce a vicious cycle. These patients suffer from a constant fear of falling and a sense of imbalance that may at times be terrifying. This causes significant prolongation of morbidity in these patients.

In our own patients with acute or chronic vertigo as a manifestation of panic and depression, who tend to develop fear of frequent falling (the 3-F phenomenon, as we like to call it), we have found encouraging results with vestibular sedatives, membrane stabilizers, and drugs like clonazepam. These drugs relieve these vestibular symptoms in many of these dizzy patients and break this vicious cycle of panic, phobia, and imbalance. Once the patient becomes asymptomatic, recurrence is prevented with vestibular and spinal exercises.

As an extrapolation to this, it may also be true that drugs for migraine prevention also reduce these symptoms of vestibulopathy, as the underlying mechanisms of migraine per se also lead to many vestibular symptoms.

A. Panagariya, MD, DM

Epicrania Fugax: Ten New Cases and Therapeutic Results

Guerrero AL, Cuadrado ML, Porta-Etessam J, et al (Hospital Clínico Universitario, Valladolid, Spain; Hospital Clínico San Carlos, Madrid, Spain)

Headache 50:451-458, 2010

Objective.—We aimed to report 10 new cases of epicrania fugax (EF), showing their clinical features and therapeutic responses.

Background.—Epicrania fugax has been recently described as a paroxysmal head pain starting in a focal area located at a posterior cranial region and rapidly spreading forward to the ipsilateral eye or nose along a linear or zigzag trajectory. In some patients the pain is followed by ocular or nasal autonomic features. In the prior series, 1 patient got pain relief with anesthetic blockades, while another patient improved with carbamazepine.

Methods.—Since the first description of EF, we have assessed 10 patients with the same clinical picture (8 women and 2 men) at the Neurology outpatient offices of our 2 centers.

Results.—The mean age at onset was 48.5 years (SD: 19.8, range: 23-83). All the patients complained of strictly unilateral pain paroxysms starting at parietal (n = 5), occipital (n = 4), or parieto-occipital locations (n = 1), and immediately spreading forward through a linear pathway toward the ipsilateral forehead (n = 3) or the ipsilateral eye (n = 7), the complete sequence lasting 1-10 seconds. No trigger was identified in any of our patients, while 5 of them suffered mild pain in the stemming area between the paroxysms. Three patients had ipsilateral lacrimation, and 2 had conjunctival injection at the end of the attacks. The frequency ranged from 1 attack per week to multiple attacks per day. Neuroimaging and laboratory tests were consistently normal. Interictal pain was responsive to acetaminophen. In 3 cases a preventive was considered in order to avoid the paroxysms. Gabapentin led to significant improvement in 2 cases. The third patient did not obtain any benefit from gabapentin or amitriptyline, but improved slightly with lamotrigine.

Conclusions.—This description reinforces the proposal of EF as a new headache variant or a new headache syndrome. Anesthetic blockades, carbamazepine, gabapentin, and lamotrigine have been apparently effective in individual patients. Further observations and therapeutic trials are needed.

▶ Neurology outpatient departments are full of patients with dubious labels whose headache characteristics cannot be categorized into any of the already described syndromes. One wonders whether these patients with weird symptoms are suffering from anxiety or there is much more to it than meets the medical eye. Finer classification of headache variants is surely required for a better and confident diagnosis.

Focal pain starting in the back of the head spreading forward in the zigzag territory lasting for a few seconds and disappearing abruptly may seem to be nonspecific to most physicians. Epicrania fugax, as described in this article, is one of the epicranial headaches that seem to occur paroxysmally in localized superficial areas occasionally associated with autonomic features. Individual patients have responded to carbamazepine, lamotrigine, and gabapentin.

I have also come across a number of patients who complain of transitory fleeting pains arising on the scalp at multiple sites that respond to carbamazepine. Literature also has reports of cephalgic seizures that present similarly with paroxysmal pains but are differentiated from this type of headache by the electroencephalographic changes and the response to anticonvulsants. Probably such entities represent border zones where vascular and ictal phenomena merge and might lead us to common molecular origins of these diverse disorders in the future.

A. Panagariya, MD, DM

Evidence of shared genetic risk factors for migraine and rolandic epilepsy

Clarke T, Baskurt Z, Strug LJ, et al (Columbia Univ Med Ctr, NY; The Hosp for Sick Children, Toronto, Ontario, Canada)

Epilepsia 50:2428-2433, 2009

Purpose.—Evidence for a specific association between migraine and rolandic epilepsy (RE) has been conflicting. Children with migraine frequently have electroencephalographic (EEG) abnormalities, including rolandic discharges, and approximately 50% of siblings of patients with RE exhibit rolandic discharges. We assessed migraine risk in RE probands and their siblings.

Methods.—We used cohort and reconstructed cohort designs to respectively assess the relative risk of migraine in 72 children with RE and their 88 siblings using International Classification of Headache Disorders (ICHD-2) criteria. Incidences were compared in 150 age and geographically matched nonepilepsy probands and their 188 siblings. We used a Cox proportional hazards model, using age as the time base, adjusting hazard ratios (HRs) for sex in the proband analysis, and for sex and proband migraine status in the sibling analysis.

Results.—Prevalence of migraine in RE probands was 15% versus 7% in nonepilepsy probands, and in siblings of RE probands prevalence was 14% versus 4% in nonepilepsy siblings. The sex-adjusted HR of migraine for an RE proband was 2.46 [95% confidence interval (CI) 1.06–5.70]. The adjusted HR of having ≥1 sibling with migraine in an RE family was 3.35 (95% CI 1.20–9.33), whereas the HR of any one sibling of a RE proband was 2.86 (95% CI 1.10–7.43).

Discussion.—Migraine is strongly comorbid in RE and independently clusters in their siblings. These results suggest shared susceptibility to migraine and RE that is not directly mediated by epileptic seizures. Susceptibility gene variants for RE may be tested as risk factors for migraine.

▶ Newer understanding of the pathogenesis of migraine has shifted in favor of migraine being a disturbance of neuronal excitability rather than a vascular disorder. Benign epilepsy of childhood with centrotemporal spikes is considered to be of genetic origin. Patients with BRE have significant family history of epilepsy or centrotemporal spikes, and migraine also has been known to have a genetic basis. Evidence of epileptiform abnormalities on electroencephalography in children with migraine and occurrence of migrainous headaches in children with rolandic epilepsy and their siblings as documented in this study, also suggest the common underlying susceptibility factors. Of course, identification of such associations is a step forward in simplifying the riddle of migraine pathogenesis.

Further studies are needed to identify whether associations between other epilepsies/epilepsy syndromes and migraine also exist or is it just that only benign variants of epilepsy may co-occur with this primary headache disorder. The therapeutic effects of anticonvulsants in migraine prophylaxis might be due to similar mechanisms involving alterations in cortical excitability.

A. Panagariya, MD, DM

Frequency of Chronic Headaches in Japanese Patients With Multiple Sclerosis: With Special Reference to Opticospinal and Common Forms of Multiple Sclerosis

Doi H, Matsushita T, Isobe N, et al (Kyushu Univ, Fukuoka, Japan)
Headache 49:1513-1520, 2009

Background.—Headache is common in Western patients with multiple sclerosis (MS), but its frequency has not been reported in Asian patients. In Asians, the opticospinal form of MS, showing similar characteristics to relapsing neuromyelitis optica in Westerners, is regarded as a different subtype from conventional MS.

Objectives.—The aim of this study was to clarify the frequency of primary and chronic secondary headaches in Japanese patients with MS and the factors associated with the emergence of such headaches.

Methods.—We investigated 127 consecutive patients with clinically definite MS. Frequencies of primary and chronic secondary headaches were compared according to clinical subtype, administration of interferon beta, and anti-aquaporin-4 antibody status.

Results.—The frequency of patients with primary and chronic secondary headaches at the time of interview was 64/127 (50.4%); the frequency of migraine was 26/127 (20.4%) and that of tension-type headache was 38/127 (29.9%). The frequencies of patients with primary and chronic secondary headaches and migraine without aura after the onset of MS were higher in patients undergoing interferon beta therapy than in those not on the therapy (42.4% vs 23.4%, $P < .05$ and 15.1% vs 4.3%, $P = .05$, respectively). There were no significant differences in the frequency of primary and chronic secondary headaches based on clinical subtype of MS. However, among patients not receiving interferon beta, the occurrence of migraine with aura after the onset of MS was significantly higher in patients with anti-aquaporin-4 antibody than in patients without the antibody (13.3% vs 0.0%, $P < .05$).

Conclusions.—In Japanese patients with MS, the frequency of primary and chronic secondary headaches, especially migraine, was higher than in the general Japanese population. Administration of interferon beta was related to a higher frequency of primary and chronic secondary headaches, especially migraine without aura, irrespective of clinical subtype of MS.

▶ An interesting area of research that might have implications on the understanding of the pathogenesis of migraine—do the primary and secondary headache disorders occur more frequently in patients with multiple sclerosis (MS) than the general population? Although we have not encountered any increased association of chronic headaches in patients with multiple sclerosis in our own clinical practice, literature has documentation of increased occurrence of headache in patients with MS—more so in patients receiving interferons.

Association of migraine has been related to even single lesion in the periaqueductal gray (PAG) matter in patients with MS. Evidence suggesting the role of PAG in the pathophysiology of migraine has been appearing in the recent literature, which has shown activation in the ventrolateral PAG during migraine episodes. The PAG may be involved through the descending modulation of nociceptive afferent information and also by its ascending projections to the pain processing centers of the thalamus. I wonder whether the usual occurrence of sensory symptoms in many migraineurs and patients with MS has basically similar pathophysiologic origins. Presence of asymptomatic white matter abnormalities in migraine with aura also implies some common pathologic substrates. The association of migraine in neuromyelitis optica with antiaquaporin 4 antibodies also has been linked to the abundance of these water channels in the periventricular regions. Interferons by way of producing neurogenic inflammation potentiate the mechanisms inducing migraine.

All these interesting facts suggest that migraine is a disorder that arises due to diffuse CNS involvement at multiple sites, although the involvement of pain modulating regions might have a greater implication in pain generation and probably also has some resemblance to CNS demyelinating diseases. Dysfunction of the normal CNS homeostasis due to either structural or functional damage leads to tipping of the critical balance in which the pain modulatory mechanisms of migraineurs are held.

A. Panagariya, MD, DM

Gray matter changes related to chronic posttraumatic headache

Obermann M, Nebel K, Schumann C, et al (Univ of Duisburg-Essen, Germany; et al)

Neurology 73:978-983, 2009

Background.—Although up to 15% of patients with whiplash injury develop chronic headache, the basis and mechanisms of this posttraumatic headache are not well understood.

Methods.—Thirty-two patients with posttraumatic headache following whiplash injury were investigated within 14 days after the accident and again after 3 months using magnetic resonance-based voxel-based morphometry. Twelve patients developed chronic headache lasting longer than 3 months and were studied a third time after 1 year.

Results.—Patients who developed chronic headache revealed decreases in gray matter in the anterior cingulate and dorsolateral prefrontal cortex after 3 months. These changes resolved after 1 year, in parallel to the cessation of headache. The same patients who developed chronic headache showed an increase of gray matter in antinociceptive brainstem centers, thalamus, and cerebellum 1 year after the accident.

Conclusion.—We demonstrate adaptive gray matter changes of pain processing structures in patients with chronic posttraumatic headache in regard to neuronal plasticity, thus providing a biologically plausible basis for this common, disabling problem.

► Neurologists often come across patients with posttraumatic headache in the outpatient department, and most of these patients receive anxiolytics, antidepressants, and repeated assurances. The mechanism of posttraumatic headache is not well understood. Trauma-induced headaches are usually heterogeneous in nature, including both chronic tension-type pain and intermittent migraine-like attacks. This article is an endeavor in demonstrating and clarifying the neurophysiological mechanisms of chronic headache that develops after trauma. The authors have demonstrated a decrease of gray matter in the anterior cingulate cortex and dorsolateral prefrontal cortex using voxel based morphometric analysis in those who developed chronic posttraumatic headache, suggesting slow adaptive processes in structures involved in the development of chronic headache. This emphasizes that the vicious mechanisms leading to development of chronic pain need to be dealt with early on, so that transformation of acute into chronic headache can be prevented .The pain cycle interrupted by therapeutic measures may help prevention of long-term suffering of these patients.

The gray matter changes in anterior cingulate cortex (ACC) and dorsolateral prefrontal cortex (DLPFC) were shown to be completely reversible, and increased gray matter was found in alternative regions like thalamus, brainstem, and cerebellum 1 year later in these patients, coinciding with relief from headache, further strengthening the hypothesis. These observations are yet another example of neuronal plasticity—a phenomenon of adaptability of neurons, reorganization of neuronal networks, and function as a result of new experiences. Use of neuroprotective agents are also known to alter neuronal adaptability and might prove useful in the future for such conditions. Further research focusing on alternative mechanisms in addition to pharmacotherapy, which enhance neuroplasticity in favor of antinociceptive mechanisms, might bring about a breakthrough in pain therapeutics.

A. Panagariya, MD, DM

Headache and Symptoms of Temporomandibular Disorder: An Epidemiological Study

Gonçalves DAG, Bigal ME, Jales LCF, et al (Sao Paulo State Univ, Brazil; Albert Einstein College of Medicine, Bronx, NY; INBIO-Instituto de Neuropsicologia e Biofeedback, Ribeirao Preto, Sao Paulo, Brazil; et al)
Headache 50:231-241, 2010

Objectives.—A population-based cross-sectional study was conducted to estimate the prevalence of migraine, episodic tension-type headaches (ETTH), and chronic daily headaches (CDH), as well as the presence of symptoms of temporomandibular disorders (TMD) in the adult population.

Background.—The potential comorbidity of headache syndromes and TMD has been established mostly based on clinic-based studies.

Methods.—A representative sample of 1230 inhabitants (51.5% women) was interviewed by a validated phone survey. TMD symptoms were assessed through 5 questions, as recommended by the American Academy of Orofacial Pain, in an attempt to classify possible TMD. Primary headaches were diagnosed based on the International Classification of Headache Disorders.

Results.—When at least 1 TMD symptom was reported, any headache happened in 56.5% vs 31.9% ($P < .0001$) in those with no symptoms. For 2 symptoms, figures were 65.1% vs 36.3% ($P < .0001$); for 3 or more symptoms, the difference was even more pronounced: 72.8% vs 37.9%. ($P < .0001$). Taking individuals without headache as the reference, the prevalence of at least 1 TMD symptom was increased in ETTH (prevalence ratio = 1.48, 95% confidence interval = 1.20-1.79), migraine (2.10, 1.80-2.47) and CDH (2.41, 1.84-3.17). At least 2 TMD symptoms also happened more frequently in migraine (4.4, 3.0-6.3), CDH (3.4; 1.5-7.6), and ETTH (2.1; 1.3-3.2), relative to individuals with no headaches. Finally, 3 or more TMD symptoms were also more common in migraine (6.2; 3.8-10.2) than in no headaches. Differences were significant for ETTH (2.7 1.5-4.8), and were numerically but not significant for CDH (2.3; 0.66-8.04).

Conclusion.—Temporomandibular disorder symptoms are more common in migraine, ETTH, and CDH relative to individuals without headache. Magnitude of association is higher for migraine. Future studies should clarify the nature of the relationship.

▶ Atypical facial pain is a less defined syndrome encompassing a variable group of facial pains often described as continuous burning, aching, or cramping on one side of the face, usually in the region of the trigeminal nerve, and can extend into the upper neck or back of the scalp; some authors also additionally report pains in one half of the body. These pains are difficult to treat, and such patients often go on consuming a cocktail of drugs, including analgesics and antidepressants.

It has been postulated to be because of infections or diseases of the paranasal sinuses or teeth for prolonged periods causing sensitization of the trigeminal nerve. Temporomandibular disorders (TMDs) too can account for these facial pains.

The interesting aspect that has emerged in recent literature is that TMDs are found to be coexisting with migraine, tension-type headaches, and chronic daily headaches. It is not very surprising, as the same trigeminovascular pathways are involved in carrying sensations from the face, head, and TM joints (TMJ), and there is a close anatomical proximity of the muscles of mastication and TMJ to the head. Moreover, these headache entities are gradually being recognized as more widespread phenomena resulting due to imbalances at the level of neurotransmitters, rather than localized entities. For example, migraine headaches have been found to have many comorbidities, including chronic fatigue syndrome, hypertension, anxiety disorders, depression, mood disorders, etc, and tension-type headaches are often associated with multiple somatic symptoms.

A significant number of patients with headache actually have TMD as one of the major causes of their pain. Recent literature has suggested that a common factor to migraine and tension-type headaches may be chronic clenching of teeth or bruxism. It is postulated that mechanical stimuli like clenching of teeth and pain of the masticatory muscles may provide the stimulus for the release of serotonin and norepinephrine from the dorsal raphe and locus ceruleus of the brain, setting off a cascade of events leading to migraine and further muscle tension. Dentists may in fact be able to add to the multidisciplinary approach to the treatment of patients with headache more effectively than previously suspected through the use of dental appliances.

Judicious treatment of TMDs might interrupt the vicious cycle of pain and muscle tension and bring about better headache control. Reassuring the patients about the benignity of the condition supported by a combination of small doses of codeine with nonsteroidal anti-inflammatory drugs, duloxetine, or amitriptyline, if tolerated, supportive jaw exercises and dental appliances in cases of bruxism may comprise a comprehensive management of these chronic patients.

A. Panagariya, MD, DM

Hemicrania Continua Responsive to Intravenous Methyl Prednisolone

Prakash S, Brahmbhatt KJ, Chawda NT, et al (Med College, Baroda, Gujarat, India)

Headache 49:604-607, 2009

Hemicrania continua (HC) is a strictly unilateral, continuous primary headache disorder with periodic exacerbations, usually accompanied by cranial autonomic disturbances. Exquisite and persistent effect of indomethacin is a fundamental property of HC. We report 2 patients of HC in which attacks were successfully eliminated by repeated infusion of methyl prednisolone.

▶ Hemicrania continua (HC) is a primary chronic daily headache disorder characterized by a continuous, fluctuating, unilateral pain without shifting sides. The pain is, typically, mild to moderate in intensity and in most patients episodes of severe pain are superimposed on the continuous baseline pain. During exacerbations, lasting from 20 minutes to several days the patient may experience a variable combination of autonomic features. The condition is usually unremitting. The etiology and pathogenesis of HC are currently unknown. The hallmark of this syndrome is the absolute positive response to indomethacin.[1,2]

However, the mechanism of the beneficial effect of indomethacin on HC, which far exceeds the effect of other nonsteroidal anti-inflammatory drugs (NSAIDs) on this disorder, remains unknown. Indomethacin can alter the cerebral hypercapnic vasodilator response involving NO generation. Whether indomethacin attenuates the facial nerve cranial parasympathetic outflow directly requires further research. Moreover, the specificity of indomethacin responsiveness for this disorder has been debated.[3]

Certain primary headaches, eg, cluster headache and status migrainosus, are steroid responsive. The basis of response to steroids in these headaches is probably by antagonizing neurogenic inflammation and the immunologic phenomena that occur in these paroxysmal headache disorders. The response of 2 cases of HC to steroids in cases not tolerating indomethacin indicates that underlying the pathophysiology of these headache disorders are common mechanisms that need to be further evaluated. It also implies that refractory cases of chronic daily headaches might respond to intravenous methylprednisolone due to certain shared pathophysiological mechanisms. It may be worthwhile to evaluate the role and efficacy of intravenous methylprednisolone in chronic daily headaches in well-designed trials.

A. Panagariya, MD, DM

References

1. Pareja JA, Antonaci F, Vincent M. The hemicrania continua diagnosis. *Cephalalgia.* 2001;21:940-946.
2. Headache Classification Subcommittee of the International Headache Society. International classification of headache disorders: 2nd edition. *Cephalalgia.* 2004;24 Suppl 1:1-160.
3. Ashkenazi A, Abbas MA, Sharma DK, Silberstein SD. Hemicrania continua-like headache associated with internal carotid artery dissection may respond to indomethacin. *Headache.* 2007;47:127-130.

Vertigo as a migraine trigger

Murdin L, Davies RA, Bronstein AM (Natl Hosp for Neurology and Neurosurgery, London, UK)
Neurology 73:638-642, 2009

Background.—It is reported in some individual patients that vestibular stimuli can trigger migraine attacks. This study used a case-control design to examine systematically the hypothesis that vertigo induced by vestibular stimulation (rotation/caloric testing) can act as a specific migraine trigger.

Methods.—A total of 123 new patients attending neuro-otology or neurology clinics were studied with questionnaires and physician interview to ascertain migraine history according to International Headache Society criteria. A total of 79 who underwent rotation/caloric vestibular testing (test group) were compared with 44 control patients in whom no such testing was carried out (control group). The principal outcome measure was the occurrence of a migraine attack within 24 hours of exposure to vestibular stimulation.

Results.—Of those participants with a past history of migraines, 19/39 (49%) of the test group experienced a migraine in the study time window, compared with 1/21 (5%) of the control group. Binary logistic regression analysis confirmed that vestibular testing was associated ($p < 0.05$) with migraine attacks.

Conclusions.—The results indicate that induced vertigo can act as a migraine trigger, a finding with implications for the diagnosis of patients with episodic vertigo and migraine headache. While such patients may well have basilar migraine or migrainous vertigo, alternatively, another disorder causing episodic vertigo (e.g., benign paroxysmal positional vertigo or Ménière disease) may be triggering migraine headaches.

▶ Previous studies have found that strong sensory stimuli can trigger a migraine headache and sometimes migraine with aura. Case reports have found that caloric stimulation can also trigger a migraine. This study determined the frequency of migraine within 24 hours of vestibular stimulation in 79 individuals. This was compared with 44 individuals in a control group who were seen but did not have vestibular stimulation. Of those who had a migraine history, 19 of 39 in the stimulated group developed migraine compared with 1 of 21 who did not receive vestibular stimulation. These findings need to be kept in mind by clinicians when seeing patients with vertigo and migraine. In those patients with both, one might attribute the cause of vertigo to the migraine, but this article suggests vertigo may cause the migraine instead and that there may be another cause for the vertigo.

R. J. Tusa, MD, PhD

Cranial autonomic symptoms in migraine: characteristics and comparison with cluster headache

Lai T-H, Fuh J-L, Wang S-J (Natl Yang-Ming Univ, Taipei, Taiwan)

J Neurol Neurosurg Psychiatry 80:1116-1119, 2009

Background.—Cranial autonomic symptoms (CAS) are distinguishing features of trigeminal autonomic cephalalgias, of which cluster headache (CH) is the most common, but they can occur in patients with migraine. For migraine with strictly unilateral headache, the presence of CAS might cause diagnostic confusion with CH. Characteristics of CAS in migraine and comparisons with those in CH have rarely been reported.

Methods.—This study prospectively recruited consecutive patients with migraine and CH treated at a headache clinic. Six CAS items were surveyed, including: conjunctival injection, lacrimation, nasal congestion, rhinorrhoea, eyelid oedema and forehead/facial sweating. The CAS characteristics recorded included: laterality, intensity, time sequence and consistency with headache attacks.

Results.—A total of 786 migraine patients (625 women/161 men, mean age 40 (13) years) and 98 CH patients (11 women/87 men, mean age 36 (11) years) were recruited. The prevalence of ≥1 CAS in migraine patients was 56% and did not differ among migraine subtypes. Except for forehead/facial sweating, the features of the other CAS differed between patients with migraine and CH: CAS in migraine tended to be bilateral (OR 5.8–23.8 among different CAS), be unrestricted to the headache sides (OR 5.0–20.4), appear with mild to moderate intensity (OR 1.7–7.7) and be inconsistent with headache attacks (OR 2.8–6.7).

Conclusions.—CAS were present in half of our migraine patients and the clinical features may help differentiate migraine from CH.

▶ International Classification of Headache Disorders (ICHD)-2 criteria use autonomic features for characterization of cluster headache (CH). The criteria for migraine do not incorporate autonomic features. The authors have documented the occurrence of autonomic features in patients fulfilling the ICHD-2 criteria for migraine. Although the periodicity, strict unilaterality, and the very severe intensity of CH seldom ever create diagnostic confusion with migraine for the experienced neurologist, it may present a dilemma in cases of chronic CH.

It may be interesting to discuss that the human body and its pathophysiologic mechanisms are not separate water tight compartments, and boundaries of related ailments keep on blurring as more and more experience and systematic documentation of various disorders is obtained. The suggestion by the author of the involvement of cranial parasympathetic pathways like CH even in migraine may be an extension of the same idea. Trigeminovascular system is involved in both the disorders, and prominence of autonomic features may be only a matter of degree to which 1 particular system is involved in these distinct yet related headache entities. As in this case series, autonomic features are more often reported by patients with severe migraine, probably it is because severe attacks are associated with more profuse and widespread abnormalities throughout the brainstem, hypothalamus, and neurovascular systems. Of course it is a preliminary clinical observation, but it paves the way for further analysis and research into the pathomechanisms of these entities.

Therapeutic relevance of this issue lies in the fact that patients of migraine with cranial autonomic symptom (CAS) are offered preventive treatment for migraine and not CH, which have entirely different lines of management.

A. Panagariya, MD, DM

5 Infectious Diseases of the Nervous System

A Novel Protective Prion Protein Variant that Colocalizes with Kuru Exposure

Mead S, Whitfield J, Poulter M, et al (Univ College London Inst of Neurology, UK; et al)

N Engl J Med 361:2056-2065, 2009

Background.—Kuru is a devastating epidemic prion disease that affected a highly restricted geographic area of the Papua New Guinea highlands; at its peak, it predominantly affected adult women and children of both sexes. Its incidence has steadily declined since the cessation of its route of transmission, endocannibalism.

Methods.—We performed genetic and selected clinical and genealogic assessments of more than 3000 persons from Eastern Highland populations, including 709 who participated in cannibalistic mortuary feasts, 152 of whom subsequently died of kuru.

Results.—Persons who were exposed to kuru and survived the epidemic in Papua New Guinea are predominantly heterozygotes at the known resistance factor at codon 129 of the prion protein gene (*PRNP*). We now report a novel *PRNP* variant — G127V — that was found exclusively in people who lived in the region in which kuru was prevalent and that was present in half of the otherwise susceptible women from the region of highest exposure who were homozygous for methionine at *PRNP* codon 129. Although this allele is common in the area with the highest incidence of kuru, it is not found in patients with kuru and in unexposed population groups worldwide. Genealogic analysis reveals a significantly lower incidence of kuru in pedigrees that harbor the protective allele than in geographically matched control families.

Conclusions.—The 127V polymorphism is an acquired prion disease resistance factor selected during the kuru epidemic, rather than a pathogenic mutation that could have triggered the kuru epidemic. Variants at codons 127 and 129 of *PRNP* demonstrate the population genetic response to an epidemic of prion disease and represent a powerful episode of recent selection in humans.

► Kuru, an incurable degenerative neurological disorder, is a type of transmissible spongiform encephalopathy found in humans. Kuru is caused by prions and is related to Creutzfeldt-Jakob disease. It is best known for the epidemic that occurred in the Eastern Highland, Papua New Guinea in the middle of the 20th century. Although it is considered a transmissible prion disease, there is evidence that the origin of the outbreak was due to consumption of an individual (cannibalism) with sporadic Creutzfeldt-Jakob disease.

Mead et al report on genetic, clinical, and genealogic assessments of more than 3000 persons from Eastern Highland populations, including 709 who participated in cannibalistic mortuary feasts, 152 of whom subsequently died of kuru. Persons who were exposed to kuru and survived the epidemic in Papua New Guinea were predominantly heterozygotes at the known resistance factor at codon 129 of the prion protein gene (*PRNP*). A novel *PRNP* variant (G127V) was exclusively found in people who lived in the region in which kuru was prevalent and that was present in half of the otherwise susceptible women from the region of highest exposure who were homozygous for methionine at *PRNP* codon 129. Although this allele was common in the area with the highest incidence of kuru, it was not found in patients with kuru and in unexposed population groups worldwide. Data support the conclusion that G127V in the heterozygous state confers resistance to kuru.

Human prion diseases have acquired, sporadic, and inherited etiologies, show wide phenotypic heterogeneity, and are associated with propagation of infectious prions of many distinct strain types. A polymorphism at codon 129 (encoding methionine or valine) of the human prion protein gene (*PRNP*) constitutes a powerful susceptibility factor in all types of prion disease. In vCJD, *PRNP* codon 129 heterozygotes generally have the longest incubation periods. This study shows that the 127V polymorphism is an acquired prion disease resistance factor.

D. van de Beek, MD, PhD

Changes in *Neisseria meningitidis* Disease Epidemiology in the United States, 1998–2007: Implications for Prevention of Meningococcal Disease

Cohn AC, MacNeil JR, Harrison LH, et al (Ctrs for Disease Control and Prevention; Atlanta, GA; Johns Hopkins Bloomberg School of Public Health, Baltimore, MD; et al)

Clin Infect Dis 50:184-191, 2010

Background.—In January 2005, a quadrivalent (serogroups A, C, Y, and W-135) meningococcal conjugate vaccine was licensed for use in adolescents. This report describes the epidemiologic features of meningococcal disease in the United States from January 1998 through December 2007, before and during implementation of adolescent quadrivalent meningococcal conjugate vaccination.

Methods.—Data were collected from active surveillance for invasive *Neisseria meningitidis* conducted through the Active Bacterial Core surveillance (ABCs) sites during 1998–2007. Isolates from cases were serogrouped at the ABCs site and confirmed at the Centers for Disease Control and Prevention. Estimates of the incidence and number of cases in the 50 states were calculated, standardizing for race and age group.

Results.—In the period 1998–2007, a total of 2262 cases of meningococcal disease were reported from ABCs sites; 11.3% of these cases were fatal. The estimated United States average annual incidence of meningococcal disease was 0.53 cases per 100,000 population (95% confidence interval, 0.51–0.55), and an estimated 1525 (95% confidence interval, 1470–1598) cases occurred annually. The annual incidence decreased 64.1%, from 0.92 cases per 100,000 population in 1998 to 0.33 cases per 100,000 population in 2007. Infants aged <1 year have the highest incidence of meningococcal disease (5.38 cases per 100,000 population). After introduction of the quadrivalent meningococcal conjugate vaccine, no significant decrease in serogroup C or Y meningococcal disease was seen among those aged 11–19 years in 2006–2007, compared with 2004–2005.

Conclusions.—Before the introduction of the quadrivalent meningococcal conjugate vaccine, the incidence of meningococcal disease in the United States decreased to a historic low. However, meningococcal disease still causes a substantial burden of disease among all age groups. Future vaccination strategies may include targeting infants and preventing serogroup B meningococcal disease.

▶ Given the significant morbidity and mortality associated with acute bacterial meningitis in the United States and throughout the world, accurate information is necessary regarding the important etiological agents and populations at risk to initiate public health measures and to ensure appropriate management. *Neisseria meningitidis* (the meningococcus), a gram-negative bacterium, is the leading cause of meningitis and severe sepsis in young adults worldwide.

Cohn et al present data collected from active surveillance for invasive *N meningitidis* conducted through the Active Bacterial Core surveillance (ABCs) sites in the United States. In the period 1998-2007, a total of 2262 cases of meningococcal disease were reported from ABCs sites; 11.3% of these cases were fatal. The estimated United States average annual incidence of meningococcal disease was 0.53 cases per 100 000 population (95% confidence interval, 0.51-0.55), and an estimated 1525 cases (95% confidence interval, 1470-1598) occurred annually. The annual incidence was decreased by 64.1%—from 0.92 cases per 100 000 population in 1998 to 0.33 cases per 100 000 population in 2007. After the introduction of the quadrivalent meningococcal conjugate vaccine, no significant decrease in serogroup C or Y meningococcal disease was seen among those aged 11 to 19 years in 2006-2007 compared with 2004-2005.

Previous recommendations for the prevention of invasive meningococcal infection included the administration of a quadrivalent meningococcal polysaccharide vaccine against serogroups A, C, Y, and W-135 in specific populations who were at an increased risk. The vaccine was not recommended for routine use in the United States because of the overall low risk of infection, the inability to protect against serogroup B disease, and the inability to provide long-lasting immunity to young children. As a result of the success of conjugate vaccines against invasive disease caused by *Haemophilus influenzae* type b and *Streptococcus* pneumoniae, conjugate vaccines against specific serogroups of *N meningitidis* were developed. These vaccines contain meningococcal polysaccharide conjugated to a protein such as tetanus toxoid, diphtheria toxoid, or CRM197 and are immunogenic and induce immunological memory in young children.

A quadrivalent meningococcal conjugate vaccine-containing serogroups A, C, Y, and W-135 conjugated to diphtheria toxoid was licensed for use in the United States in January 2005 and was initially recommended for routine immunization starting at the age of 11 to 12 years and for catch-up vaccination for 15-year-old adolescents and those entering high school; these recommendations were later changed to include the routine vaccination of all persons aged 11 to 18 years, with 1 dose and revaccination for those at a prolonged, increased risk of meningococcal disease (ie, persistent complement component deficiencies, anatomical or functional asplenia, and prolonged exposure, such as microbiologists working with *N meningitidis* or travelers to or residents of countries where meningococcal disease is hyperendemic or epidemic). A recent trial also demonstrated that another novel tetravalent meningococcal conjugate vaccine, conjugated to CRM197, was well tolerated and immunogenic in infants when vaccination was initiated for those as young as 2 months of age. This vaccine was also well tolerated and generated a strong immune response in adolescents. Licensure of the CRM197 conjugate for adolescents in the United States is currently pending. However, further surveillance data are needed to determine the effectiveness of these vaccines in preventing meningococcal meningitis.

D. van de Beek, MD, PhD

Delayed cerebral thrombosis after initial good recovery from pneumococcal meningitis

Schut ES, Brouwer MC, de Gans J, et al (Academic Med Ctr, Amsterdam, the Netherlands)

Neurology 73:1988-1995, 2009

Objective.—To report an unusual clinical course in 6 patients with community-acquired acute bacterial meningitis and to compare clinical features with cases reported in the literature.

Methods.—Case series from Dutch hospitals from 2003 to 2008.

Results.—Five out of six patients were male, age ranged from 30 to 73 years (mean age, 47 years). All patients had pneumococcal meningitis, received adjunctive dexamethasone treatment on admission, and made a good or excellent initial recovery. After 7 to 19 days, patients suddenly deteriorated, developing headache, fever, a decreased level of consciousness, brainstem signs, or hemiparesis. Imaging studies showed infarctions involving the thalamus or brainstem in all patients. Repeated lumbar puncture showed a pleocytosis, but CSF cultures were sterile. Five patients were treated with high-dose steroids on deterioration. Outcome was poor: 4 patients died and 2 remained disabled. Autopsies, performed in 2 patients, showed infarctions predominantly involving the posterior circulation territory, thrombosis in penetrating arteries, but no evidence of vasculitis. We identified 5 meningitis cases with delayed vasculopathy in the literature, but these patients did not exactly resemble the clinical course of our patients.

Conclusions.—Delayed cerebral thrombosis may occur in patients with excellent recovery from pneumococcal meningitis. All patients were treated initially with adjunctive dexamethasone therapy, suggesting a dexamethasone-associated effect. Pathology suggests an immunologic reaction targeting cerebral blood vessels.

▶ Bacterial meningitis is a severe infection of the central nervous system and is associated with high morality and morbidity.[1] Transient or permanent deafness, or other neurological sequelae arise in up to one-third of survivors.[1]

Studies in animals have shown that adjuvant treatment with anti-inflammatory agents, such as dexamethasone, reduces both cerebrospinal fluid inflammation and neurological sequelae. A *Cochrane* review on adjunctive dexamethasone in bacterial meningitis showed an overall reduction in mortality, severe hearing loss, and neurological sequelae.[2]

This article reports an unusual clinical course in community-acquired acute bacterial meningitis. All 6 patients had pneumococcal meningitis, received adjunctive dexamethasone treatment on admission, and made a good or excellent initial recovery (Table 1 in the original article). After 7 to 19 days, patients suddenly deteriorated, developing headache, fever, a decreased level of consciousness, brainstem signs, or hemiparesis. Imaging studies showed infarctions involving the thalamus or brainstem in all patients. Repeated lumbar puncture showed a pleocytosis, but cerebrospinal fluid cultures were sterile. All patients were treated initially with adjunctive dexamethasone therapy, suggesting a dexamethasone-associated effect. Pathology suggested an immunologic reaction targeting cerebral blood vessels.

The authors of previous large series of bacterial meningitis are prompted to re-review their records in order to find similar cases. This might shed further light on the possible cause of this devastating complication and its relation to the use of adjuvant dexamethasone therapy.

D. van de Beek, MD, PhD

References

1. van de Beek D, de Gans J, Tunkel AR, Wijdicks EFM. Community-acquired bacterial meningitis in adults. *N Engl J Med.* 2006;354:46-55.
2. van de Beek D, de Gans J, McIntyre P, Prasad K. Corticosteroids in acute bacterial meningitis. *Cochrane Database Syst Rev.* 2007;1:CD004305.

Determinants of survival in progressive multifocal leukoencephalopathy

Marzocchetti A, Tompkins T, Clifford DB, et al (Harvard Med School, Boston, MA; Washington Univ School of Medicine, St Louis, MO; et al)

Neurology 73:1551-1558, 2009

Background.—We sought to characterize the role of immunologic, virologic, and radiologic determinants of survival in patients with progressive multifocal leukoencephalopathy (PML).

Methods.—We recorded the clinical outcome of 60 patients with PML (73% HIV+) who were prospectively evaluated between 2000 and 2007 for the presence of JC virus (JCV)-specific CD8+ cytotoxic T-lymphocytes (CTL) in blood.

Results.—Estimated probability of survival at 1 year was 52% for HIV ± PML and 58% for HIV− patients with PML. Patients with PML with detectable CTL within 3 months of diagnosis had a 1-year estimated survival of 73% compared to 46% for those without CTL (hazard ratio [HR] for death = 0.47, 95% confidence interval [CI] 0.13–1.75, $p = 0.26$). Patients with CTL response had an increased likelihood of having contrast enhancement of PML lesions and immune reconstitution inflammatory syndrome (odds ratio 3.7 and 7.8). Estimated 1-year survival was 48% in HIV+ patients with PML with CD4 count <200/μL at PML diagnosis compared to 67% in those with CD4 >200/μL (HR for death 1.41, 95% CI 0.27–7.38, $p = 0.68$). JCV DNA was detected in the urine of 48% and in the blood of 56% of patients with PML, but viruria and viremia were not associated with survival.

Conclusions.—The presence of JC virus (JCV)-specific cytotoxic T-lymphocytes (CTL) was associated with a trend toward longer survival in patients with progressive multifocal leukoencephalopathy (PML), which was more pronounced than the impact of CD4 count in HIV+ patients with PML early after diagnosis. Despite the association of contrast enhancement and immune reconstitution inflammatory syndrome with JCV-specific CTL, these cannot be considered as surrogate markers for the prognostic value of the CTL. Strategies aiming at improving the cellular immune response may improve the course of PML.

▶ Progressive multifocal leukoencephalopathy (PML) is a rare central nervous system demyelinating disease caused by the reactivation of JC virus (JCV). Although more than 90% of adults have been infected with JCV, only certain populations are susceptible to the rare and devastating consequences of virus reactivation that can lead to PML. PML has been reported in multiple conditions, almost always associated with immunosuppression, including human immunodeficiency virus infection, rheumatologic disorders, multiple sclerosis treated with natalizumab and rituximab, and more rarely in other conditions.

Marzocchetti et al describe clinical, immunologic, virologic, and radiologic determinants in 60 patients with PLM. Sixty patients with virologic, histologic, or clinical-radiologic diagnosis of PML, including 44 HIV-positive (73%) and 16 HIV-negative (27%) patients, were recruited between 2000 and 2007.

PML was diagnosed by experienced clinicians and defined by typical clinical and imaging findings and supported by JCV DNA detection in cerebrospinal fluid or biopsy. One-year survival rates were 52% in the HIV-positive and 58% in the HIV-negative patients. The presence of JCV-specific cytotoxic T lymphocytes (CTL) was associated with a trend toward longer survival in patients with PML, which was more pronounced than the impact of CD4 count in HIV-positive patients with PML early after diagnosis.

D. van de Beek, MD, PhD

Effect of Pneumococcal Conjugate Vaccine on Pneumococcal Meningitis

Hsu HE, Shutt KA, Moore MR, et al (Univ of Pittsburgh, PA; Ctrs for Disease Control and Prevention, Atlanta, GA; et al)

N Engl J Med 360:244-256, 2009

Background.—Invasive pneumococcal disease declined among children and adults after the introduction of the pediatric heptavalent pneumococcal conjugate vaccine (PCV7) in 2000, but its effect on pneumococcal meningitis is unclear.

Methods.—We examined trends in pneumococcal meningitis from 1998 through 2005 using active, population-based surveillance data from eight sites in the United States. Isolates were grouped into PCV7 serotypes (4, 6B, 9V, 14, 18C, 19F, and 23F), PCV7-related serotypes (6A, 9A, 9L, 9N, 18A, 18B, 18F, 19B, 19C, 23A, and 23B), and non-PCV7 serotypes (all others). Changes in the incidence of pneumococcal meningitis were assessed against baseline values from 1998–1999.

Results.—We identified 1379 cases of pneumococcal meningitis. The incidence declined from 1.13 cases to 0.79 case per 100,000 persons between 1998–1999 and 2004–2005 (a 30.1% decline, $P<0.001$). Among persons younger than 2 years of age and those 65 years of age or older, the incidence decreased during the study period by 64.0% and 54.0%, respectively ($P<0.001$ for both groups). Rates of PCV7-serotype meningitis declined from 0.66 case to 0.18 case (a 73.3% decline, $P<0.001$) among patients of all ages. Although rates of PCV7-related–serotype disease decreased by 32.1% ($P = 0.08$), rates of non-PCV7–serotype disease increased from 0.32 to 0.51 (an increase of 60.5%, $P<0.001$). The percentages of cases from non-PCV7 serotypes 19A, 22F, and 35B each increased significantly during the study period. On average, 27.8% of isolates were nonsusceptible to penicillin, but fewer isolates were nonsusceptible to chloramphenicol (5.7%), meropenem (16.6%), and cefotaxime (11.8%). The proportion of penicillin-nonsusceptible isolates decreased between 1998 and 2003 (from 32.0% to 19.4%, $P = 0.01$) but increased between 2003 and 2005 (from 19.4% to 30.1%, $P = 0.03$).

Conclusions.—Rates of pneumococcal meningitis have decreased among children and adults since PCV7 was introduced. Although the overall effect of the vaccine remains substantial, a recent increase in meningitis caused by non-PCV7 serotypes, including strains nonsusceptible to antibiotics, is a concern.

▶ The article by Hsu et al describes the changes in epidemiology of pneumococcal meningitis after the introduction of the 7-valent pneumococcal conjugate vaccine (PCV7) in the United States in 2000. Data were gathered by the active bacterial core surveillance network, a component of the Centers for Disease Control and Prevention (CDC) Emerging Infectious Disease Programs Network, in 8 US states. Pneumococcal meningitis cases were identified by positive cerebrospinal fluid culture or clinical diagnosis of meningitis, with pneumococci isolated from another normally sterile site (mostly blood).

A previous report on pneumococcal disease did not show an effect on the incidence of pneumococcal meningitis in elderly (>50 years old) through herd immunity. This report showed a decrease in all cases of pneumococcal disease, due to a strong decline in vaccine serotypes. Furthermore, serotype replacement was found with nonvaccine-related serotypes. The current report focuses on pneumococcal meningitis in all age groups and can thereby evaluate the true effect on pneumococcal meningitis incidence.

A total of 1379 cases were identified in a period of 8 years (Jan 1998-Dec 2005), of which 369 cases occurred in children (<18 years) and 1010 cases occurred in adults. The incidence rate declined from 1.13 cases to 0.79 per 100 000 persons. The decline was strongest in PCV7 serotypes (−73%), a nonsignifcant decrease was found in PCV7-related serotypes (−32%), and non-PCV7 serotypes increased by 61%. In children <2 years, the total incidence of pneumococcal meningitis decreased by 64%.

One of the aims of the vaccine program was to decrease the incidence of antibiotic-resistant *Streptococcus pneumoniae* strains. This study shows no decrease in nonsusceptible strains.

This study provides evidence for a decrease in the incidence of pneumococcal meningitis through PCV7 vaccination in children and through herd immunity in adults. However, the introduction of the PCV7 vaccine has not led to a major decrease in the antibiotic susceptibility of pneumococcal strains.

Further surveillance studies will remain important, as the trend of serotype replacement might lead to an increase in incidence and other vaccination strategies.

D. van de Beek, MD, PhD

Immune responses to JC virus in patients with multiple sclerosis treated with natalizumab: a cross-sectional and longitudinal study

Jilek S, Jaquiéry E, Hirsch HH, et al (Centre Hospitalier Universitaire Vaudois, Lausanne, Switzerland; Univ Hosp Basel, Switzerland)

Lancet Neurol 9:264-272, 2010

Background.—Natalizumab is used to prevent relapses and progression of disability in patients with multiple sclerosis but has been associated with progressive multifocal leukoencephalopathy (PML). We aimed to better understand the associations between JC virus, which causes PML, and natalizumab treatment.

Methods.—We prospectively assessed patients with multiple sclerosis who started treatment with natalizumab. Blood and urine samples were tested for the presence of JC virus DNA with quantitative real-time PCR before treatment and at regular intervals after treatment onset for up to 18 months. At the same timepoints, by use of proliferation and enzyme-linked immunospot assays, the cellular immune responses against JC virus, Epstein-Barr virus, cytomegalovirus, myelin oligodendrocyte glycoprotein, and myelin oligodendrocyte basic protein (MOBP) were assessed. Humoral immune response specific to JC virus was assessed with an enzyme immunoassay. The same experiments were done on blood samples from patients with multiple sclerosis before and 10 months after the start of interferon beta treatment.

Findings.—We assessed 24 patients with multiple sclerosis who received natalizumab and 16 who received interferon beta. In patients treated with natalizumab, JC virus DNA was not detected in the blood at any timepoint. However, JC virus DNA was present in the urine of six patients and in most of these patients the concentrations of JC virus DNA were stable over time. Compared with pretreatment values, the cellular immune response was increased to cytomegalovirus at 6 months, to JC virus at 1, 9, and 12 months, and to Epstein-Barr virus and MOBP at 12 months. Humoral responses remained stable. There were no increases in cellular immune responses specific to the viruses or myelin proteins in the 16 patients treated with interferon beta.

Interpretation.—Natalizumab increases cellular immune responses specific to viruses and myelin proteins in the peripheral blood after 1 year, without evidence of viral reactivation.

▶ The article by Jilek et al describes the monitoring of the JC virus and other viruses in a cohort of patients with multiple sclerosis (MS) treated with natalizumab. Treatment with this monoclonal antibody is associated with an increased risk of progressive multifocal leukoencephalopathy (PML). This demyelinating central nervous system disorder caused by the JC virus is untreatable and therefore usually fatal. The study addresses an important clinical problem, and the recognition of risk factors for PML would be an important step forward.

JC virus titers in blood and urine were monitored in 24 patients with MS treated with natalizumab and compared with 16 patients with MS treated with interferon beta. To assess whether a dysregulated immune response during natalizumab treatment is specific for JC virus, Epstein-Barr virus (EBV) and cytomegalovirus (CMV) were also monitored. The study aims to unravel the association of natalizumab treatment with JC virus infection. A previous study showed JC viruria in a large proportion of patients treated with natalizumab and also showed JC viremia. However, patients in this study were already treated with natalizumab when included in the study, and a causal relation between the drug and the detection of the virus was unclear.

No patients treated with natalizumab or interferon developed JC viremia during the study period (18 months). JC virus was detected in urine of 25% of patients treated with natalizumab, which is comparable with the healthy population. The number of virus copies varied during treatment but did not consistently increase. An increased response of memory T cells specific to JC, EBV, CMV, and myelin oligodendrocyte basic protein was detected after starting natalizumab. This response was absent in patients treated with interferon beta. No patients in this study developed PML. The authors conclude that natalizumab enhances the T-cell response, independent of their antigen specificity, and the risk of PML might be higher in patients without JC virus-specific T-cell response.

The strength of the study lies in the detailed analysis of viral presence and markers of inflammation. However, the sample size of the study is small, and none of the patients developed PML. Therefore, no solid conclusions can be drawn for the effect of natalizumab on JC virus replication and immunity against JC virus. It remains unclear which patients with MS treated with natalizumab are at risk for PML, and what pathophysiological mechanism leads to JC infection.

New prospective studies should aim to identify clinical or laboratory markers that can be used to identify patients at increased risk for PML. As PML is a rare complication of natalizumab treatment, large studies are needed to solve this problem.

D. van de Beek, MD, PhD

Infectious Encephalitis in France in 2007: A National Prospective Study

Mailles A, on behalf of the Steering Committee and the Investigators Group (Univ Hosp of Grenoble, France)

Clin Infect Dis 49:1838-1847, 2009

Background.—Encephalitis is associated with significant mortality and morbidity, but its cause remains largely unknown. We designed a national prospective study in France in 2007 to describe patients with encephalitis, investigate the etiologic diagnosis of encephalitis, and assess risk factors associated with death.

Methods.—Patients were enrolled by attending physicians according to case definition, and data were collected with a standardized questionnaire. The etiologic diagnosis was investigated after a standardized procedure. Risk factors associated with death during hospitalization were assessed by multivariate logistic regression.

Results.—A total of 253 patients with acute infectious encephalitis from 106 medical units throughout France were included in the study. Their ages ranged from 1 month to 89 years (median age, 54 years); 61% were male. Cause of the encephalitis was determined in 131 patients (52%). Herpes simplex virus 1 (42%), varicella-zoster virus (15%), *Mycobacterium tuberculosis* (15%), and *Listeria monocytogenes* (10%) were the most frequently identified agents. Twenty-six patients (10%, all adults) died, 6 of them with tuberculosis and 6 with listeriosis. Risk factors independently associated with death during hospitalization identified by the multivariable analysis were age (odds ratio [OR], 1.2; 95% confidence interval [CI], 1.0–1.4; for 5-year increase), cancer (OR, 17; 95% CI, 2.3122.6), immunosuppressive treatment before onset (OR, 24; 95% CI, 1.3–426.0), percentage of hospitalized patients receiving mechanical ventilation (OR, 2.0; 95% CI, 1.4–3.0; for 10% increase), the etiologic agent, coma on day 5 after admission (OR, 16; 95% CI, 2.8–92.3), and sepsis on day 5 after admission (OR, 94; 95% CI, 4.9–1792.2).

Conclusions.—Our prospective study provides an overview of the clinical and etiologic patterns of acute infectious encephalitis in adults in France. Herpes simplex virus 1 remains the main cause of encephalitis, but bacteria accounts for the highest case-fatality rates.

► Infections of the central nervous system can be caused by a wide variety of infectious agents, including bacteria, viruses, fungi, parasites, and prions. The diagnosis of encephalitis is often considered. Clinical findings, such as fever, headache, and altered level of consciousness, are common but fail to distinguish among various pathogens and can be seen with a variety of noninfectious conditions that mimic encephalitis, such as autoimmune disease or vasculitis. The etiologic origin remains undetermined in most patients, despite a wide range of diagnostic tools.

Mailles et al report on a prospective multicenter cohort study of patients from infectious diseases units, neurologic units, pediatric units, and intensive care units throughout France. To avoid including patients with aseptic meningitis without brain involvement, the study design encompassed the exclusion of surviving patients with a hospital stay of fewer than 5 days. Additional exclusion criteria were positive human immunodeficiency virus status, meningitis without clinical brain involvement, brain abscess, prion diseases, cerebral malaria, and noninfectious CNS diseases. All medical files were reviewed by a single multidisciplinary, national panel of senior experts from the Steering Committee, who validated the diagnosis and classified patients as having confirmed, probable, or possible cases of encephalitis according to clinical data, imaging findings, and biological test results.

Two hundred ninety-five patients were enrolled by 106 hospital units in 44 of 95 French mainland districts. Patients were enrolled in infectious diseases units (43%), ICUs (29%), neurologic units (17%), pediatric units (10%), or miscellaneous units (1%). On admission, 240 patients (95%) presented with an altered mental status, 94 patients (37%) presented with focal neurologic signs, 76 patients (30%) presented with seizures, 64 patients (25%) presented with decreased consciousness, and 13 patients (5%) presented with coma.

The study identified an infectious cause in slightly > 50% of cases; herpes simplex virus (HSV) and varicella zoster virus were the most commonly identified infections, similar to other studies. An unexpectedly high number of patients were diagnosed as having *Mycobacterium tuberculosis* and *Listeria monocytogenes*. Arboviruses were rarely identified (eg, tick-borne encephalitis virus or Toscana virus). These findings are consistent with the available data in

France, indicating that arboviruses' circulation is rare and limited to specific areas, such as tick-borne encephalitis at the German and Swiss borders and Toscana virus along the Mediterranean coast. A fatal outcome occurred in 26 patients (10%) during hospitalization. The highest case fatality rates were found in patients with listeriosis (46%) and in patients with tuberculosis (30%).

This study shows that surveillance and regional guidelines play an important role in optimizing diagnostic testing and identifying pathogens, and stresses the need for well-structured nationwide surveillance infrastructures for encephalitis.

D. van de Beek, MD, PhD

Predictors of mortality and impact of aminoglycosides on outcome in listeriosis in a retrospective cohort study

Mitjà O, Pigrau C, Ruiz I, et al (Universitat Autònoma, Barcelona, Spain)

J Antimicrob Chemother 64:416-423, 2009

Objectives.—Gentamicin is often used to treat listeriosis, particularly in patients with meningitis; nonetheless, some clinicians question this practice because of the drug's associated nephrotoxicity and inability to cross the blood–brain barrier. The aim of this study was to evaluate predictors of mortality and the impact of aminoglycosides on outcome in patients with listeriosis.

Methods.—We conducted a retrospective study of all non-pregnant adult patients with *Listeria monocytogenes* infection detected in sterile body fluids between 1983 and 2006. Early mortality was defined as death occurring between days 3 and 14 after admission, and late mortality as in-hospital death after 14 days.

Results.—Of 118 episodes, 16 were excluded because patients died in the first 48 h. Among the 102 patients analysed, 33 (32%) had received combined β-lactam and aminoglycoside therapy and 69 (68%) β-lactam monotherapy. Both groups had similar demographic and clinical features, and rate of appropriate initial therapy. Overall mortality was 21/102 (20.6%). Early overall mortality was 11.8%: 27.3% (9/33) in the combined group and 4.3% (3/69) in the monotherapy group ($P = 0.003$). Late mortality was 8.8%. In the multivariate analysis, the factors predicting early mortality were renal failure, previous corticosteroid therapy and age >65 years, whereas neoplastic disease and coma were associated with late mortality. Gentamicin administration did not decrease early mortality, but seemed to increase it. In the late mortality analysis, gentamicin use had no impact. In an analysis with the propensity score method for the use of aminoglycosides, combined therapy with this antibiotic was associated with an increasing trend for early mortality (OR 3.40, 95% CI 0.82–14.07).

Conclusions.—The addition of aminoglycosides to treatment for listeriosis did not improve the patients' outcome.

► The article by Mitjà et al describes a large retrospective cohort study of 118 episodes of invasive infections with *Listeria monocytogenes* and evaluates predictors of mortality and the impact of aminoglycoside treatment on outcomes. Listeriosis is often treated with gentamicin, as in vitro studies have shown synergy and a bactericidal effect when gentamicin is added. However, the value of aminoglycosides is questioned in listeriosis treatment, as these drugs are unable to cross the blood-brain barrier, and animal studies have shown conflicting results with regard to synergy.

The study included all nonpregnant adult patients with infection by *L monocytogenes*, confirmed by culture of blood, cerebrospinal fluid, or other sterile body fluids, between January 1983 and December 2006 in a tertiary referral center. Mortality was defined as death from any cause during hospitalization. Early mortality was defined as death occurring 3 to 14 days after admission, and late mortality was defined as death occurring after day 14. Patients who died on days 1 and 2 were excluded, as deaths occurring that early were unlikely to be related to the treatment modality.

Among the 102 patients who survived past day 2, 32% of them had received combined β-lactam and aminoglycoside therapy, and 68% of them had received β-lactam monotherapy. Demographic features, clinical features, and rate of appropriate initial therapy were similar between groups. Overall mortality was 21%. Early overall mortality was 12%, 28% in the combined group and 4% in the monotherapy group. Late mortality was 9%. The factors predicting early mortality in the multivariate analysis were renal failure, previous corticosteroid therapy, and age > 65 years, whereas cancer and coma were associated with late mortality. Gentamicin administration did not decrease mortality in the early mortality group but appeared to increase it. In the late mortality analysis, gentamicin use had no impact. In an analysis with a propensity score method for the use of aminoglycosides, an increased trend for early mortality in the combined therapy group (OR 3.40, 95% CI 0.82-14.07) was seen.

These findings clearly show that aminoglycosides do not improve outcomes in listeriosis. The evidence to support the use of aminoglycosides in listeriosis is less convincing than the presented results. Therefore, aminoglycosides should be held back in invasive *L monocytogenes* infections.

The strength of the study lies in its sample size, detailed clinical information, and sound statistical methods. Its weakness lies in the retrospective design, as patients might have been missed. However, a randomized clinical trial is unlikely to be performed in this rather rare disease. Other retrospective series could confirm the results of this study and could add to the evidence to withhold aminoglycosides.

D. van de Beek, MD, PhD

6 Miscellaneous

Age-related Iron Deposition in the Basal Ganglia: Quantitative Analysis in Healthy Subjects

Aquino D, Bizzi A, Grisoli M, et al (C. Besta Neurological Inst, Italy)

Radiology 252:165-172, 2009

Purpose.—To determine the values of iron accumulation in the basal ganglia of healthy volunteers of different ages with R2* and raw signal intensity measurements from T1-weighted magnetic resonance (MR) images, supported by voxel-based relaxometry (VBR), and to compare them with previously reported iron concentrations found in autopsy material.

Materials and Methods.—The ethics committee approved the study, and the participants or their parents gave written informed consent. Eighty subjects (41 female and 39 male subjects; age range, 1–80 years) were examined at 1.5 T. For each subject, R2* values were calculated. Curves for R2* versus age were obtained for globus pallidus (GP), putamen, caudate nucleus, substantia nigra (SN), and frontal white matter (FWM). To highlight possible differences in iron concentration among the age decades, VBR was applied. Signal intensity values were estimated on T1-weighted fast low-angle shot images, and regions of interest were drawn in each nucleus. R2* values were also compared with iron concentrations reported in a postmortem study. Statistical analysis was performed (t test), and a difference with $P < .05$ (FDR corrected) was significant.

Results.—The curves for R2* versus age showed an exponential increase with increasing age in all the basal ganglia. VBR demonstrated significant differences ($P < .05$, corrected) in the comparison between the 2nd and the following decades for lenticular nuclei. Good correlation coefficients were found for GP ($R^2 = 0.64$), putamen ($R^2 = 0.51$), and SN ($R^2 = 0.53$) when compared with findings in the post-mortem study. Signal intensity curves were similar to the R2* curves.

Conclusion.—R2* measurements can be used to quantify brain iron accumulation and thus may allow better evaluation of neurodegenerative diseases associated with iron deposition.

► In this study, Aquino et al set out to determine the concentrations of iron in various nuclei of the basal ganglia via the use of T2* gradient echo (GRE) and T1-weighted magnetization prepared rapid acquisition gradient echo (MPRAGE) imaging at 1.5 T. This is based on previous studies which have found that iron deposition can be detected by T2* GRE imaging, and that this concentration increases with age both on T2* images (measured by a measurement called "R2*") and on histopathologic sectioning, akin to the concept that the greater the amount of dark signal on T2 or T2* GRE imaging, the greater the amount of iron.[1,2] As there are a number of technical details of this article, a brief albeit incomplete explanation of technique is probably warranted to understand the implications for future research: the authors used voxel-based relaxometry (VBR) to stereotactically smooth, warp, and conform to a R2* template (from the Montreal Neurological Institute ICBM152; International Consortium for Brain Mapping, Montreal Neurological Institute, McGill University, Montreal, Quebec, Canada).[3] The resulting R2* measurements in various basal ganglia nuclei were then plotted versus age and calculated estimates for age using an equation by Hallgren and Sourander.[4]

The authors found that the R2* values (and thereby iron) and signal intensity on T1 MPRAGE increased with age to the greatest degree in the substantia nigra, followed by the globus pallidus, putamen, caudate nucleus, and periventricular frontal white matter; notably, both the caudate and frontal white matter had a scarce iron load at any age. The authors point out that patients within the first decade were excluded because there are no R2* templates of that age group, and that they found significant interindividual fluctuations in patients > 50 years. However, their confirmation of the plateau of iron levels in the globus pallidus and substantia nigra in early adulthood with later variability (after about the age of 50) corresponds with susceptibility weighted imaging (SWI) studies[5] and previous data documenting that this age-related increasing mineralization can be measured using R2* (via T2* GRE images). The authors also document the expected progression of mineralization within the globus pallidus (ie, medial to lateral and posterior to anterior). The gradual decreasing signal on T1 MPRAGE in the globus pallidus and putamen were similar to that observed with R2*, while the R2* moderate strongly correlated with iron load from a previous postmortem study.[4]

The significance of this article is that the R2* measurements appear to be valid and produce results that may be a tentative, although incomplete, reference for future noninvasive studies. Given the significance of brain iron in various neurodegenerative and metabolic disorders (iron is not normally present in measurable quantities at birth), these preliminary values and their method of measurement can possibly be reproduced. Future studies will hopefully use a 3.0 T or higher field strength magnet, use SWI in combination with T2* GRE (and correlate the 2 measurements), and contain both control patients and those with neurodegenerative diseases.

A. M. McKinney IV, MD

References

1. Drayer B, Burger P, Darwin R, Riederer S, Herfkens R, Johnson GA. MRI of brain iron. *AJR Am J Roentgenol.* 1986;147:103-110.
2. Gelman N, Gorell JM, Barker PB, et al. MR imaging of human brain at 3.0 T: preliminary report on transverse relaxation rates and relation to estimated iron content. *Radiology.* 1999;210:759-767.

3. Pell GS, Briellmann RS, Waites AB, Abbott DF, Jackson GD. Voxel-based relaxometry: a new approach for analysis of T2 relaxometry changes in epilepsy. *Neuroimage*. 2004;21:707-713.
4. Hallgren B, Sourander P. The effect of age on the non-haemin iron in the human brain. *J Neurochem*. 1958;3:41-51.
5. Harder SL, Hopp KM, Ward H, Neglio H, Gitlin J, Kido D. Mineralization of deep gray matter with age: a retrospective review with susceptibility-weighted MR imaging. *AJNR Am J Neuroradiol*. 2008;29:176-183.

APP overexpression prevents neuropathic pain and motoneuron death after peripheral nerve injury in mice

Kotulska K, Larysz-Brysz M, LePecheur M, et al (The Children's Memorial Health Inst, Warsaw, Poland; Med Univ of Silesia, Medyków, Katowice, Poland; et al)

Brain Res Bull 81:378-384, 2010

Despite general capacity of peripheral nervous system to regenerate, peripheral nerve injury is often followed by incomplete recovery of function and sometimes burdened by neuropathic pain. Amyloid precursor protein (APP) was suggested to play a role in neuronal growth, however, its role in peripheral nerve repair was not studied. The aim of this study was to examine the role of APP overexpression in peripheral nerve regeneration and neuropathic pain-related behavior in mice. Sciatic nerves of APP overexpressing and FVB/N wild-type mice were transected and immediately resutured. Evaluation of motor and sensory function and autotomy was carried out during 4-week follow up. We found no autotomy behavior as well as less significant atrophy of denervated muscles in APP overexpressing animals when compared to wild-type ones. Sciatic nerve function index outcome did not differ between groups. Histological evaluation revealed that the intensity of regeneration features, including GAP-43-positive growth cones and Schwann cells number in the distal stump of the transected nerve, was also similar in both groups. However, the regenerating fibers were organized more chaotically in wild-type mice and neuromas were much more often seen in this group. The number of macrophages infiltrating the injury site was significantly higher in control group. The number of surviving motoneurons was higher in transgenic mice than in control animals. Taken together, our findings suggest that APP overexpression is beneficial for nerve regeneration processes due to better organization of regenerating fibers, increased survival of motoneurons after autotomy and prevention of neuropathic pain.

► This provocative article from Poland suggests that Alzheimer amyloid precursor protein (APP) has a beneficial role in recovery from peripheral nerve injury in mice. The evidence presented has at least 2 interesting implications. One is that APP secretion is a protective response. Of course, a protective response can overshoot and then become damaging, as often happens for instance with chronic inflammation. The second possibility is that the accumulation of APP and of its side product, amyloid β peptides, is a response to and therefore a marker of ongoing chronic or repetitive injury. That leaves open the question of what the primary insult(s) is or are. One candidate, of course, is cardiovascular insufficiencies, which so often accompany arterial disease and cardiac arrhythmias in older people.

J. P. Blass, MD, PhD

Asymmetric Hearing Loss: Rule 3,000 for Screening Vestibular Schwannoma

Saliba I, Martineau G, Chagnon M (Montreal Univ, Quebec, Canada)
Otol Neurotol 30:515-521, 2009

Objective.—To assess the diagnostic yield of audiograms associated to electronystagmography (ENG) for screening vestibular schwannomas (VSs), to determine what definition of asymmetric sensorineural hearing loss (ASNHL) fits best for the diagnosis of VS, and to determine if cochleovestibular symptoms and atherosclerotic potential risk factors play a role in the VS screening.

Study Design.—Retrospective chart review in a tertiary care center.

Methods.—One hundred twenty-two patients were included in the study and divided into 2 groups: 1) patients presenting a VS (n = 74) and 2) patients without VS (n = 48). They had received an audiometry assessment, an ENG, and a posterior fossa magnetic resonance imaging (MRI). In addition, a variety of risk factors and clinical data were collected. Mean hearing threshold by frequency, mean asymmetries by frequency, speech discrimination score (SDS), ENG results, and presence or absence of vertigo are studied. Cochleovestibular symptoms and atherosclerotic potential risk factors were collected. Characteristics were studied with analysis of variance, χ^2 test, or a paired t test. A receiver operating characteristic curve was obtained. A logistic regression with a step-wise selection based on the likelihood ratio was used to identify the best subgroup of predictors of the VS.

Results.—The most revealing data were the mean ASNHL at 3,000 Hz ($p < 0.001$), the interaural SDS asymmetry ($p < 0.001$), the vestibular deficit ($p < 0.049$), and the absence of vertigo ($p < 0.001$). The ASNHL at 3,000 Hz was the most representative value of all the frequencies and for the SDS asymmetry. Interaural difference of 15 dB or more at 3,000 Hz is sufficient to consider hearing loss as asymmetric. When the cutoff for a positive test was placed at 50% probability, the receiver operating characteristic curve shows a sensitivity of 73%. The grade of the tumor was also related with the degree of ASNHL at 3,000 Hz. Caloric test does not predict the localization or the grade of the VS. Tinnitus and atherosclerotic potential risk factors were not considered significantly linked with VS.

Conclusion.—To reduce the number of negative MRI performed in the investigation of an ASNHL, we propose the "rule 3,000," ASNHL of 15 dB or more at the 3,000-Hz frequency. In this case, an investigation with MRI is crucial. If this ASNHL is less than 15 dB, we recommend a biannual audiometric follow-up.

▶ Vestibular schwannoma (VS) is a common slow-growing brain tumor that arises from the transition zone between Schwann cells and oligodendrocytes of the vestibular nerve within the internal auditory meatus. The most frequent clinical sign is asymmetric sensorineural hearing loss with or without tinnitus. MRI scan with gadolinium that includes the eighth nerve sections is the most sensitive diagnostic test; yet, this is a very costly test to do, especially when 98% of patients with asymmetric hearing loss will not have this tumor. This retrospective study examined the diagnostic yield of a number of auditory tests in 176 patients who also had an MRI scan of the head. One hundred twenty-two patients were selected for the study (74 with VS and 48 without VS). The authors found that asymmetric sensorineural hearing loss of 15 db or more at 3000 Hz was the most diagnostic with a sensitivity of 73% and

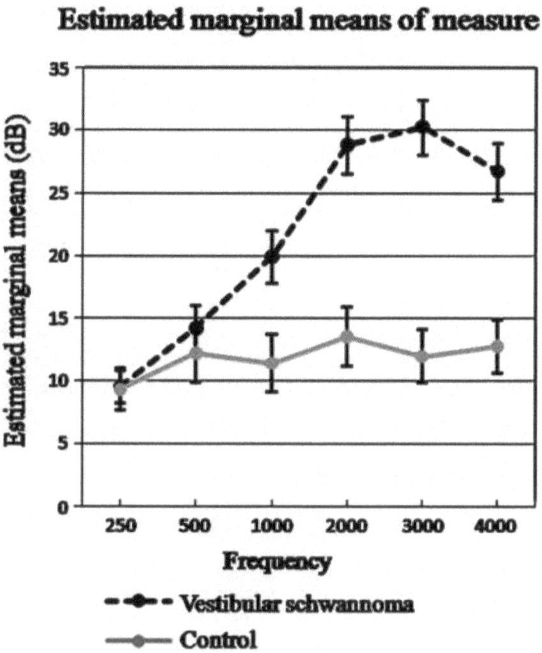

FIGURE 1.—Mean asymmetries of sensorineural hearing loss by frequency for vestibular schwannoma and control groups; (Mean ± standard error of mean). (Courtesy of Saliba I, Martineau G, Chagnon M. Asymmetric hearing loss: Rule 3,000 for screening vestibular schwannoma. *Otol Neurotol.* 2009;30: 515-521.)

specificity of 76% (Fig 1). They recommend biannual audiometric testing if the asymmetry is less than 15 db at this frequency.

R. J. Tusa, MD, PhD

Bruns' Nystagmus in Patients With Vestibular Schwannoma

Lloyd SKW, Baguley DM, Butler K, et al (Cambridge Univ Hosps NHS Trust, UK)

Otol Neurotol 30:625-628, 2009

Objectives.—To determine the prevalence of Bruns' nystagmus in patients undergoing surgical treatment for unilateral sporadic vestibular schwannomas (VSs), identify the clinical characteristics of patients with Bruns' nystagmus and compare these characteristics with those of VS patients with no nystagmus and other types of nystagmus, and determine the long-term impact of having preoperative Bruns' nystagmus.

Study Design.—A retrospective review using a prospectively updated database of patients who had undergone surgical removal of a VS. Patients were divided into 3 groups: Bruns' nystagmus, other types of nystagmus, or no nystagmus. Statistical comparison of each group was undertaken.

Patients.—Nine hundred eighty-four patients were included consisting of 492 men and 492 women with a mean age of 59 years (range, 11–86 yr).

Results.—Bruns' nystagmus was present in 11% of patients. Bruns' nystagmus was associated with larger tumor size ($p < 0.001$). Beyond 3.5-cm maximum diameter, 92% of patients had nystagmus, 67% of which had Bruns' nystagmus. Preoperative balance impairment was present in 95% of patients with Bruns' nystagmus compared with 59% with no nystagmus. The balance status of all groups improved considerably postoperatively, but the patients with Bruns' nystagmus had a relatively greater improvement in balance status.

Conclusion.—Bruns' nystagmus occurs in patients with large VSs. These patients tend to have greater balance impairment pre\operatively, but after surgery, long-term balance outcomes are similar to those of patients with no nystagmus or other forms of nystagmus.

▶ Vestibular schwannoma (VS) is a benign tumor that usually originates at the junction of schwann cells and myelin around the superior vestibular nerve (cranial nerve VIII). This portion of the nerve lies within the internal auditory canal. As it grows it can compress the vestibular nerve, which leads to vestibular hypofunction. This peripheral nerve defect leads to the loss of tone to the vestibular nucleus. For discussion sake, assume the tumor is on the right side. Reduced fibers and myelin of the vestibular nerve will cause a nystagmus that beats to the left (left beat nystagmus). As the tumor continues to grow, it extends into the cerebellopontine angle to compress the cerebellum (flocculus and paraflocculus). This central defect leads to an additional type of nystagmus that is central in nature and labeled gaze-holding or gaze-paretic nystagmus. When these peripheral and central types of nystagmus are added together, Bruns' nystagmus occurs. In this type of nystagmus, when the patient is asked to hold their eyes to the left or straight ahead, there is a left beat nystagmus and when the patient is asked to hold their eyes to the right, there is a right beat nystagmus. In the article by Lloyd et al, they did a retrospective review of 984 patients that had VS. The 3 conclusions were as follows: (1) the larger the tumor, the more likely nystagmus would occur, ranging from 3% for tumors <1.5 cm to 100% for tumors >4.5 cm (Fig 1 in the original article); (2) the larger the tumor, the more likely the nystagmus would be Bruns', ranging from 0% for tumors <1.5 cm to 45% for tumors >4.5 cm (Fig 2 in the original article); (3) Bruns' nystagmus was more likely to be associated with imbalance (positive Romberg test) than those without nystagmus (95% vs 59%). The results are to be expected based on our understanding of the causes of Bruns' and non-Bruns' nystagmus, but this is the first study of this size that actually provides a distribution of the number of patients with and without Bruns' nystagmus. The data suggest that a simple bedside exam can help determine the size of the tumor simply based on the pattern of nystagmus.

R. J. Tusa, MD, PhD

Gene–environment interactions in Leber hereditary optic neuropathy

Kirkman MA, Yu-Wai-Man P, Korsten A, et al (Newcastle Univ, UK; Univ Med Ctr Rotterdam, The Netherlands; et al)

Brain 132:2317-2326, 2009

Leber hereditary optic neuropathy (LHON) is a genetic disorder primarily due to mutations of mitochondrial DNA (mtDNA). Environmental factors are thought to precipitate the visual failure and explain the marked incomplete penetrance of LHON, but previous small studies have failed to confirm this to be the case. LHON has no treatment, so identifying environmental triggers is the key to disease prevention, whilst potentially revealing new mechanisms amenable to therapeutic manipulation. To address this issue, we conducted a large, multicentre epidemiological study of 196 affected and 206 unaffected carriers from 125 LHON pedigrees known to harbour one of the three primary pathogenic mtDNA mutations: m.3460G>A, m.11778G>A and m.14484T>C. A comprehensive history of exposure to smoking, alcohol and other putative environmental insults was collected using a structured questionnaire. We identified a strong and consistent association between visual loss and smoking, independent of gender and alcohol intake, leading to a clinical penetrance of 93% in men who smoked. There was a trend towards increased visual failure with alcohol, but only with a heavy intake.

Based on these findings, asymptomatic carriers of a LHON mtDNA mutation should be strongly advised not to smoke and to moderate their alcohol intake.

► This was a survey study that canvassed 196 patients with Lebers hereditary optic neuropathy (LHON) and 206 unaffected carriers from 125 different pedigrees using a standardized questionnaire. The questionnaire covered basic demographic information as well as visual symptoms and possible environmental triggers. The factors included smoking, alcohol, recreational drugs, toxins, as well as trauma, diet, medications (including vitamins and herbal remedies), exercise, and medical comorbidities.

As expected, most LHON symptomatic cases were male (74.5%) with carriers predominantly female (70.9%). The mean age of onset of vision loss was 27.9 years. They were able to conclude that smoking was associated with an increased risk of vision loss in LHON carriers. They also found that the risk of vision loss was related to the cumulative amount of smoking and the maximum intensity of smoking. Of males with LHON, 93% who smoked developed vision loss. The statistics for alcohol consumption and vision loss were not as strong, only suggesting that heavy alcohol use correlated with vision loss.

Despite this correlation with smoking, the study also included 15 LHON cases with vision loss before age 10 who had never smoked nor consumed alcohol. They conclude that the disease is likely multifactorial, but as there is currently no treatment for LHON all asymptomatic carriers should be encouraged not to smoke and to moderate their alcohol intake.

J. Leavitt, MD

Treatment of Neuromyelitis Optica With Mycophenolate Mofetil: Retrospective Analysis of 24 Patients

Jacob A, Matiello M, Weinshenker BG, et al (Mayo Clinic College of Medicine, Rochester, MN; et al)

Arch Neurol 66:1128-1133, 2009

Background.—Neuromyelitis optica (NMO) is the first inflammatory autoimmune demyelinating disease of the central nervous system for which a specific antigenic target has been identified; the marker autoantibody NMO-IgG specifically recognizes the astrocytic water channel aquaporin 4. Current evidence strongly suggests that NMO-IgG may be pathogenic. Since disability accrues incrementally related to attacks, attack prevention with immunosuppressive therapy is the mainstay of preventing disability.

Objective.—To evaluate the efficacy and safety of mycophenolate mofetil therapy in NMO spectrum disorders.

Design.—Retrospective case series with prospective telephone follow-up.

Setting.—Mayo Clinic Health System.

Patients.—Twenty-four patients with NMO spectrum disorders (7 treatment-naive).

Intervention.—Mycophenolate mofetil (median dose of 2000 mg per day).

Main Outcome Measures.—Annualized relapse rates and disability (Expanded Disability Status Scale).

Results.—At a median follow-up of 28 months (range, 18-89 months), 19 patients (79%) were continuing treatment. The median duration of treatment was 27 months (range, 1-89 months). The median annualized posttreatment relapse rate was lower than the pretreatment rate (0.09; range, 0-1.5; and 1.3; range, 0.23-11.8, respectively; $P < .001$). Disability stabilized or decreased in 22 of 24 patients (91%). One patient died of disease complications during follow-up. Six patients (25%) noted adverse effects during treatment with mycophenolate.

Conclusion.—Mycophenolate is associated with reduction in relapse frequency and stable or reduced disability in patients with NMO spectrum disorders.

▶ This was a retrospective medical record review study of 24 patients with neuromyelitis optica (NMO) or NMO spectrum disorder who had been treated with mycophenolate mofetil. Fifteen were diagnosed with NMO (fulfilling the 2006 NMO diagnostic criteria), 7 with relapsing longitudinally extensive transverse myelitis, 1 with relapsing optic neuritis, 1 with a single episode of longitudinally extensive transverse myelitis. Seven of the patients had not received any therapy before the initiation of mycophenolate mofetil, whereas the other 17 had received immunosuppressive therapy (6), immunomodulatory therapy (2) or both (9) before the mycophenolate mofetil.

This was not prospective so the dose of mycophenolate mofetil ranged from 750 mg/day to 3000 mg/day with a median of 2000 mg/day. Follow-up ranged from 18 to 89 months with a median of 28 months. Treatment with mycophenolate mofetil ranged from 1 to 89 months with a median of 27.4 months. At the last follow-up, 19 patients (79%) were still on mycophenolate mofetil (range 20-89 months, median 29.4 months). Five patients (2%) stopped mycophenolate mofetil—1 died, 1 had adverse effects, 1 chose to switch to rituximab after 1 month, and 2 had relapses and were switched to rituximab or azathioprine.

They analyzed the efficacy of treatment with mycophenolate mofetil by comparing the annual relapse rate posttreatment to pretreatment using the Wilcoxon signed-rank test. They did 3 different analyses—(1) excluding patients treated for less than 6 months (2 patients); (2) excluding patients treated for less than 6 months and the 1 patient who died (3); (3) excluding patients treated for less than 6 months, the 1 patient who died, and any patients who received additional therapy (9). In the first subgroup 77% had an improvement in the annualized relapse rate. The second and third subgroups also had reductions in the relapse rate but the percentages were not reported for each group, however, overall they reported a 79% reduction in the annualized relapse rate after treatment with mycophenolate mofetil. They also looked at the disability using the expanded disability status scale (EDSS) scores as a measure of treatment effect. Before mycophenolate mofetil treatment the median EDSS score was 6. The posttreatment score was stable in 15 and improved in 7 (for a median of 1 point).

Mycophenolate mofetil acts to inhibit inosine monophosphate dehydrogenase which is involved in the conversion of inosine monophosphate to guanosine monophosphate which is then converted to GDP, GTP, and dGTP. Mycophenolate mofetil thereby reduces GTP and dGTP in lymphocytes decreasing lymphocyte proliferation and antibody synthesis. Mycophenolate mofetil is currently used in a variety of posttransplant conditions and autoimmune entities. The drug is felt to have fewer adverse effects than other immunosuppressive agents and is given orally.

This is a preliminary study showing improvement in NMO and NMO spectrum disorder patients with the use of mycophenolate mofetil. It will be important to follow this with a well-designed, randomized, case-controlled, double-masked study of mycophenolate mofetil in NMO and NMO spectrum disorder patients to see if the improvement in therapy is consistently found. Given the poor prognosis with NMO (50% wheelchair dependent and 62% blind within 5 years[1,2]), better treatment modalities are needed.

J. Leavitt, MD

References

1. Wingerchuk DM, Hogancamp WF, O'Brien PC, Weinshenker BG. The clinical course of neuromyelitis optica (Devic's syndrome). *Neurology.* 1999;53: 1107-1114.
2. Wingerchuk DM, Pittock SJ, Lucchinetti CF, Lennon VA, Weinshenker BG. A secondary progressive clinical course in uncommon in neuromyelitis optica. *Neurology.* 2007;68:603-605.

7 Movement Disorders

A Double-Blind, Delayed-Start Trial of Rasagiline In Parkinson's Disease

Olanow CW, Rascol O, Hauser R, et al (Mount Sinai School of Medicine, NY; Centre Hospitalier Universitaire and Univ of Toulouse, France; Univ of South Florida, Tampa; et al)

N Engl J Med 361:1268-1278, 2009

Background.—A therapy that slows disease progression is the major unmet need in Parkinson's disease.

Methods.—In this double-blind trial, we examined the possibility that rasagiline has disease-modifying effects in Parkinson's disease. A total of 1176 subjects with untreated Parkinson's disease were randomly assigned to receive rasagiline (at a dose of either 1 mg or 2 mg per day) for 72 weeks (the early-start group) or placebo for 36 weeks followed by rasagiline (at a dose of either 1 mg or 2 mg per day) for 36 weeks (the delayed-start group). To determine a positive result with either dose, the early-start treatment group had to meet each of three hierarchical end points of the primary analysis based on the Unified Parkinson's Disease Rating Scale (UPDRS, a 176-point scale, with higher numbers indicating more severe disease): superiority to placebo in the rate of change in the UPDRS score between weeks 12 and 36, superiority to delayed-start treatment in the change in the score between baseline and week 72, and noninferiority to delayed-start treatment in the rate of change in the score between weeks 48 and 72.

Results.—Early-start treatment with rasagiline at a dose of 1 mg per day met all end points in the primary analysis: a smaller mean (±SE) increase (rate of worsening) in the UPDRS score between weeks 12 and 36 (0.09±0.02 points per week in the early-start group vs. 0.14±0.01 points per week in the placebo group, P = 0.01), less worsening in the score between baseline and week 72 (2.82±0.53 points in the early-start group vs. 4.52±0.56 points in the delayed-start group, P = 0.02), and noninferiority between the two groups with respect to the rate of change in the UPDRS score between weeks 48 and 72 (0.085±0.02 points per week in the early-start group vs. 0.085±0.02 points per week in the delayed-start group, P < 0.001). All three end points were not met with rasagiline at a dose of 2 mg per day, since the change in the UPDRS score between baseline and week 72 was not significantly different in the two groups (3.47±0.50 points in the early-start group and 3.11±0.50 points in the delayed-start group, P = 0.60).

Conclusions.—Early treatment with rasagiline at a dose of 1 mg per day provided benefits that were consistent with a possible disease-modifying effect, but early treatment with rasagiline at a dose of 2 mg per day did not. Because the two doses were associated with different outcomes, the study results must be interpreted with caution. (ClinicalTrials.gov number, NCT00256204.)

▶ The article by Olanow and colleagues presents the results of the Attenuation of Disease Progression with Azilect Given Once-daily (ADAGIO) trial of rasagiline for the treatment of Parkinson disease (PD). The investigators used a delayed-start/delayed wash-in trial design, which generally follows regulatory agency guidelines for a trial designed to show benefits beyond symptom improvement.

In delayed-start trials, patients are randomized to either placebo or study drug (phase A), and then after a period of treatment, those originally assigned to receive placebo are also switched to study drug (phase B).

Differences between the 2 groups at the end of phase A could be because of symptomatic and/or disease-modifying effects. If the difference observed at the end of phase A disappears at the end of phase B, this indicates a purely symptomatic effect. Conversely, if the difference is sustained and the group that received placebo does not catch up with the early-start group, this means that early treatment conferred a benefit that may not be readily explained by a symptomatic effect.

The authors of the ADAGIO trial suggest that rasagiline might have disease-modifying effects. The ADAGIO trial investigated the effects of 1 and 2 mg doses of rasagiline. The lower, 1 mg dose met all primary endpoints. However, the 2 mg dose did not. Hence, the results are mixed and their interpretation challenging.

The ADAGIO authors suggest, given the mixed message of the trial, there are no immediate new implications for clinical practice. However, the implications for clinical research also remain uncertain. Disease modification trials are usually long, require thousands of participants, and therefore can be extremely costly. Trial sponsors, regulators, and the medical community may revisit critical elements of disease modification and further discuss study design approaches.

S. Papapetropoulos, MD, PhD

A Randomized, Placebo-Controlled Trial of Latrepirdine in Huntington Disease

Kieburtz K, The Dimebon in Subjects with Huntington Disease (DIMOND) Investigators of the Huntington Study Group (Univ of Rochester, NY; et al)
Arch Neurol 67:154-160, 2010

Objectives.—To evaluate the safety and tolerability of latrepirdine in Huntington disease (HD) and explore its effects on cognition, behavior, and motor symptoms.

Design.—Double-blind, randomized, placebo-controlled trial.

Setting.—Multicenter outpatient trial.

Participants.—Ninety-one participants with mild to moderate HD enrolled at 17 US and UK centers from July 18, 2007, through July 16, 2008.

Intervention.—Latrepirdine, 20 mg 3 times daily (n = 46), or matching placebo (n = 45) for a 90-day treatment period.

Main Outcome Measures.—The primary outcome variable was tolerability, defined as the ability to complete the study at the assigned drug dosage. Secondary outcome variables included score changes from baseline to day 90 on the Unified Huntington's Disease Rating Scale (UHDRS), the Mini-Mental State Examination (MMSE), and the Alzheimer Disease Assessment Scale-cognitive subscale (ADAS-cog).

Results.—Latrepirdine was well tolerated (87% of the patients given latrepirdine completed the study vs 82% in the placebo group), and adverse event rates were comparable in the 2 groups (70% in the latrepirdine group and 80% in the placebo group). Treatment with latrepirdine resulted in improved mean MMSE scores compared with stable performance in the placebo group (treatment effect, 0.97 points; 95% confidence interval, 0.10-1.85; P = .03). No significant treatment effects were seen on the UHDRS or the ADAS-cog.

Conclusions.—Short-term administration of latrepirdine is well tolerated in patients with HD and may have a beneficial effect on cognition. Further investigation of latrepirdine is warranted in this population with HD.

Trial Registration.—clinicaltrials.gov Identifier: NCT00497159.

▶ Huntington disease (HD) affects movement, behavior, and cognition and may lead to death within 20 years of disease onset. Cognitive decline occurs early in the disease and significantly affects activities of daily living. The pathophysiology of HD is unknown, but the authors postulate that it may involve abnormal mitochondrial depolarization, causing collapse of the mitochondrial membrane and resulting in neuronal death.

Latrepirdine is a synthetic molecule currently in late stage of clinical development for the treatment of Alzheimer disease (AD). Latrepirdine's success in improving cognitive, behavioral, and functional outcomes in mild-to-moderate AD in a single-country phase 2 study[1] was not replicated in a large phase 3 international study.[2]

Latrepirdine's mechanism of action is unknown, but it has been postulated that it stabilizes the mitochondrial membrane and may increase neurite outgrowth in cultured neurons. The goal of this double-blind, randomized, placebo-controlled trial was to assess the safety and tolerability of latrepirdine in HD as well as its effects on cognitive, behavioral, and motor symptoms.

From July 18, 2007 through July 16, 2008, 91 subjects with mild-to-moderate HD were enrolled at 17 US and UK centers and randomly received either latrepirdine 20 mg 3 times daily (n = 46) or placebo (n = 45) for a 90-day treatment period. The primary outcome variable was tolerability, defined as the ability to complete the study at the assigned drug dosage. Secondary outcome variables included score changes from baseline to day 90 on the

Unified Huntington Disease Rating Scale (UHDRS), the Mini-Mental State Examination (MMSE), and the Alzheimer Disease Assessment Scale-cognitive subscale (ADAS-cog).

The main study endpoint of tolerability, which was defined as the ability to complete study treatment at the assigned dosage, occurred in 87% of patients in the latrepirdine group and in 82% of patients in the placebo group. In addition, rates of adverse events were similar in both groups (70% and 80%, respectively). Headache and somnolence were seen more often in those taking latrepirdine than in those taking placebo.

MMSE score improved from baseline to day 90 in the latrepirdine group but remained stable in the placebo group (treatment effect, 0.97 points; 95% confidence interval, 0.10-1.85; $P = .03$). The significant finding on the MMSE is surprising, given that the MMSE is generally considered a relatively insensitive measure of cognitive function and has to be interpreted with caution, given the limitations of the study and lack of significant treatment effects noted on UHDRS or ADAS-cog.

Limitations of this study include relatively small sample size, limited duration of treatment, and the study design, which does not allow for a comfortable detection of a minimal clinically significant effect on any of the efficacy measures. Nonetheless, results from this controlled trial suggest that in the short term, latrepirdine is well tolerated in patients with HD and has shown some interesting but difficult-to-interpret trends on cognition, warranting further study.

S. Papapetropoulos, MD, PhD

References

1. Doody RS, Gavrilova SI, Sano M, et al. Dimebon Investigators. Effect of dimebon on cognition, activities of daily living, behaviour, and global function in patients with mild-to-moderate Alzheimer's disease: a randomised, double-blind, placebo-controlled study. *Lancet.* 2008;372:207-215.
2. Press release: Pfizer and medivation announce results from two phase 3 studies in dimebon (latrepirdine*) Alzheimer's disease clinical development program. http://investors.medivation.com/releasedetail.cfm?ReleaseID=448818. Accessed April 6, 2010.

Children With Tourette Disorder: A Follow-Up Study in Adulthood

Altman G, Staley JD, Wener P (Univ of Manitoba, Winnipeg, Canada; St Boniface General Hosp Child and Adolescent Mental Health Program, Winnipeg, Manitoba, Canada)

J Nerv Ment Dis 197:305-310, 2009

This study intended to examine the impact of TD on adult psychosocial functioning. A 29-item self-report questionnaire was mailed to 180 former and current adult TD patients. Adult TD patients reported relatively good psychosocial adjustment although many continued to be dependent upon their families for living and financial support. For adults with TD, personal acceptance and medication use were the most important factors in coping with the disorder. The severity of vocal tics had a much greater influence on adult functioning than the severity of motor tics. Although TD continued to interfere with patient's lives in adulthood, the impact was relatively modest. Most patients were able to cope utilizing family and medical support. Clinicians need to be aware of the greater influence of vocal tics on adult functioning compared with motor tics.

▶ Tourette syndrome is diagnosed in childhood. What becomes of these patients in adulthood? This article analyzes 58/180 patients with Tourette syndrome, 19 to 55 years of age, who completed a 29-item questionnaire. Forty-one percent were living with their parents; 53% reported improvement of their tics; 40% were taking medication for tics or for symptoms associated with Tourette syndrome; 41% reported some degree of interference with their lives by Tourette syndrome; and 19% reported marked interference. Patients with severe vocal tics had greater difficulty making friends and generally greater interference in their lives than those with moderate or mild vocal tics. Motor tic severity had only a marginal effect on adult functioning. Vocal tic severity also correlated with problems with concentration, anxiety, depression, and emotional lability.

G. N. Breningstall, MD

Clinical Features in Early Parkinson Disease and Survival

Lo RY, Tanner CM, Albers KB, et al (The Parkinson's Inst and Clinical Ctr, Sunnyvale, CA; Kaiser Permanente, Oakland, CA; et al)

Arch Neurol 66:1353-1358, 2009

Objective.—To examine the association between demographic and clinical features in early Parkinson disease (PD) and length of survival in a multiethnic population.

Design.—Clinical features within 2 years of diagnosis were determined for an inception cohort established during 1994-1995. Vital status was determined through December 31, 2005. Predictor variables included age at diagnosis, sex, race/ethnicity, as well as clinical subtype (modified tremor dominant, postural instability gait difficulty), symmetry, cognitive impairment, depression, dysphagia, and hallucinations. Cox proportional hazards regression analysis was used to identify factors associated with shorter survival.

Setting.—Kaiser Permanente Medical Care Program, northern California.

Patients.—Five hundred seventy-three men and women with newly diagnosed PD.

Results.—Three hundred fifty-two participants in the PD cohort (61.4%) had died in the follow-up period. Older age at diagnosis (hazard ratio [HR], 1.1; 95% confidence interval [CI], 1.09-1.12), modified postural instability gait difficulty subtype (HR, 1.8; 95% CI, 1.3-2.7), symmetry of motor signs (HR, 2.0; 95% CI, 1.1-3.7), mild (HR, 1.7; 95% CI, 1.3-2.2) and severe (HR, 2.7; 95% CI, 1.9-3.9) cognitive impairment, dysphagia (HR, 1.4; 95% CI, 1.1-1.9), and hallucinations (HR, 2.1; 95% CI, 1.3-3.2) were associated with increased all-cause mortality, after adjusting for age, sex, and race/ethnicity. None of the other factors altered mortality risk. In an empirical predictive analysis, most previous significant predictors remained associated with shorter survival.

Conclusions.—Both motor and nonmotor features in early PD predict increased mortality risk, particularly postural instability gait difficulty, cognitive impairment, and hallucinations. These predictors may be useful in clinical practice and when designing clinical trials.

▶ Lo et al examine the association between demographic and clinical features in early Parkinson disease (PD) and the length of survival. Several studies have found that increased mortality is associated with older age, male gender, dementia, and the postural instability/gait difficulty disease subtype.

The study database was drawn from the Parkinsonism Epidemiology at Kaiser Study, which identified patients with newly diagnosed PD from the Kaiser Permanente Medical Care Program (KPMCP) of northern California (3 million persons) during a 2-year period between 1994 and 1995. Five hundred seventy-three men and women with newly diagnosed PD were identified.

Three hundred fifty-two participants in the PD cohort (61.4%) had died in the follow-up period. Older age at diagnosis, postural instability gait difficulty subtype, symmetry of motor signs (hazard ratio [HR], 2.0; 95% confidence interval [CI], 1.1-3.7), mild and severe cognitive impairment, dysphagia, and hallucinations were associated with increased all-cause mortality, after adjusting for age, sex, and race/ethnicity.

The elegantly conducted study utilizes a unique population identified through a health maintenance organization that may be considered more typical of the general population in northern California compared with populations participating in clinical trials. Another important feature of the study is the adequate sample size and the systematic collection of relevant longitudinal clinical data. The relative uniformity of care is likely to minimize variation in treatment. Importantly, no medication or surgical modality has yet been shown to prolong survival in PD.

With effective clinical predictors, we can improve understanding of the disease process, refine risk stratification in designing clinical trials, and guide decision making in clinical practice.

S. Papapetropoulos, MD, PhD

Effects of a Dopamine Agonist on the Pharmacodynamics of Levodopa in Parkinson Disease

Brodsky MA, Park BS, Nutt JG (Oregon Health & Science Univ, Portland)
Arch Neurol 67:27-32, 2010

Background.—Treatment of Parkinson disease commonly includes levodopa and dopamine agonists; however, the interaction of these 2 drugs is poorly understood.

Objective.—To examine the effects of a dopamine agonist on the motor response to levodopa.

Design.—Double-blind, randomized, placebo-controlled, crossover clinical trial.

Setting.—Ambulatory academic referral center.

Patients.—Thirteen patients with idiopathic Parkinson disease taking levodopa and experiencing motor fluctuations and dyskinesia.

Interventions.—Eligible individuals were randomly assigned to receive pramipexole dihydrochloride or placebo for 4 weeks followed by a 2-hour intravenous levodopa infusion on consecutive days at 2 rates and with blinded assessments. They were then crossed over to the alternate oral therapy for 4 weeks followed by levodopa infusion and reassessment.

Main Outcome Measures.—Change in finger-tapping speed, measured using the area under the curve (AUC) for finger taps per minute across time; peak fingertapping speed; duration of response; time to "ON" (defined as a 10% increase in finger-tapping speed above baseline); walking speed; and dyskinesia AUC.

Results.—Pramipexole with levodopa infusion increased finger-tapping speed beyond the change in baseline by a mean (SE) of 170 (47.2) per minute × minutes ($P = .006$) and more than doubled the AUC for finger-tapping speed. Pramipexole increased peak finger-tapping speed by a mean (SE) of 18 (8.5) taps per minute ($P = .02$) and improved mean (SE) walking speed (15.9 [0.70] vs 18.9 [0.70] seconds, $P = .004$). Pramipexole prolonged duration of response after levodopa infusion and shortened time to ON. Pramipexole increased mean (SE) baseline dyskinesia scores (26.0 [5.85] vs 12.1 [5.85] points, $P = .05$) and peak dyskinesia scores with levodopa infusion.

Conclusions.—Pramipexole augmented the motor response to levodopa beyond a simple additive effect and increased the severity of levodopa-induced dyskinesia. When considering a combination of these therapies, an appropriate balance should be maintained regarding gain of motor function vs worsening of dyskinesia.

Trial Registration.—clinicaltrials.gov Identifier: NCT00666653.

► Pharmacological treatment of Parkinson disease (PD) commonly includes L-dopa in combination with a dopamine agonist (DA). DA are used either as monotherapy in early disease stages to delay the onset of motor complications (motor fluctuations and dyskinesias) or as adjunct therapy that allows a reduction of L-dopa dose and ultimately a reduction of motor fluctuations.

The article by Brodsky and colleagues presents a small double-blind, randomized, placebo-controlled, crossover study of patients taking a stable dose of pramipexole for 4 weeks or placebo for 4 weeks. Responses to 2-hour L-dopa infusions at 0.5 mg/kg/h (threshold) and 1.0 mg/kg/h (suprathreshold) were examined at the end of each 4-week treatment period.

The primary outcome was change in finger-tapping speed, as measured by the area under the curve (AUC) for finger taps per minute across time. Secondary outcomes included the AUC for dyskinesia and effects of L-dopa infusion on the motor score of the unified Parkinson disease rating scale (mUPDRS) (Part III).

Pramipexole augmented the motor response to L-dopa beyond a simple additive effect but increased the severity of L-dopa-induced dyskinesia. When considering a combination of these therapies, an appropriate balance should be maintained regarding gain of motor function versus worsening of dyskinesia.

S. Papapetropoulos, MD, PhD

Multicenter Analysis of Glucocerebrosidase Mutations in Parkinson's Disease

Sidransky E, Nalls MA, Aasly JO, et al (Natl Insts of Health, Bethesda, MD; St Olav's Hosp, Trondheim, Norway; et al)

N Engl J Med 361:1651-1661, 2009

Background.—Recent studies indicate an increased frequency of mutations in the gene encoding glucocerebrosidase (*GBA*), a deficiency of which causes Gaucher's disease, among patients with Parkinson's disease. We aimed to ascertain the frequency of *GBA* mutations in an ethnically diverse group of patients with Parkinson's disease.

Methods.—Sixteen centers participated in our international, collaborative study: five from the Americas, six from Europe, two from Israel, and three from Asia. Each center genotyped a standard DNA panel to permit comparison of the genotyping results across centers. Genotypes and phenotypic data from a total of 5691 patients with Parkinson's disease (780 Ashkenazi Jews) and 4898 controls (387 Ashkenazi Jews) were analyzed, with multivariate logistic-regression models and the Mantel-Haenszel procedure used to estimate odds ratios across centers.

Results.—All 16 centers could detect two *GBA* mutations, L444P and N370S. Among Ashkenazi Jewish subjects, either mutation was found in 15% of patients and 3% of controls, and among non-Ashkenazi Jewish subjects, either mutation was found in 3% of patients and less than 1% of controls. *GBA* was fully sequenced for 1883 non-Ashkenazi Jewish patients, and mutations were identified in 7%, showing that limited mutation screening can miss half the mutant alleles. The odds ratio for any *GBA* mutation in patients versus controls was 5.43 across centers. As compared with patients who did not carry a *GBA* mutation, those with a *GBA* mutation presented earlier with the disease, were more likely to have affected relatives, and were more likely to have atypical clinical manifestations.

Conclusions.—Data collected from 16 centers demonstrate that there is a strong association between *GBA* mutations and Parkinson's disease.

▶ This study explored the role of glucocerebrosidase (GBA) mutations in Parkinson disease (PD) development by pooling clinical and genotypic data for 5691 PD patients and 4898 unaffected individuals from 16 international centers. Genotyping was performed for either 2 mutations (N370S and L444P) or for 3 to 8 GBA mutations. One of the N370S and L444P mutations was found in 15% and 3% of PD patients of Ashkenazi and non-Ashkenazi Jewish origin, respectively. Whole gene sequencing performed in a subgroup of these patients revealed a combined odds ratio of carrying any GBA mutation of 5.43. Genotype-phenotype correlations confirm previously published studies showing that GBA mutations, besides being panethnic, seem to effectively influence specific clinical PD manifestations, including earlier age at disease onset, increased incidence of family history, and cognitive changes, but decreased occurrence of resting tremor and bradykinesia.[1-5] Important methodological pitfalls that might have influenced the accuracy of estimations include variable case-ascertainment protocols among centers, incomplete phenotypic profiles, and missed genotypes due to limited whole GBA gene sequencing data. In spite of few obstacles in standardizing data collection, the large cohort sizes and ethnic diversity lend robustness to the presented findings and highlights the importance of adequate sample power for the detection of rare variants (ie, less than 5% frequency in the general population) of small effect sizes. Sidransky and colleagues clearly demonstrate a significant association between GBA mutations and PD and provide a wealth of evidence that unequivocally substantiate the role of these sequence alterations as the most common genetic risk factor to date for the development of this complex disorder. The study, however, highlights the need for further studies using large number of patients and controls to elucidate the effect(s) of GBA mutations on PD clinical manifestations and the role of the mutated enzyme in the molecular mechanisms of PD pathogenesis.

S. Papapetropoulos, MD, PhD

References

1. Lwin A, Orvisky E, Goker-Alpan O, LaMarca ME, Sidransky E. Glucocerebrosidase mutations in subjects with parkinsonism. *Mol Genet Metab.* 2004;81:70-73.
2. Ziegler SG, Eblan MJ, Gutti U, et al. Glucocerebrosidase mutations in Chinese subjects from Taiwan with sporadic Parkinson disease. *Mol Genet Metabol.* 2007;91:195-200.
3. Gan-Or Z, Giladi N, Rozovski U, et al. Genotype-phenotype correlations between GBA mutations and Parkinson disease risk and onset. *Neurology.* 2008;70: 2277-2283.
4. Nichols WC, Pankratz N, Marek DK, et al. Mutations in GBA are associated with familial Parkinson disease susceptibility and age at onset. *Neurology.* 2009;72: 310-316.
5. Neumann J, Bras J, Deas E, et al. Glucocerebrosidase mutations in clinical and pathologically proven Parkinson's disease. *Brain.* 2009;132:1783-1794.

Nonmotor symptoms in de novo Parkinson disease before and after dopaminergic treatment

Kim H-J, Park S-Y, Cho Y-J, et al (Seoul Natl Univ Hosp, Republic of Korea; Dong-eui Med Ctr, Busan, Republic of Korea; Inje Univ Ilsan Paik Hosp, Goyang-si, Gyeonggi-do, Republic of Korea)

J Neurol Sci 287:200-204, 2009

Background.—Nonmotor symptoms (NMSs) are common in patients with Parkinson disease (PD), but little is known about the burden of the full range of NMSs in de novo PD patients.

Objectives.—NMSs in untreated de novo PD patients were evaluated both quantitatively and qualitatively using the Non-Motor Symptoms Assessment Scale (NMSS); the findings were compared to those of control subjects. The effects of dopaminergic treatment on NMSs were also determined.

Methods.—NMSs were evaluated in 23 patients with untreated de novo PD and 23 healthy controls. The motor section of the Unified Parkinson Disease Rating Scale (mUPDRS) and the Hoehn and Yahr (HY) stage were also checked in the PD patients. The number of NMSs and the NMSS scores of the PD patients were compared with those of the controls. Three months after the start of dopaminergic medication, 16 PD patients were reevaluated with respect to the NMSS and mUPDRS, and the HY stage.

Results.—The number of NMSs and the NMSS scores were significantly higher in the PD patients than in the controls. The three most prevalent NMSs among the PD patients were 'nocturia,' 'forget things or events,' and 'restless legs.' In the PD group, the number of NMSs was correlated with the HY stage but not with age, disease duration, or mUPDRS score. Follow-up of 16 patients at 3 months after commencing PD medication revealed no changes in either the number of NMSs or the NMSS score, despite improvement in motor symptoms.

Conclusions.—Untreated de novo PD patients have more nonmotor problems than controls, and these NMSs are not ameliorated by dopaminergic medication.

▶ Nonmotor symptoms (NMSs) are common in patients with Parkinson disease (PD) and can be more disabling than the motor symptoms like tremor, bradykinesia, and rigidity. NMSs in PD encompass a wide clinical spectrum, including neuropsychiatric symptoms, sleep disturbances, autonomic impairments, and sensory dysfunctions. Some NMSs increase with disease duration; others can present in the premotor stage of PD.

In their article, Kim et al evaluated the types and severity of NMSs in 23 consecutive patients with untreated, newly diagnosed de novo PD and 23 healthy controls. Sixteen out of 23 patients were re-evaluated 3 months after the initiation of dopaminergic medication. NMSs were evaluated using the Non-Motor Symptom Assessment Scale (NMSS). The NMSS has been validated in an international cohort that included Japanese PD patients. The

NMSS includes 30 items in 9 domains, and the score for each item is based on a product of severity (0-3) and frequency (1-4); the maximum score for each item is 12, and the maximum score for the total NMSS is 360.

The authors found that the number of NMSs and the NMSS scores were significantly higher in the PD patients than in the controls. The 3 most prevalent NMSs among the PD patients were nocturia, forgetting things or events, and restless legs. In the PD group, the number of NMSs was only weakly correlated with the HY stage ($r = 0.426$, $P = .043$) but not with age, disease duration, or mUPDRS score. Follow-up of 16 patients at 3 months after commencing PD medication revealed no changes in either the number of NMSs or the NMSS score, despite improvement in motor symptoms.

The major limitation of this study is its small sample size, which limits the generalizability of its findings. Another important limitation is the duration of nondopaminergic treatment, which was limited to 3 months and may not fully support the conclusion that medicated patients revealed no changes in the number or severity of NMSs. There is also some uncertainty around the validation of the NMMS in Korean populations. Confirmation of these preliminary results is warranted.

S. Papapetropoulos, MD, PhD

The Clinically Important Difference on the Unified Parkinson's Disease Rating Scale

Shulman LM, Gruber-Baldini AL, Anderson KE, et al (Univ of Maryland School of Medicine, Baltimore)

Arch Neurol 67:64-70, 2010

Objective.—To determine the estimates of minimal, moderate, and large clinically important differences (CIDs) for the Unified Parkinson's Disease Rating Scale (UPDRS).

Design.—Cross-sectional analysis of the CIDs for UPDRS total and motor scores was performed on patients with Parkinson disease (PD) using distribution- and anchor-based approaches based on the following 3 external standards: disability (10% on the Schwab and England Activities of Daily Living Scale), disease stage (1 stage on the Hoehn and Yahr Scale), and quality of life (1 SD on the 12-Item Short Form Health Survey).

Setting.—University of Maryland Parkinson Disease and Movement Disorders Center.

Patients.—Six hundred fifty-three patients with PD.

Results.—A minimal CID was 2.3 to 2.7 points on the UPDRS motor score and 4.1 to 4.5 on the UPDRS total score. A moderate CID was 4.5 to 6.7 points on the UPDRS motor score and 8.5 to 10.3 on the UPDRS total score. A large CID was 10.7 to 10.8 points on the UPDRS motor score and 16.4 to 17.8 on the UPDRS total score.

Conclusions.—Concordance among multiple approaches of analysis based on subjective and objective data show that reasonable estimates for the CID on the UPDRS motor score are 2.5 points for minimal, 5.2

for moderate, and 10.8 for large CIDs. Estimates for the UPDRS total score are 4.3 points for minimal, 9.1 for moderate, and 17.1 for large CIDs. These estimates will assist in determining clinically meaningful changes in PD progression and response to therapeutic interventions.

▶ A clinically important difference (CID) is the amount of change on a clinical research measure that patients can recognize a value. Shulman et al attempt to determine the minimal, moderate, and large CIDs for the Unified Parkinson Disease Rating Scale (UPDRS). The UPDRS is widely used as a clinical endpoint in a variety of clinical research studies, including randomized clinical trials, as a part of the experimental drug development. The definition of CID is supported by regulatory agencies, such as the FDA, for labeling claims of medicinal products.

This study used 2 different key methods of CID determination—the distribution- and anchor-based approaches. Cross-sectional analysis of the CIDs for UPDRS total and motor scores was performed on a sample of 653 subjects with Parkinson disease (PD) based on 3 external standards: disability (10% on the Schwab and England Activities of Daily Living Scale), disease stage (1 stage on the Hoehn and Yahr Scale), and quality of life (1 SD on the 12-Item Short Form Health Survey).

The article very elegantly describes the mean motor and total UPDRS scores by Hoehn and Yahr stages and by 10% change on the Schwab and England Scale. Using multiple approaches, the CID scores were: (a) minimal CID was 2.3 to 2.7 points on the UPDRS motor score and 4.1 to 4.5 on the UPDRS total score; (b) moderate CID was 4.5 to 6.7 points on the UPDRS motor score and 8.5 to 10.3 on the UPDRS total score; and (c) large CID was 10.7 to 10.8 points on the UPDRS motor score and 16.4 to 17.8 on the UPDRS total score.

Limitations of this study include its cross-sectional and single-center nature hinder generalization. The scientific and medical communities anticipate similar definitions for the new version of the UPDRS, the MDS-UPDRS, before fully implementing the new and clinimetrically improved scale in clinical research. Establishing CID values for UPDRS is critical; CID values may not only influence patient management and clinical trials but also influence decision making by government and industry. Further validation of the CID values in longitudinal studies is warranted for both new and old versions of the UPDRS.

S. Papapetropoulos, MD, PhD

8 Neoplastic Disease

A "Vascular Normalization Index" as Potential Mechanistic Biomarker to Predict Survival after a Single Dose of Cediranib in Recurrent Glioblastoma Patients

Sorensen AG, Batchelor TT, Zhang W-T, et al (Massachusetts General Hosp, Boston, MA; et al)

Cancer Res 69:5296-5300, 2009

Early imaging or blood biomarkers of tumor response are desperately needed to customize antiangiogenic therapy for cancer patients. Anti–vascular endothelial growth factor (VEGF) therapy can "normalize" brain tumor vasculature by decreasing vessel diameter and permeability, and thinning the abnormally thick basement membrane. We hypothesized that the extent of vascular normalization will be predictive of outcome of anti-VEGF therapy in glioblastoma. We used advanced magnetic resonance imaging methods to monitor vascular parameters and treatment response in 31 recurrent glioblastoma patients enrolled in a phase II trial of cediranib, an oral pan-VEGF receptor tyrosine kinase inhibitor. We evaluated the correlation between clinical outcome and magnetic resonance imaging–measured changes in vascular permeability/flow (i.e., K^{trans}) and in microvessel volume, and the change of circulating collagen IV levels, all after a single dose of cediranib. Here, we show that evaluation of biomarkers as early as after one day of anti-VEGF therapy with cediranib is predictive of response in patients with recurrent glioblastoma. Changes in K^{trans}, microvessel volume, and circulating collagen IV correlated with duration of overall survival and/or progression-free survival ($P < 0.05$). When we combined these three parameters into a "vascular normalization index," we found that it closely associated with overall survival ($\rho = 0.54$; $P = 0.004$) and progression-free survival ($\rho = 0.6$; $P = 0.001$). The vascular normalization index described here should be validated in randomized clinical trials.

▶ One of the challenges in neuro-oncology clinical trials is following therapy administration, we typically need to wait 1 to 2 months to determine whether the tumor has shrunk or not in response to the study drug. An area of intense research has been to identify laboratory markers that could be assayed at a much earlier time point that would predict patient outcomes.

In a previous report,[1] the authors had evaluated cediranib, a small molecule inhibitor of the receptor for vascular endothelial growth factor and showed that a change in the vascular permeability/flow (K^{trans}, as assessed by MRI) 1 day after drug dosing correlated with tumor response. In this report, the authors build upon that finding by adding 2 other prognostic markers—microvessel volume (as assessed by dynamic contrast MRI) and circulating collagen IV levels.

Together, these 3 variables (K^{trans} or vascular permeability, microvessel volume, and serum levels of collagen type IV) constitute the vascular normalization index.

J. Uhm, MD

Reference

1. Batchelor TT, Sorensen AG, di Tomaso E, et al. AZD2171, a pan-VEGF receptor tyrosine kinase inhibitor, normalizes tumor vasculature and alleviates edema in glioblastoma patients. *Cancer Cell.* 2007;11:83-95.

Bevacizumab Safety in Patients with Central Nervous System Metastases

Besse B, Lasserre SF, Compton P, et al (Institut Gustave Roussy, Villejuif, France; F. Hoffmann-La Roche, Basel, Switzerland; Genentech, Inc, San Francisco, CA)

Clin Cancer Res 16:269-278, 2010

Purpose.—Patients with central nervous system (CNS) metastases were excluded from bevacizumab trials following a case of fatal cerebral hemorrhage in a patient with hepatocellular carcinoma in 1997. Safety information for bevacizumab-treated patients with CNS metastases was reviewed to determine whether general exclusion of these patients from bevacizumab treatment is still justified.

Experimental Design.—A retrospective exploratory analysis was conducted using datasets from 13 randomized controlled phase II/III trials (dataset A), two open-label single-arm safety trials (dataset B), and two prospective studies including patients with treated CNS metastases (dataset C). In datasets A and B, known CNS metastasis was an exclusion criterion; patients with CNS metastasis had unrecognized CNS metastases at study entry or developed them during the trial. All reported cerebral hemorrhage grades in patients with CNS metastases were quantified.

Results.—In dataset A, occult brain metastases were identified in 187 of 8,443 patients (91 in bevacizumab arms and 96 in non-bevacizumab arms). Three bevacizumab-treated patients (3.3%) developed grade 4 cerebral hemorrhage, whereas one control-arm patient (1.0%) developed grade 5 cerebral hemorrhage. In dataset B, 321 of 4,382 patients had initially occult CNS metastases, in whom two grade 1 and one grade 3 cerebral hemorrhage (0.9%) were reported. In 131 patients with treated CNS metastases in dataset C, one bevacizumab-treated patient (0.8%) developed grade 2 cerebral hemorrhage.

Conclusions.—In this selected population, patients with CNS metastases are at similar risk of developing cerebral hemorrhage, independent of bevacizumab therapy. Consequently, such patients with CNS metastases from advanced/metastatic breast cancer, non–small cell lung carcinoma, and renal and colorectal cancer should not be generally excluded from bevacizumab therapy or clinical trials.

► While angiogenesis inhibitors have shown much promise in the treatment of a variety of cancer types, the remodeling of vasculature affected by such therapies has led to concerns of hemorrhagic transformation of the tumor mass. Nowhere has this concern been more evident than in the context of brain metastases, in which a bleeding complication can have devastating consequences.

In this article, the authors reviewed a dataset of almost 13 000 patients, in which brain metastases were identified in approximately 500 patients. Review of the data showed that the incidence of intracranial hemorrhage was similar between the patients who received bevacizumab compared with those who did not receive bevacizumab.

Clinicians still need to exercise caution in that angiogenesis inhibitor therapy should be avoided in patients whose scans show bleeding in a metastatic lesion. However, this report indicates that patients with brain metastases should not be excluded from clinical trials (or off-protocol therapies) that use bevacizumab.

J. Uhm, MD

Cancer-associated IDH1 mutations produce 2-hydroxyglutarate

Dang L, White DW, Gross S, et al (Agios Pharmaceuticals, Cambridge, MA)
Nature 462:739-744, 2009

Mutations in the enzyme cytosolic isocitrate dehydrogenase 1 (IDH1) are a common feature of a major subset of primary human brain cancers. These mutations occur at a single amino acid residue of the IDH1 active site, resulting in loss of the enzyme's ability to catalyse conversion of isocitrate to α-ketoglutarate. However, only a single copy of the gene is mutated in tumours, raising the possibility that the mutations do not result in a simple loss of function. Here we show that cancer-associated IDH1 mutations result in a new ability of the enzyme to catalyse the NADPH-dependent reduction of a-ketoglutarate to *R*(−)-2-hydroxyglutarate (2HG). Structural studies demonstrate that when arginine 132 is mutated to histidine, residues in the active site are shifted to produce structural changes consistent with reduced oxidative decarboxylation of isocitrate and acquisition of the ability to convert α-ketoglutarate to 2HG. Excess accumulation of 2HG has been shown to lead to an elevated risk of malignant brain tumours in patients with inborn errors of 2HG metabolism. Similarly, in human malignant gliomas harbouring IDH1 mutations, we find markedly elevated levels of 2HG. These data demonstrate that the IDH1 mutations result in production of the onco-metabolite 2HG, and

indicate that the excess 2HG which accumulates *in vivo* contributes to the formation and malignant progression of gliomas.

▶ A very important recent advance in molecular neuro-oncology is the identification of isocitrate dehydrogenase (*IDH1*) gene mutations in gliomas.[1] In summary, *IDH1* mutations are (1) associated with a better prognosis; and (2) occur as an early genetic event in gliomagenesis, as the mutations are seen in low-grade gliomas.

While the discovery of *IDH1* mutations in gliomas has led to tremendous focus on this genetic alteration as a prognostic variable, an important question is the mechanism by which this mutation affects glioma behavior. In this article by Dang et al, the authors show that *IDH1* mutation leads to increased levels of 2-hydroxyglutarate (2HG). Is the overproduction of 2HG important in gliomagenesis? Based on the following points, several data from others and from this group indicate that this may be so:

(1) 2HG accumulation in inborn errors of metabolism is associated with an increased risk of brain tumors.
(2) 2HG levels are elevated in human glioma samples, as shown in this article.
(3) The mutation of arginine at codon 132 of *IDH1* is found in gliomas, but mutations that affect other residues of *IDH1* are not found in brain tumors. Interestingly, codon 132 mutation leads to the increased ability to catalyze the conversion of α-ketoglutarate to 2HG (mutations at other codons do not confer this activity).

So if *IDH1* leads to increased 2HG, then how does 2HG impact upon gliomagenesis? This clearly constitutes an area of intense research. In the meantime, the important clinical implications of this article are as follows:

(1) Measurement of 2HG in glioma patients. This may identify patients with *IDH1* mutant gliomas, which may serve as a prognostic variable.
(2) Would the inhibition of 2HG production negate the ability of a low-grade glioma to a high-grade counterpart and thereby change the course of the disease?

The last couple of years have seen a tremendous amount of data regarding *IDH1*—the current article represents an important milestone in leading the field toward the mechanism by which this mutation contributes to gliomagenesis.

J. Uhm, MD

Reference

1. Parsons DW, Jones S, Zhang X, et al. An integrated genomic analysis of human glioblastoma multiforme. *Science*. 2008;321:1807-1812.

Intrinsic Gene Expression Profiles of Gliomas Are a Better Predictor of Survival than Histology

Gravendeel LAM, Kouwenhoven MCM, Gevaert O, et al (Erasmus Univ Med Ctr, Rotterdam, The Netherlands; Katholieke Universiteit Leuven, Belgium; et al)

Cancer Res 69:9065-9072, 2009

Gliomas are the most common primary brain tumors with heterogeneous morphology and variable prognosis. Treatment decisions in patients rely mainly on histologic classification and clinical parameters. However, differences between histologic subclasses and grades are subtle, and classifying gliomas is subject to a large interobserver variability. To improve current classification standards, we have performed gene expression profiling on a large cohort of glioma samples of all histologic subtypes and grades. We identified seven distinct molecular subgroups that correlate with survival. These include two favorable prognostic subgroups (median survival, >4.7 years), two with intermediate prognosis (median survival, 1–4 years), two with poor prognosis (median survival, <1 year), and one control group. The intrinsic molecular subtypes of glioma are different from histologic subgroups and correlate better to patient survival. The prognostic value of molecular subgroups was validated on five independent sample cohorts (The Cancer Genome Atlas, Repository for Molecular Brain Neoplasia Data, GSE12907, GSE4271, and Li and colleagues). The power of intrinsic subtyping is shown by its ability to identify a subset of prognostically favorable tumors within an external data set that contains only histologically confirmed glioblastomas (GBM). Specific genetic changes (epidermal growth factor receptor amplification, IDH1 mutation, and 1p/19q loss of heterozygosity) segregate in distinct molecular subgroups. We identified a subgroup with molecular features associated with secondary GBM, suggesting that different genetic changes drive gene expression profiles. Finally, we assessed response to treatment in molecular subgroups. Our data provide compelling evidence that expression profiling is a more accurate and objective method to classify gliomas than histologic classification. Molecular classification therefore may aid diagnosis and can guide clinical decision making.

► Tumor cell morphology, mitotic index, cellular density, and vascularity comprised the key factors used in determining the prognosis of patients with glioma. While these factors maintain their relative importance as prognostic variables, the last decade or 2 have witnessed the emergence of data implicating molecular genetic factors that influence prognosis. These include 1p/19q deletion, methylguanylmethyltransferase (MGMT) promoter methylation, and isocitrate dehydrogenase (*IDH1*) gene mutation, all of which are associated with improved survival.

In this article, the authors evaluated gliomas of all histologic/grade types and performed an extensive molecular analysis based on 5000 most variable genes. The study identified 7 distinct molecular subgroups associated with different survival. These molecular subgroups appear to be independent of histology. Moreover, the data were validated in 5 other independent sample cohorts, underscoring the validity of this work.

As this vein of research continues to evolve and gain momentum, the field of neuro-oncology will likely witness a gradual transition toward molecular classification of patients with glioma.

J. Uhm, MD

NOA-04 Randomized Phase III Trial of Sequential Radiochemotherapy of Anaplastic Glioma With Procarbazine, Lomustine, and Vincristine or Temozolomide

Wick W, Hartmann C, Engel C, et al (Univ of Tübingen, Germany; Heinrich-Heine-Univ, Düsseldorf, Germany; Univ of Heidelberg, Germany; et al)

J Clin Oncol 27:5874-5880, 2009

Purpose.—The standard of care for anaplastic gliomas is surgery followed by radiotherapy. The NOA-04 phase III trial compared efficacy and safety of radiotherapy followed by chemotherapy at progression with the reverse sequence in patients with newly diagnosed anaplastic gliomas.

Patients and Methods.—Patients (N = 318) were randomly assigned 2:1:1 (A:B1:B2) to receive conventional radiotherapy (arm A); procarbazine, lomustine (CCNU), and vincristine (PCV; arm B1); or temozolomide (arm B2) at diagnosis. At occurrence of unacceptable toxicity or disease progression, patients in arm A were treated with PCV or temozolomide (1:1 random assignment), whereas patients in arms B1 or B2 received radiotherapy. The primary end point was time to treatment failure (TTF), defined as progression after radiotherapy and one chemotherapy in either sequence.

Results.—Patient characteristics in the intention-to-treat population (n = 274) were balanced between arms. All histologic diagnoses were centrally confirmed. Median TTF (hazard ratio [HR] = 1.2; 95% CI, 0.8 to 1.8), progression-free survival (PFS; HR = 1.0; 95% CI, 0.7 to 1.3, and overall survival (HR = 1.2; 95% CI, 0.8 to 1.9) were similar for arms A and B1/B2. Extent of resection was an important prognosticator. Anaplastic oligodendrogliomas and oligoastrocytomas share the same, better prognosis than anaplastic astrocytomas. Hypermethylation of the O^6-methylguanine DNA-methyltransferase (*MGMT*) promoter (HR = 0.59; 95% CI, 0.36 to 1.0), mutations of the isocitrate dehydrogenase (*IDH1*) gene (HR = 0.48; 95% CI, 0.29 to 0.77), and oligodendroglial histology (HR = 0.33; 95% CI, 0.2 to 0.55) reduced the risk of progression. Hypermethylation of the *MGMT* promoter was associated with prolonged PFS in the chemotherapy and radiotherapy arm.

Conclusion.—Initial radiotherapy or chemotherapy achieved comparable results in patients with anaplastic gliomas. *IDH1* mutations are a novel positive prognostic factor in anaplastic gliomas, with a favorable

impact stronger than that of 1p/19q codeletion or *MGMT* promoter methylation.

▶ What is the optimal up-front treatment for glioma—chemotherapy or radiotherapy? This question has been a core focus of debate in neuro-oncology. On one hand, a tremendous literature base exists for the role of radiotherapy as the mainstay of therapy, enhancing both progression-free and overall survival. However, an apprehension shared by many clinicians in the field with respect to radiotherapy is the potential for decline in cognitive abilities as a consequence of radiation. This apprehension has led some in the field to consider chemotherapy up front.

The NOA-04 randomized study addresses the question of chemotherapy versus radiotherapy as the frontline therapy in patients with grade 3 glioma. One group starts with chemotherapy (procarbazine/CCNU/vincristine or temozolomide) and at the time of progression switches to radiotherapy, while the other group starts with radiotherapy and at the time of progression switches to chemotherapy.

The key finding in this study was that whether patients were treated up front with chemotherapy or radiotherapy overall survival was similar between the 2 groups. Other key findings include the observation that isocitrate dehydrogenase (*IDH1*) mutations conferred the most favorable impact on survival, stronger than that of 1p/19q deletion or O6-methylguanine DNA-methyltransferase (MGMT) promoter methylation.

So how is this study to be interpreted?

(1) Radiotherapy is inevitable, so it should be used up front. This is the position put forth by the authors and is most definitely tenable, as every patient who was started on chemotherapy up front ultimately progressed and required radiotherapy.

(2) Chemotherapy as up-front treatment is very reasonable, as it did not reduce the overall survival. Clinicians who were apprehensive about radiotherapy as the up-front therapy before this study's results were available may likely still continue to use chemotherapy up front based on the results of this study. One of the rationales for using chemotherapy up front may be that should the tumor undergo shrinkage, then perhaps the reduction in the target for radiation may translate into a reduction in the risk of cognitive and other adverse effects related to radiation.

Hence, the study, while definitive in its findings, will likely not change the practices of clinicians in the field. However, it does provide affirmation by way of a well-conducted, high-quality, randomized study to give each clinician—regardless of his/her bias—the knowledge that their own approach to the patient (up-front chemotherapy or radiotherapy) will not compromise the patient's overall survival.

J. Uhm, MD

The transcriptional network for mesenchymal transformation of brain tumours

Carro MS, Lim WK, Alvarez MJ, et al (Columbia Univ Med Ctr, NY; et al)

Nature 463:318-325, 2010

The inference of transcriptional networks that regulate transitions into physiological or pathological cellular states remains a central challenge in systems biology. A mesenchymal phenotype is the hallmark of tumour aggressiveness in human malignant glioma, but the regulatory programs responsible for implementing the associated molecular signature are largely unknown. Here we show that reverse-engineering and an unbiased interrogation of a glioma-specific regulatory network reveal the transcriptional module that activates expression of mesenchymal genes in malignant glioma. Two transcription factors (C/EBPβ and STAT3) emerge as synergistic initiators and master regulators of mesenchymal transformation. Ectopic co-expression of C/EBPβ and STAT3 reprograms neural stem cells along the aberrant mesenchymal lineage, whereas elimination of the two factors in glioma cells leads to collapse of the mesenchymal signature and reduces tumour aggressiveness. In human glioma, expression of C/EBPβ and STAT3 correlates with mesenchymal differentiation and predicts poor clinical outcome. These results show that the activation of a small regulatory module is necessary and sufficient to initiate and maintain an aberrant phenotypic state in cancer cells.

▶ While there is no doubt that age, performance status, and diagnosis (eg, tumor cell type and tumor grade) constitute key prognostic factors in patients with glioma, the last decade has seen a tremendous surge in data that point toward molecular prognostic variables. Of these, the classification of high-grade gliomas into the proneural and mesenchymal categories based upon gene expression profiles[1] represented a landmark advance in the field, where transcriptomes predicted the patient outcomes.

In that original collaborative report by Phillips et al, another important finding was that the transformation of a proneural transcriptome (better prognosis) tumor to a mesenchymal type (worse prognosis, treatment resistance) occurred at a relatively high frequency. In the current article, the authors pursued the hypothesis that the expression of specific genes may turn on this proneural-to-mesenchymal transition. In summary, the authors show that C/EBPβ and STAT3 expression correlates with this mesenchymal transition. In addition to the importance of having identified these regulators of the mesenchymal transition, another key finding is the observation that only a small number of genes—2 in this instance—is sufficient to drive this process.

J. Uhm, MD

Reference

1. Phillips HS, Kharbanda S, Chen R, et al. Molecular subclasses of high-grade glioma predict prognosis, delineate a pattern of disease progression, and resemble stages in neurogenesis. *Cancer Cell.* 2006;9:157-173.

Tumor invasion after treatment of glioblastoma with bevacizumab: radiographic and pathologic correlation in humans and mice

de Groot JF, Fuller G, Kumar AJ, et al (The Univ of Texas M. D. Anderson Cancer Ctr, Houston)

Neuro Oncol 12:233-242, 2010

Patients with recurrent malignant glioma treated with bevacizumab, a monoclonal antibody to vascular endothelial growth factor (VEGF), alone or in combination with irinotecan have had impressive reductions in MRI contrast enhancement and vasogenic edema. Responses to this regimen, as defined by a decrease in contrast enhancement, have led to significant improvements in progression-free survival rates but not in overall survival duration. Some patients for whom this treatment regimen fails have an uncharacteristic pattern of tumor progression, which can be observed radiographically as an increase in hyperintensity on T2-weighted or fluid-attenuated inverse recovery (FLAIR) MRI. To date, there have been no reports of paired correlations between radiographic results and histopathologic findings describing the features of this aggressive tumor phenotype. In this study, we correlate such findings for 3 illustrative cases of gliomas that demonstrated an apparent phenotypic shift to a predominantly infiltrative pattern of tumor progression after treatment with bevacizumab. Pathologic examination of abnormal FLAIR areas on MRI revealed infiltrative tumor with areas of thin-walled blood vessels, suggesting vascular "normalization," which was uncharacteristically adjacent to regions of necrosis. High levels of insulin-like growth factor binding protein-2 and matrix metalloprotease-2 expression were seen within the infiltrating tumor. In an attempt to better understand this infiltrative phenotype associated with anti-VEGF therapy, we forced a highly angiogenic, noninvasive orthotopic U87 xenograft tumor to become infiltrative by treating the mice with bevacizumab. This model mimicked many of the histopathologic findings from the human cases and will augment the discovery of alternative or additive therapies to prevent this type of tumor recurrence in clinical practice.

▶ In another article that I reviewed,[1] I discussed how the advent of angiogenesis inhibitors has led to the identification of a novel method of treatment resistance. Specifically, gliomas that become resistant to the angiogenesis inhibitor, bevacizumab, may grow more as an infiltrative/invasive mass tracking along white matter tracts rather than as an expansion of the contrast-enhancing tumor. As discussed in that review, this invasive phenotype of tumor cells resistant to bevacizumab is an important driver behind the revised/updated imaging criteria in the evaluation of patients with glioma.

In this article, the authors address the question of how tumor cells become invasive after treatment with bevacizumab. They describe 2 key findings:

(1) Expression of insulin like growth factor binding protein type 2 (IGFBP2) and matrix metalloproteinase-2 (MMP2) at the invasive edges of in patient

tumors resistant to bevacizumab. This data corroborates the reports by other groups.

(2) Recapitulation of the patient-sample findings (infiltrative behavior of tumor cells and expression of MMP2) in an animal model. In a mouse model, the authors were able to transform an otherwise noninvasive glioma xenograft (U87) to become invasive upon treatment of the animal with bevacizumab. Moreover, the invasive tumor cells expressed elevated levels of MMP2 similar to what was seen in the human tumor samples.

The importance of this report lies in the fact that the animal model may be a platform for identifying other molecular factors that underlie this transition to invasive phenotype, which, in turn, may lead to therapeutic strategies to block this method of escaping angiogenesis inhibitor therapy (eg, inhibitors of MMP2).

J. Uhm, MD

Reference

1. Wen PY, MacDonald DR, Reardon DA, et al. Updated response assessment criteria for high-grade gliomas: response assessment in Neuro-Oncology Working Group. *J Clin Oncol.* 2010;28:1963-1972.

Updated Response Assessment Criteria for High-Grade Gliomas: Response Assessment in Neuro-Oncology Working Group

Wen PY, Macdonald DR, Reardon DA, et al (Dana-Farber/Brigham and Women's Cancer Ctr, Boston, MA; Brigham and Women's Hosp, Boston, MA; Massachusetts General Hosp, Boston; et al)

J Clin Oncol 28:1963-1972, 2010

Currently, the most widely used criteria for assessing response to therapy in high-grade gliomas are based on two-dimensional tumor measurements on computed tomography (CT) or magnetic resonance imaging (MRI), in conjunction with clinical assessment and corticosteroid dose (the Macdonald Criteria). It is increasingly apparent that there are significant limitations to these criteria, which only address the contrast-enhancing component of the tumor. For example, chemoradiotherapy for newly diagnosed glioblastomas results in transient increase in tumor enhancement (pseudoprogression) in 20% to 30% of patients, which is difficult to differentiate from true tumor progression. Antiangiogenic agents produce high radiographic response rates, as defined by a rapid decrease in contrast enhancement on CT/MRI that occurs within days of initiation of treatment and that is partly a result of reduced vascular permeability to contrast agents rather than a true antitumor effect. In addition, a subset of patients treated with antiangiogenic agents develop tumor recurrence characterized by an increase in the nonenhancing component depicted on T2-weighted/fluid-attenuated inversion recovery sequences. The recognition that contrast enhancement is nonspecific and may not always be a true surrogate of tumor response and the need to account for the nonenhancing component of the tumor mandate that new criteria be developed and validated to permit accurate assessment of the efficacy of novel therapies. The Response Assessment in Neuro-Oncology Working Group is an international effort to develop new standardized response criteria for clinical trials in brain tumors. In this proposal, we present the recommendations for updated response criteria for high-grade gliomas.

▶ This is a key article that details the updated imaging criteria in the assessment of patients with high-grade glioma. Since 1990, the MacDonald Criteria[1] had been the convention and was based upon measurements of the contrast-enhancing dimensions of the tumor mass on MRI or CT. While the MacDonald Criteria represented the first standardized measure of brain tumor assessment and has served the field of neuro-oncology so very well, its key limitation is that it measures only the contrast-enhancing lesion and does not provide a way by which the nonenhancing tumor can be included in the assessment of response to therapeutics. This limitation has become even more apparent with the advent of angiogenesis inhibitors in neuro-oncology, as tumors that become resistant to agents such as bevacizumab (angiogenesis inhibitor that neutralizes vascular endothelial growth factor) often grow as nonenhancing lesions. Hence, should the contrast-enhancing mass stay stable but the nonenhancing portion grow, that patient's tumor, according to MacDonald Criteria, may be labeled as stable, as only the enhancing lesion is measured by this method.

In this article, Wen leads an international panel encompassing the various subdisciplines of neuro-oncology to announce the updated response criteria that now includes quantitating both the enhancing and nonenhancing tumor burden. Furthermore, in addition to recognizing the importance of nonenhancing tumor, the updated criteria address the issue of pseudoprogression. Pseudoprogression is a situation in which the first postradiation imaging shows worsening of MRI lesion(s), and yet instead of due to actual tumor growth, the MRI worsening is caused by a transient increase in the size of enhancement and/or edema, which subsides with no change in therapy. The updated criteria in this article make special reference to pseudoprogression and present a specific radiographic criterion for evaluating the first postradiation scan.

This is an important article that redefines imaging evaluation of patients with brain tumor. Its conception reflects the evolution of the field of neuro-oncology as a whole in terms of advances in therapy and how our use of technology to evaluate patients must advance and evolve in kind. No doubt the updated criteria will undergo further evolution with time; however, as it stands, the current form represents a landmark report.

J. Uhm, MD

Reference

1. MacDonald DR, Cascino TL, Schold SC Jr, et al. Response criteria for phase II studies of supratentorial malignant glioma. *J Clin Oncol.* 1990;8:1277-1280.

9 Neuromuscular Disease

A Novel Recessive *NEFL* Mutation Causes a Severe, Early-Onset Axonal Neuropathy

Yum SW, Zhang J, Mo K, et al (Drexel Univ College of Medicine, Philadelphia, PA; Univ of Pennsylvania School of Medicine, Philadelphia)

Ann Neurol 66:759-770, 2009

Objective.—To report the first cases of a homozygous recessive mutation in *NEFL*, the gene that encodes the light subunit of neurofilaments.

Methods.—Clinical and electrophysiologic data were evaluated, and a sural nerve biopsy from one affected child was examined by immunohistochemistry and electron microscopy. The ability of the mutant protein to form filaments was characterized in an established cell culture system.

Results.—Four of five siblings developed of a severe, progressive neuropathy beginning in early childhood. Serial nerve conduction studies showed progressively reduced amplitudes with age and pronounced slowing at all ages. Visual-evoked responses were slowed in three children, indicating that central nervous system axons were subclinically involved. All four affected children were homozygous for a nonsense mutation at glutamate 210 (E210X) in the *NEFL* gene; both parents were heterozygous carriers. A sural nerve biopsy from an affected patient showed markedly reduced numbers of myelinated axons; the remaining myelinated axons were small and lacked intermediate filaments. The E210X mutant protein did not form an intermediate filament network and did not interfere with the filament formation by wild-type human light subunit of neurofilaments in SW-13 vim^- cells.

Interpretation.—This is the first demonstration of a recessive *NEFL* mutation, which appears to cause a simple loss of function, resulting in a severe, early-onset axonal neuropathy with unique features. These results confirm that neurofilaments are the main determinant of axonal caliber and conduction velocity, and demonstrate for the first time that neurofilaments are required for the maintenance of myelinated peripheral nervous system axons.

▶ One of the increasing challenges to clinicians and scientists working in hereditary neuropathy research is the increasing complex classification of

Charcot-Marie-Tooth disease (CMT). Traditionally, CMT is classified into CMT1 (demyelinating) and CMT2 (axonal) based chiefly on upper limb motor conduction velocities less than or more than 38 m/sec. As our molecular genetic knowledge in this field is unfolding, it is becoming increasingly clear that many CMT genes can cause a spectrum of phenotypes, for example, myelin protein zero can cause CMT1, CMT2, and intermediate CMT.[1-3] Yum and colleagues now report a novel recessive mutation (E210X) in the NEFL gene causing severe early onset axonal CMT2E. Mutations in NEFL gene were initially reported to cause autosomal dominant axonal CMT21, autosomal dominant demyelinating CMT12, and autosomal recessive intermediate CMT3. It is obvious that in current genomic era, it is particularly important to recognize the broad spectrum of CMT phenotypes and inheritance such as with NEFL gene mutation to ensure that first, clinicians consider screening for these genes in appropriate settings and second, to help in genetic counseling.

A. Verma, MD, DM, MBA

References

1. Mersiyanova IV, Perepelov AV, Polyakov AV, et al. A new variant of Charcot-Marie-Tooth disease type 2 is probably the result of a mutation in the neurofilament-light gene. *Am J Hum Genet.* 2000;67:37-46.
2. Jordanova A, De Jonghe P, Boerkoel CF, et al. Mutations in the neurofilament light chain gene (NEFL) cause early onset severe Charcot-Marie-Tooth disease. *Brain.* 2003;126:590-597.
3. Abe A, Numakura C, Saito K, et al. Neurofilament light chain polypeptide gene mutations in Charcot-Marie-Tooth disease: nonsense mutation probably causes a recessive phenotype. *J Hum Genet.* 2009;54:94-97.

Autoantibody-Mediated Dysfunction of Sympathetic Neurons in Guillain-Barré Syndrome

Lehmann HC, Jangouk P, Kierysch EK, et al (Heinrich-Heine-Univ, Düsseldorf, Germany)

Arch Neurol 67:203-210, 2010

Objective.—To investigate a pathologic immune response to autonomic nerve fibers in Guillain-Barré syndrome (GBS).

Design.—We compared the effects of purified IgG from patients with GBS, multiple sclerosis, and chronic inflammatory demyelinating polyneuropathy on transmitter synthesis and synaptic transmission in an in vitro model of sympathetic neurons and cardiomyocytes.

Subjects.—Three patients with GBS, 2 with chronic inflammatory demyelinating polyradiculoneuropathy, and 2 with relapsing-remitting multiple sclerosis.

Results.—Incubation of sympathetic neurons with GBS-IgG resulted in an upregulation of tyrosine hydroxylase and caused a relative increase of noradrenaline levels. In cocultures of sympathetic neurons and cardiomyocytes, GBS-IgG altered the synaptic transmission, as assessed by changes in the average cardiomyocyte beat rate. These effects could be neutralized by preincubation of sympathetic neurons with intravenous immunoglobulins.

Conclusion.—Our findings indicate that in GBS, circulating antibodies directed against sympathetic neurons may contribute to autonomic dysfunction via functionally relevant changes in the noradrenaline synthesis.

▶ Significant autonomic disturbances occur in rare patients with Guillain-Barré syndrome (GBS) in the acute stage of illness, and they are often harbingers of higher morbidity and mortality. The authors demonstrate humoral factors as the underlying cause of sympathetic dysautonomia in GBS in 3 cases. The finding is important but requires duplication in larger number of GBS cases before it can be used as diagnostic and prognostic index. It is currently unclear whether severe cases of GBS that require ventilatory support show greater degree of autonomic dysfunction and seropositivity and whether their course can be favorably modified by earlier therapy with intravenous immunoglobulin.

A. Verma, MD, DM, MBA

Effect of Alemtuzumab (CAMPATH 1-H) in patients with inclusion-body myositis

Dalakas MC, Rakocevic G, Schmidt J, et al (Natl Inst of Neurological Disorders and Stroke, Bethesda, MD; et al)

Brain 132:1536-1544, 2009

Sporadic inclusion-body myositis (sIBM) is the most common disabling, adult-onset, inflammatory myopathy histologically characterized by intense inflammation and vacuolar degeneration. In spite of T cell-mediated cytotoxicity and persistent, clonally expanded and antigen-driven endomysial T cells, the disease is resistant to immunotherapies. Alemtuzumab is a humanized monoclonal antibody that causes an immediate depletion or severe reduction of peripheral blood lymphocytes, lasting at least 6 months. We designed a proof-of-principle study to examine if one series of Alemtuzumab infusions in sIBM patients depletes not only peripheral blood lymphocytes but also endomysial T cells and alters the natural course of the disease. Thirteen sIBM patients with established 12-month natural history data received 0.3 mg/kg/day Alemtuzumab for 4 days. The study was powered to capture ≥ 10% increase strength 6 months after treatment. The primary end-point was disease stabilization compared to natural history, assessed by bi-monthly Quantitative Muscle Strength Testing and Medical Research Council strength measurements. Lymphocytes and T cell subsets were monitored concurrently in the blood and the repeated muscle biopsies. Alterations in the mRNA expression of inflammatory, stressor and degeneration-associated molecules were examined in the repeated biopsies. During a 12-month observation period, the patients' total strength had declined by a mean of 14.9% based on Quantitative Muscle Strength Testing. Six months after therapy, the overall decline was only 1.9% ($P < 0.002$), corresponding to a 13% differential gain. Among those patients, four improved by a mean of 10% and six reported improved performance of daily activities. The benefit was more evident by the Medical Research Council scales, which demonstrated a decline in the total scores by 13.8% during the observation period but an improvement by 11.4% ($P < 0.001$) after 6 months, reaching the level of strength recorded 12 months earlier. Depletion of peripheral blood lymphocytes, including the naive and memory $CD8_+$ cells, was noted 2 weeks after treatment and persisted up to 6 months. The effector $CD45RA^+$ $CD62L^-$ cells, however, started to increase 2 months after therapy and peaked by the 4th month. Repeated muscle biopsies showed reduction of CD3 lymphocytes by a mean of 50% ($P < 0.008$), most prominent in the improved patients, and reduced mRNA expression of stressor molecules Fas, Mip-1a and αB-crystallin; the mRNA of desmin, a regeneration-associated molecule, increased. This proof-of-principle study provides insights into the pathogenesis of inclusion-body myositis and concludes that in sIBM one series of Alemtuzumab infusions can slow down disease progression up to 6 months, improve the strength of some patients, and reduce endomysial inflammation and stressor molecules. These encouraging results, the first in sIBM, warrant a future study with repeated infusions.

▶ This single-center, nonrandomized, nonblinded clinical therapeutic study was done to determine whether a monoclonal antibody against CD52 (Alemtuzumab or CAMPATH) would have an effect in sporadic inclusion-body myositis (sIBM). The theory was that a reduction in T cells peripherally and in the muscle of sIBM patients would lead to stabilization or improvement in clinical parameters.

The authors studied 13 patients followed in their natural history study, such that standardized data for the preceding 12 to 24 months were available before study drug administration. The average age of patients was 60; they had been diagnosed on average 10 years previously with sIBM based on typical criteria. These patients were ambulatory (no mention made of whether they required assistive devices such as braces, canes, etc). None were taking immunomodulating medications for at least a year. The study drug was given every other day over 4 doses. Importantly, no adverse effects were noted other than transient hypotension in 3 instances of the intravenous infusion. Patients were given coverage with trimethoprim/sulfamethoxazole (TMP/SMZ), clotrimazole troches, and valganciclovir.

Clinical outcome measures showed positive effect in the 6 months following treatment. The quantitative muscle strength testing (QMT) and manual muscle testing (MMT) scores were stable and improved, respectively, compared with 12 to 24 months before treatment. The QMT score worsened, though, in the time 6 to 12 months after treatment such that patients were near their baseline level. No data were given on the 6- to 12-month interval for the MMT measurement, which was perplexing as the data were collected (based on the study design). Patient self reporting revealed that 5/13 felt no change; 3/13 felt a moderate, but clear benefit; and 5/13 felt there was a clear improvement.

The patient report of improvement started at 2 months and lasted for 5 to 8 months.

As expected, there was a reduction in lymphocyte counts and repeat biopsies revealed less reduction in $CD3^+$ T cells, which appeared to correlate to those patients who improved the most. Muscle cytoarchitecture was improved.

Importantly, in this protocol, patients did not suffer any significant complications, such as infections.

Overall, this study does show that Alemtuzumab exerts an affect in sIBM, namely in slowing disease progression based on standard muscle testing and patient self-reporting. The study was not a placebo controlled study nor was it blinded or randomized, so we await the results of a follow-up study to determine whether this medication regimen is useful. As the authors allude to, this is a chronic condition and repeated infusions may be necessary, the safety, cost, and efficacy of which needs to be proven.

B. A. Crum, MD

Ganglionic Acetylcholine Receptor Autoantibody: Oncological, Neurological, and Serological Accompaniments

McKeon A, Lennon VA, Lachance DH, et al (Mayo Clinic, Rochester, MN)
Arch Neurol 66:735-741, 2009

Objective.—To describe the clinical utility of the nicotinic ganglionic acetylcholine receptor (α3-AChR) autoantibody as a marker of neurological autoimmunity and cancer.

Design.—Case-control study.

Setting.—Mayo Clinic, Rochester, Minnesota.

Patients.—A total of 15 000 patients seen at Mayo Clinic (2005-2007) and evaluated on a service basis for paraneoplastic neurological autoimmunity for whom clinical information was obtained retrospectively by medical record review as well as 457 neurologically asymptomatic patients or control subjects of whom 173 were healthy, 245 had lung cancer, and 39 had systemic lupus erythematosus or Sjögren syndrome.

Outcome Measures.—Neurological, oncological, and serological associations of α3-AChR autoantibody seropositivity.

Results.—Of 15 000 patients tested on a service basis, 1% were seropositive (median, 0.12 nmol/L; range, 0.03-18.8 nmol/L; normal, ≤0.02 nmol/L), 55% were male, and the median age was 65 years. Cancer was found (new or by history) in 24 of 78 patients evaluated for cancer while at Mayo Clinic (30%); 43% had adenocarcinoma (more patients had breast cancer than prostate, lung, and gastrointestinal cancers; each of the latter groups had about the same number of patients). Of 12 patients with high antibody values (≥1.00 nmol/L), 83% had pandysautonomia. Of 85 patients with medium antibody values (0.10-0.99 nmol/L), neurological presentations were more diverse and included peripheral neuropathies (36%), dysautonomia (20%, usually limited), and encephalopathy (13%). Of 58 patients with low antibody values (0.03-0.09 nmol/L),

54% had a nonautoimmune neurological disorder or no neurological disorder. Of 245 control patients with lung cancer, 7.8% were seropositive. Only 1 of 212 control patients without cancer (0.5%) was seropositive ($P < .001$).

Conclusion.—The detection of α3-AChR autoantibody aids the diagnosis of neurological autoimmunity and cancer.

▶ In this retrospective analysis on a total of 15 000 patients suspected for neurological autoimmunity and cancer, the authors extend their earlier observations on the relationship between α3-AChR Ab and dysautonomia in experimental animals and patients. Of these 15 000 patients, 1% were found to be α3-AChR seropositive. Approximately one third of seropositive patients had cancer, mostly adenocarcinoma—in contrast to patients with other paraneoplastic syndromes in whom small cell lung cancer is the most common systemic malignancy. The authors demonstrate that the neurologic manifestations in α3-AChR seropositive patients depend on the titer of antibodies; patients with high titers have pandysautonomia and patients with medium titers have limited dysautonomia with or without somatic neuropathy and encephalopathy. Patients with low titers had either nonimmune neurological symptoms or they were neurologically asymptomatic. The shortcomings in this study include drawbacks of retrospective analysis, limited follow-ups of patients, and uncertain importance of low titer serology in asymptomatic patients with lung cancer and collagen vascular diseases. Many of these patients also had other autoantibodies (glutamic acid decarboxylase 65-isoform [GAD65], muscle AChR, N- and P/Q-type calcium channels, potassium channel, striational, antineuronal nuclear antibody-1 [ANNA-1], and collapsin response-mediator protein-5 [CRMP-5] IgG) of which detailed work-up is unavailable in this report. On balance, α3-AChR Ab seems to be frequent in patients with dysautonomia, and its presence should trigger a search for the underlying cause (including cancer) for this potentially treatable neurological syndrome.

A. Verma, MD, DM, MBA

Pharmacokinetics of Intravenous Immunoglobulin and Outcome in Guillain-Barré Syndrome

Kuitwaard K, de Gelder J, Tio-Gillen AP, et al (Erasmus Med Ctr, Rotterdam, The Netherlands)

Ann Neurol 66:597-603, 2009

Objective.—Intravenous immunoglobulin (IVIg) is the first choice treatment for Guillain-Barré syndrome (GBS). All patients initially receive the same arbitrary dose of 2 g per kg body weight. Not all patients, however, show a good recovery after this standard dose. IVIg clearance may depend on disease severity and vary between individuals, implying that this dose is suboptimal for some patients. In this study, we determined whether the pharmacokinetics of IVIg is related to outcome in GBS.

Methods.—We included 174 GBS patients who had previously participated in 2 randomized clinical trials. At entry, all patients were unable to walk unaided and received a standard dose of IVIg. Total IgG levels in serum samples obtained immediately before and 2 weeks after the start of IVIg administration were determined by turbidimetry and related to clinical outcome at 6 months.

Results.—The increase in serum IgG (ΔIgG) 2 weeks after IVIg treatment varied considerably between patients (mean, 7.8g/L; standard deviation, 5.6g/L). Patients with a low ΔIgG recovered significantly more slowly, and fewer reached the ability to walk unaided at 6 months (log-rank $p < 0.001$). In multivariate analysis adjusted for other known prognostic factors, a low ΔIgG was independently associated with poor outcome ($p = 0.022$).

Interpretation:.—After a standard dose of IVIg treatment, GBS patients show a large variation in pharmacokinetics, which is related to clinical outcome. This may indicate that patients with a small increase in serum IgG level may benefit from a higher dosage or second course of IVIg.

▶ Approximately 25% of patients with GBS have significant respiratory muscle weakness requiring ventilatory support and 5% succumb to complications. Although standard dose intravenous immunoglobulin (IVIg) therapy at 2 g/kg over 5 days improves the outcome in Guillain-Barré syndrome (GBS), it is not known if more severe cases require higher IVIg dosage and if the outcome can be improved overall by higher initial or booster IVIg dosage in those severe cases. The authors in this study present pharmacokinetic data from nearly 300 patients who received IVIg in earlier clinical trials and attempt to correlate IgG levels with clinical outcome. First, as expected, they demonstrate that the largest variability in IgG levels occurred at 2 weeks after IVIg infusion. The IgG levels reached to near base line at 4 weeks after infusion in these patients (Fig 1 in the original article). Second, patients with low IgG levels at 2 weeks after IVIg had a more severe clinical course and the less favorable clinical outcome. The latter observation was compelling even after taking into account other variables that are known to be associated with poor outcome (such as age, preceding diarrhea, initial severity) in multivariate analysis. Finally, serum IgG levels at 2 weeks predicted the ability of patients who regained ability to walk unaided at 6-month follow-up (Fig 3 in the original article). It all indicates that a subgroup of patients of GBS with more severe illness stand to further improve after initial higher or a booster IVIg dose during the acute phase of the disease. This seminal observation should trigger a prospective study to determine if monitoring of serum IgG levels in the first few days can be used to optimize the use in IVIg in GBS.

A. Verma, MD, DM, MBA

Pregabalin for painful HIV neuropathy: A randomized, double-blind, placebo-controlled trial

Simpson DM, Schifitto G, Clifford DB, et al (Mount Sinai School of Medicine, NY; Univ of Rochester, NY; Washington Univ School of Medicine, St Louis, MO; et al)

Neurology 74:413-420, 2010

Objective.—Pregabalin is effective in several neuropathic pain syndromes. This trial evaluated its efficacy, safety, and tolerability for treatment of painful HIV-associated neuropathy.

Methods.—This randomized, double-blind, placebo-controlled, parallel-group trial included a 2-week double-blind dose-adjustment (150-600 mg/day BID) phase, a 12-week double-blind maintenance phase, and an optional 3-month open label extension phase. The primary efficacy measure was the mean Numeric Pain Rating Scale (NPRS) score, an 11-point numeric rating scale. Secondary measures included Patient Global Impression of Change (PGIC) and sleep measurements.

Results.—Baseline mean NPRS score was 6.93 for patients randomized to pregabalin (n = 151) and 6.72 for those to placebo (n = 151). Pregabalin average daily dosage (SD) was 385.7 (160.3) mg/d. At endpoint, pregabalin and placebo showed substantial reductions in mean NPRS score from baseline:−2.88 vs −2.63, $p = 0.3941$. Pregabalin had greater improvements in NPRS score relative to placebo at weeks 1 (−1.14 vs −0.69, $p = 0.0131$) and 2 (−1.92 vs −1.43, $p = 0.0393$), and at weeks 7 (−3.22 vs −2.53 $p = 0.0307$) and 8 (−3.33 vs −2.53, $p = 0.0156$). At all other time points, differences between groups were not significant. Sleep measurements and 7-item PGIC did not differ among treatment groups; however, collapsed PGIC scores showed 82.8% of pregabalin and 66.7% of placebo patients rated themselves in 1 of the 3 "improved" categories ($p = 0.0077$). Somnolence and dizziness were the most common adverse events with pregabalin.

Conclusions.—Pregabalin was well-tolerated, but not superior to placebo in the treatment of painful HIV neuropathy. Factors predicting analgesic response in HIV neuropathy warrant additional research.

Classification of Evidence.—This Class II trial showed that pregabalin is not more effective than placebo in treatment of painful HIV neuropathy.

▶ HIV-associated distal sensory polyneuropathy (HIV-DSP) is the most common form of painful and often disabling neuropathy in HIV-infected individuals. The prevalence of HIV-DSP has significantly increased in post-HAART era, as patients with HIV/AIDS live longer with effective antiretroviral therapy. Effective pain control in folks with HIV-DSP is urgently needed. The 1066 HIV Neuropathy Study Group has added new information regarding the use of pregabalin in HIV-DSP. Pregabalin exerts analgesic effect by binding to voltage-gated calcium channels on primary sensory afferent neurons, and it has been found effective in diabetic painful neuropathy, postherpetic neuralgia, and other painful neuropathies. The results of this class II trial are overall statistically negative, but the trend seems to favor pregabalin reaching significance at certain points during the study period (Fig 3 in the original article). Interestingly, the absolute effect of pregabalin in pain control was not different from that reported in diabetic neuropathy; however, the parallel placebo effect was greater in this study. Greater placebo effect in this study is reminiscent of similar reports in other HIV-DSP drug trials.[1,2] What predicts analgesic effects in HIV-DSP requires additional research to better design future trials.

A. Verma, MD, DM, MBA

References

1. Kieburtz K, Simpson D, Yiannoutsos C, et al. A randomized trial of amitriptyline and mexiletine for painful neuropathy in HIV infection. AIDS Clinical Trial Group 242 Protocol Team. *Neurology.* 1998;51:1682-1688.
2. Simpson DM, McArthur JC, Olney R, et al. Lamotrigine HIV Neuropathy Study Team. Lamotrigine for HIV-associated painful sensory neuropathies: a placebo-controlled trial. *Neurology.* 2003;60:1508-1514.

Rituximab for polyneuropathy with IgM monoclonal gammopathy

Niermeijer JMF, Eurelings M, Lokhorst HL, et al (Univ Med Ctr, Utrecht, The Netherlands)

J Neurol Neurosurg Psychiatry 80:1036-1039, 2009

Background.—Polyneuropathy with IgM monoclonal gammopathy can be a disabling disorder necessitating treatment.

Methods.—In a prospective open label trial, 17 patients with disabling IgM MGUS polyneuropathy were treated with rituximab, a chimeric anti-CD-20 monoclonal antibody.

Results.—Rituximab induced an improvement of ≥1 point on the Overall Disability Sum Score in 2/17 patients, an improvement of ≥5% of the distal MRC sum score in 4/17 and the sensory sum score in 9/17 patients. Bone marrow investigations showed CD 20 B cell depletion in all patients. There were no serious adverse events. Compared with treatment with intermittent cyclophosphamide with prednisone or treatment with fludarabine, it shows a comparable response percentages but fewer side effects. The presence of anti-MAG and a disease duration shorter than 10 years may predict treatment response.

Conclusion.—Rituximab is a candidate for treatment of IgM MGUS polyneuropathy and should be further investigated in a double-blind randomised trial.

▶ One form of subacute and predominantly motor polyneuropathy has a high concordance with IgM monoclonal gammopathy, monoclonal gammopathy of uncertain significance (MGUS) or GM1, directed against ganglioside components of peripheral myelin. For this reason, some view it related to the class of paraproteinemic neuropathies. IgM MUGS-related polyneuropathy is also distinctive in the sense that conventional immunosuppressant drugs effective in other immune-mediated polyneuropathies are generally ineffective in IgM monoclonal gammopathy-related predominantly motor neuropathies. Plasma pheresis or IVIg infusion therapies are mostly ineffective or only temporarily effective in these cases. Some authoritative clinicians favor early addition of cyclophosphamide in treatment-resistant cases or when the frequency of plasma exchange or IVIg infusions is unsustainable. Other immune modulating agents that decrease IgM titer, such as rituximab, should be a logical choice in recalcitrant cases. The favorable findings in this small open label prospective study bring us a step closer to a larger double-blind rituximab trial in IgM MGUS polyneuropathy for a more definitive answer.

A. Verma, MD, DM, MBA

Sarcoplasmic redistribution of nuclear TDP-43 in inclusion body myositis

Salajegheh M, Pinkus JL, Taylor JP, et al (Brigham and Women's Hosp, Boston, MA; St Jude Children's Research Hosp, Memphis, TN; et al)

Muscle Nerve 40:19-31, 2009

The nucleic acid binding protein TDP-43 was recently identified in normal myonuclei and in the sarcoplasm of inclusion body myositis (IBM) muscle. Here we found TDP-43 sarcoplasmic immunoreactivity in 23% of IBM myofibers, while other reported IBM biomarkers were less frequent, with rimmed vacuoles in 2.8%, fluorescent Congo red material in 0.57%, SMI-31 immunoreactivity in 0.83%, and focal R1282 beta-amyloid immunoreactivity in 0.00% of myofibers. The presence of as little as >1% of myofibers with nonnuclear sarcoplasmic TDP-43 was highly sensitive (91%) and specific (100%) to IBM among 50 inflammatory myopathy patient samples, although some patients with hereditary inclusion body myopathies and myofibrillar myopathy also had sarcoplasmic TDP-43. TDP-43 mutations were sought, and none were identified. TDP-43 could be one of many nucleic acid binding proteins that are abnormally present in IBM sarcoplasm. They could potentially interfere with the normal function of extranuclear RNAs that maintain myofiber protein production.

▶ Sporadic inclusion body myositis (sIBM) is the most common form of inflammatory muscle disease in older patients. IBM is diagnosed on light microscopy based on the presence of rimmed vacuoles on routine histology and amyloid and other inclusions in immunohistology in occasional muscle fibers (less than 1% fibers). The findings in this report confirm and extend other recent observations of excessive TDP-43 in IBM muscle fibers. As reported in the accompanying editorial,[1] the fact that TDP-43-positive inclusions are present in nearly 25% of muscle fibers makes it the most reliable histologic marker in IBM so far. The presence of similar TDP-43 inclusions in other myopathies, such as hereditary IBM, and myofibrillar myopathies, indicates some common element in pathogenesis of these disorders. It is currently unknown whether TDP-43 inclusions are just trashed proteins or they are pathogenic through either gain of some toxic property or loss of normal function from its sequestration in protein aggregates. Likewise, it also remains unclear whether TDP-43, normally an intranuclear protein, abnormally escapes into the cytoplasm or it represents impaired trafficking from cytoplasm back to nucleus in these disorders. A better understanding of the role of TDP-43 in IBM may pave the way to the development of targeted therapy for this hitherto incurable disease.

A. Verma, MD, DM, MBA

Reference

1. Verma, Tandan R. TDP-43: a reliable immunohistochemistry marker for inclusion body myositis? *Muscle Nerve.* 2009;40:8-9.

Selective T-Type Calcium Channel Blockade Alleviates Hyperalgesia in *ob/ob* Mice

Latham JR, Pathirathna S, Jagodic MM, et al (Univ of Virginia Health System, Charlottesville; et al)
Diabetes 58:2656-2665, 2009

Objective.—Morbid obesity may be accompanied by diabetes and painful diabetic neuropathy, a poorly understood condition that is manifested by mechanical or thermal allodynia and hyperalgesia. Recent studies have highlighted the importance of T-type calcium channels (T-channels) in peripheral nociception; therefore, our goal was to examine the function of these channels in the pathophysiology and development of painful diabetic neuropathy.

Research Design and Methods.—In vivo testing of mechanical and thermal sensation, morphometric peripheral nerve studies, and electrophysiological and biochemical measurements were used to characterize the role of T-channels and the development of painful diabetic neuropathy in leptin-deficient (*ob/ob*) mice.

Results.—We found that *ob/ob* mice developed significant mechanical and thermal hypersensitivity early in life that coincided with hyperglycemia and was readily reversed with insulin therapy. These disturbances were accompanied by significant biophysical and biochemical modulation of T-channels in dorsal root ganglion neurons as measured by a large increase in the amplitude of T-currents and the expression of mRNA. The most prevalent subtype, α1H ($Ca_v3.2$), was most strongly affected. Moreover, (3β,5α,17β)-17-hydroxyestrane-3-carbonitrile (ECN), a novel neuroactive steroid and selective T-channel antagonist, provided dose-dependent alleviation of neuropathic thermal and mechanical hypersensitivity in diabetic *ob/ob* mice.

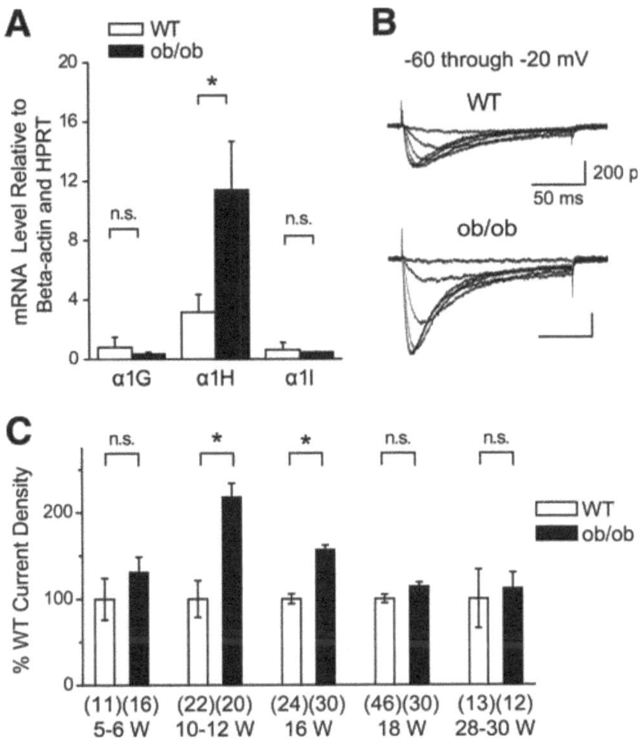

FIGURE 3.—Upregulation of T-current in smaller DRG cells after the development of hyperglycemia in *ob/ob* mice. *A*: qRT-PCR analysis of the relative expression of mRNA for three isoforms of T-channels in lumbar DRGs and from *ob/ob* mice and age-matched wild-type controls at 10–12 weeks of age. There was a fourfold upregulation of α1H isoform but no significant change in α1G and α1I isoforms in lumbar DRG tissues from *ob/ob* mice compared with wild-type mice (*$P < 0.001$). *B*: Raw current traces evoked in DRG cells from wild-type (*top panel*) and *ob/ob* (*bottom panel*) mice 10–12 weeks old by voltage steps from −90 mV (V_h [holding potential]) to V_t (test potential) from −60 through −20 mV in 10-mV increments. Calibrations on top bars pertain to both panels. *Ob/ob* mouse had increased absolute amplitude of isolated T-current more than twofold at a range of test potentials from −50 to −20 mV. C: Histograms indicate average T-current amplitudes (V_t −30 mV) in DRG cells from wild-type (open bars) and *ob/ob* mice (filled bars) expressed as percent current density normalized to wild type. The size of each sample is in parentheses; vertical bars are SE of multiple determinations. Weeks of age for each of the five groups are indicated at the bottom. In each group, recordings were made from at least three mice. At the peak of hyperglycemia and sensory hypersensitivity (age 10–12 weeks), peak T-current density averaged 20 ± 4 pA/pF in the wild-type group and 44 ± 7 pA/pF in the *ob/ob* group. At 16 weeks of age, T-currents were still significantly upregulated in the *ob/ob* group by about 1.5-fold, with normalization occurring at 18 weeks of age. Before the onset (5–6 weeks) and at the outset of hyperglycemia (28–30 weeks of age), peak T-current density was not different between the wild-type group and the *ob/ob* group ($P > 0.05$). Asterisk indicates significant value by Mann-Whitney test ($P < 0.01$); n.s. indicates $P > 0.05$. HPRT, hypoxanthine-guanine-phosphoribosyltransferase; WT, wild type. (Reprinted from Latham JR, Pathirathna S, Jagodic MM, et al. Selective T-type calcium channel blockade alleviates hyperalgesia in *ob/ob* mice. *Diabetes*. 2009;58:2656-2665, with permission from The American Diabetes Association.)

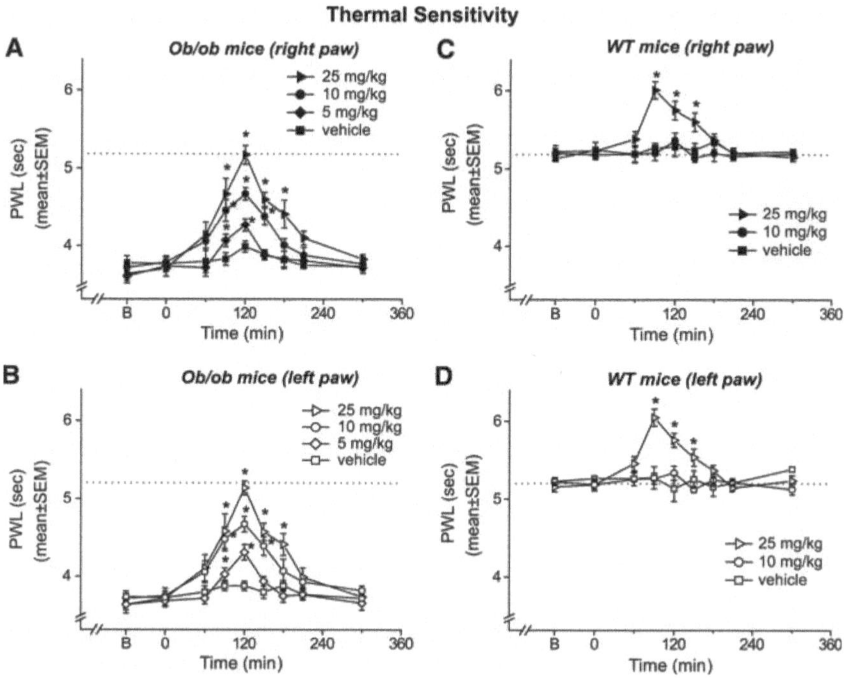

FIGURE 5.—ECN, a selective T-channel blocker and neuroactive steroid, induced greater dose-dependent alleviation of heat hypersensitivity in *ob/ob* mice (*A* and *B*) than in wild-type mice (*C* and *D*). For all dose-response experiments, 10- to 12-week-old mice (at the peak of thermal hypersensitivity) were used. ECN (5 mg/kg i.p.) caused small but significant increases in PWLs in right (*A*) and left paws (*B*) of *ob/ob* mice, with the peak effect at 120 min after injection ($*P < 0.001$). When 10 mg/kg of ECN was administered, the peak effect still occurred at 120 min but lasted longer; that is, the increase in PWLs was still significant at 150 min compared with those at 0 min (immediately before the injection) ($*P < 0.001$) in both right (*A*) and left paws (*B*). Injection of 25 mg/kg of ECN caused a profound increase in PWLs that remained significant 180 min after injection ($*P < 0.001$). At the peak effect, the highest dose of ECN caused complete reversal of mechanical hypersensitivity; that is, PWLs were similar to the baseline PWLs recorded in wild-type mice (dotted line). When ECN was administered to wild-type mice at 10 mg/kg, a dose that was effective in *ob/ob* mice, there was no effect on PWLs at any time in either right (C) or left paws (*D*); that is, PWLs remained at the baseline level (dotted line). Only at 25 mg/kg did ECN cause a significant increase in PWLs in wild-type mice, with a peak effect at 90 min. However, this effect was not as robust as that in *ob/ob* mice ($*P < 0.001$) ($n = 6$ *ob/ob* mice per group; $n = 6$ wild-type mice per group). WT, wild type. (Reprinted from Latham JR, Pathirathna S, Jagodic MM, et al. Selective T-type calcium channel blockade alleviates hyperalgesia in *ob/ob* mice. *Diabetes.* 2009;58:2656-2665, with permission from The American Diabetes Association.)

Conclusions.—Our results indicate that pharmacological antagonism of T-channels is potentially an important novel therapeutic approach for the management of painful diabetic neuropathy.

▶ Diabetes mellitus is the most common cause of painful neuropathy in clinical practice. Approximately 15% of patients with diabetes have clinical polyneuropathy, and nearly half of cross-sectional population samples exhibit evidence of peripheral nerve damage on nerve conduction studies. The importance of effective remedy to control neuropathic pain in patients with diabetes cannot be overestimated. The earlier evidence in Cav3.2 knockout mice that T-type calcium channels on dorsal root ganglia (DRG) modulate pain impulse in painful polyneuropathy is confirmed in this rodent model of obesity and type 2 diabetes. The researchers demonstrate that morbidly obese hyperglycemic *ob/ob* mice develop painful polyneuropathy in conjunction with upregulation of T-type calcium channels in DRG (Fig 3), and that selective blockade of them with T-channel antagonist alleviates pain in a predictable dose-dependent fashion (Fig 5), It is interesting that in this mice model, the behavioral and biophysical aspects of neuropathic pain spontaneously decrease as the animal advances in age, a finding that is not observed in diabetic patients with painful neuropathy. It is nonetheless hoped that designed safe and effective T-channel calcium blockers will find its way in human clinical trials to eventually develop reliable treatment for painful and disabling diabetic neuropathy.

A. Verma, MD, DM, MBA

The diagnostic pathway and prognosis in bulbar-onset amyotrophic lateral sclerosis

Turner MR, Scaber J, Goodfellow JA, et al (Oxford Univ, UK)
J Neurol Sci 2010 [Epub ahead of print]

Background.—Despite the inevitability of disease progression in amyotrophic lateral sclerosis, there is a high degree of prognostic heterogeneity in all subtypes. Some bulbar-onset (BO) patients may develop rapid anarthria yet remain ambulant for a prolonged period, whereas others progress rapidly, with early generalisation of motor weakness to the limbs and respiratory muscles. Diagnostic delay is a common occurrence in ALS, and many BO patients report having attended other specialist clinics prior to diagnosis.

Methods.—A retrospective descriptive study of BO ALS patients seen in a tertiary clinic over a six year period.

Results.—Forty-nine BO ALS patients were studied. Median survival from symptom onset was 27 months (range 6–84). 63% of subjects were female and the mean age at symptom onset was 68 years. Half had been referred to another speciality prior to diagnosis, either otolaryngology or stroke clinics, but this did not influence diagnostic latency or survival. Emotionality was reported in 45% of patients. Neurophysiological assessment was performed in 80%, brain imaging recorded in 69%, and antibody testing for myasthenia gravis in 22%. The median time to symptomatic progression beyond the bulbar region was approximately 1 year, with equal proportions progressing to the upper or lower limbs. The median interval from onset to anarthria was 18 months, and to loss of ambulation 22 months. There was a close correlation between the two ($r^2 = 0.6$) and median survival from loss of ambulation was only 3 months. Gastrostomy was carried out in 78% of patients with a median time of 13 months from symptom onset, and 3 months from diagnosis. Median survival from gastrostomy was 10 months.

Conclusions.—Survival in bulbar-onset ALS is highly variable. Half of the patients were referred to an inappropriate clinic prior to diagnosis. The time interval to the development of anarthria predicted the timing of subsequent loss of ambulation accurately from which survival may then be only a few months.

▶ This is a retrospective study of patients with bulbar amyotrophic lateral sclerosis (ALS) seen in an ALS clinic in Oxford, United Kingdom. A standardized database is used in this clinic, allowing review of important clinical information. This study attempted to outline the diagnostic pathway in patients with ALS and some contributors to progression (or not) in bulbar onset ALS as well as provides information on time to progression to important time points in these patients. While many studies have assessed the factors of progression of ALS, this study gives practicing neurologists useful information regarding actual time to progression to anarthria, loss of ambulation, etc.

Forty-nine patients were reviewed. These patients were compared with a subset of patients with lower limb-onset ALS. Not surprisingly, patients with bulbar onset were older (mean age at onset: 68 years vs 60 years in patients with lower limb-onset ALS) and more commonly female. Time from symptom onset to diagnosis was on average 10 months. In retrospective studies, this time can be tricky to measure, given the reliance on the patient and/or family to indicate the onset of symptoms. Mean survival was 33 months, though 10% lived longer than 4 years and the range was 6 to 84 months.

One point of this article was to outline the diagnostic pathway to get a diagnosis of ALS. Nearly half of the patients consulted an ENT physician, and 42% were seen in a stroke clinic before being referred to the ALS specialists. This did not influence the overall diagnostic latency or survival.

In terms of progression, the following median times were noted: time from onset to progression outside the bulbar region was 11 months (this was split equally between progression to the arms and the legs). In 18 months, the patients became anarthric. In 4 more months, patients lost the ability to ambulate (though the article does not specify whether this means with or without any assistive devices like walkers).

Interestingly, there was no correlation between time to anarthria and time to progression outside the bulbar region, though there was a correlation between the time to anarthria and the time to lose ambulation.

A feeding tube was placed in 78% of patients on average 13 months from onset. There was no comment regarding the difference in survival comparing those with and without feeding tubes other than the note that females lived longer than males with the feeding tube (16 months vs 6 months).

Riluzole was taken by 43% of patients, and there was no relationship to survival.

For the practicing neurologist, this study is useful in providing some general guidelines on how long it takes for patients with bulbar onset ALS to reach certain milestones. There are always exceptions; however, many patients ask how long it takes to reach these events. In this group of patients, the following can be said: It takes 10 months to make a diagnosis of bulbar onset ALS. Overall survival is just under 3 years from onset. Progression into the limbs (can be arms or legs) takes about a year from onset, with loss of ambulation about a year after that. Progression of bulbar symptoms to anarthria takes 1.5 years from onset and a feeding tube is usually placed before that, about a year from onset. Death is linked to the time one loses ambulation (follows by 3 months) and the time one loses speech (follows by 10 months). Another way to display this would be that once a diagnosis is made, the need for a feeding tube comes first (~3 months), then anarthria (~8 months after diagnosis), then loss of ambulation (~12 months after diagnosis), and then death (~15-18 months after diagnosis). It is not clear whether a feeding tube or riluzole lengthens the survival.

The strength of this article involves the standardized data collection at 1 ALS clinic, though this may have introduced some tertiary referral bias. It is not clear whether all patients with ALS in this region are cared for by this ALS clinic. There was no mention of noninvasive ventilation, which could have impacted the survival data. Also, there was no mention of the first symptom the patients presented with (ie, to the ENT or stroke clinic), but experience would dictate that this was likely dysarthria. It is very uncommon for a patient with ALS to present with dysphagia before dysarthria. Despite difficult speech being the first symptom in most, this study shows that most patients lose their ability to swallow safely before they become anarthric.

In summary, this article gives important information that speaks about educating our colleagues in medicine regarding the early signs of ALS. Given the hope of intervening in this disease early on with some effective treatment, making a diagnosis as early as possible will be vital. In addition, this article assists those of us seeing ALS patients in counseling them on average times to reach important clinical milestones.

B. A. Crum, MD

Triplet-repeat oligonucleotide-mediated reversal of RNA toxicity in myotonic dystrophy

Mulders SAM, van den Broek WJAA, Wheeler TM, et al (Radboud Univ Nijmegen Med Centre, The Netherlands; Univ of Rochester, NY; et al)

Proc Natl Acad Sci U S A 106:13915-13920, 2009

Myotonic dystrophy type 1 (DM1) is caused by toxicity of an expanded, noncoding (CUG)n tract in DM protein kinase (DMPK) transcripts. According to current evidence the long (CUG)n segment is involved in entrapment of muscleblind (Mbnl) proteins in ribonuclear aggregates and stabilized expression of CUG binding protein 1 (CUGBP1), causing aberrant premRNA splicing and associated pathogenesis in DM1 patients. Here, we report on the use of antisense oligonucleotides (AONs) in a therapeutic strategy for reversal of RNA-gain-of-function toxicity. Using a previously undescribed mouse DM1 myoblast–myotube cell model and DM1 patient cells as screening tools, we have identified a fully 2′-O-methyl-phosphorothioate-modified (CAG)7 AON that silences mutant

DMPK RNA expression and reduces the number of ribonuclear aggregates in a selective and (CUG)n-length-dependent manner. Direct administration of this AON in muscle of DM1 mouse models in vivo caused a significant reduction in the level of toxic (CUG)n RNA and a normalizing effect on aberrant premRNA splicing. Our data demonstrate proof of principle for therapeutic use of simple sequence AONs in DM1 and potentially other unstable microsatellite diseases.

► Myotonic dystrophy type 1 (DM1) was the first RNA toxic-gain-of-function disorder described. A potential therapeutic strategy for DM1 is explored in this article, using an antisense RNA oligonucleotide (AON) to silence mutant DM protein kinase RNA expression and to reduce the number of ribonuclear aggregates and the aberrant premRNA splicing caused by the toxic RNA. A variety of in vitro and in vivo studies, the latter using direct injection of the AON with electroporation protocols, demonstrate a significant reduction in the level of toxic RNA and a normalizing effect on aberrant premRNA splicing. The chemical nature of the antinucleotide used precludes efficient uptake in tissues. As the authors indicate, more sophisticated delivery techniques to promote uptake in vivo are necessary before this type of intervention will have clinical applicability. Other RNA toxic-gain-of-function disorders showing potential for this form of treatment include myotonic dystrophy type 2, spinocerebellar atrophy 8 and 10, fragile X ataxia, and Huntington disease-like 2.

G. N. Breningstall, MD

Vitamin E neuroprotection for cisplatin neuropathy: A randomized, placebo-controlled trial

Pace A, Giannarelli D, Galiè E, et al (Regina Elena Natl Cancer Inst, Rome, Italy; et al)

Neurology 74:762-766, 2010

Objective.—The clinical use of cisplatin chemotherapy is limited by severe peripheral neurotoxicity reported in up to 90% of patients receiving a cumulative dose higher than 300 mg/m^2. The present study evaluates the neuroprotective effect of antioxidant supplementation (vitamin E) in patients treated with cisplatin chemotherapy.

Methods.—A total of 108 patients treated with cisplatin chemotherapy were randomly assigned to receive vitamin E supplementation (α-tocopherol 400 mg/day) or placebo. Treatment was started orally before chemotherapy and continued for 3 months after the suspension of cisplatin.

Results.—Of 108 randomized patients, 68 received at least one clinical and neurophysiologic examination after cisplatin CT; 41 patients received a cumulative dose of cisplatin higher than 300 mg/m^2 and were eligible for statistical analysis: 17 in the vitamin E group (group 1) and 24 in the placebo group (group 2). The incidence of neurotoxicity was significantly lower in group 1 (5.9%) than in group 2 (41.7%) ($p < 0.01$). The severity of neurotoxicity, measured with a validated neurotoxicity score (Total Neuropathy Score [TNS]), was significantly lower in patients receiving vitamin E than those receiving placebo (mean TNS 1.4 vs 4.1; $p < 0.01$).

Conclusions.—This phase III study confirms the neuroprotective role of vitamin E against cisplatin peripheral neurotoxicity. Vitamin E supplementation should be adopted in patients receiving cisplatin-based chemotherapy.

Classification of Evidence.—This study provides Class II evidence that vitamin E supplementation significantly reduces the relative risk of developing signs or symptoms of neurotoxicity (relative risk = 0.14) (95% confidence interval = 0.02–1.00, $p < 0.05$).

▶ Therapeutic dosage of platinum-based chemotherapeutic agents almost always gives rise to some degree of toxic neuropathy. Neuropathic deficit following cisplatin can be particularly debilitating in persons with pre-existent neuropathy, such as hereditary or diabetic neuropathy. Thus, finding a way to protect or curtail the neurotoxicity caused by platinum-based chemotherapy would be a major advance, particularly as more cancer patients are now living longer after chemotherapy. The findings in this study corroborate results of previous research[1] that vitamin E can protect against nerve damage caused by cisplatin-based chemotherapy without diminishing the chemotherapeutic efficacy. However, the small size of the patient population in this study does not make it possible to draw definite conclusions. Also, the study suffered from a high dropout rate, though researchers claim they had expected that to happen and they had planned for it by enrolling more people at study initiation than statistically needed. Although vitamin E supplementation is relatively safe and there seems to be promising evidence of the benefit of vitamin E in capsulation-induced neuropathy, a larger phase 3 study is needed to establish definite efficacy. The working hypothesis of vitamin E efficacy in prevention of capsulation-induced neurotoxicity is its antioxidant activity, and it will be worth exploring the benefit of other antioxidants, such as glutathione and alpha-lipoic acid, along with vitamin E in blinded controlled clinical studies.

A. Verma, MD, DM, MBA

Reference

1. Argyriou AA, Chroni E, Koutras A, et al. A randomized controlled trial evaluating the efficacy and safety of vitamin E supplementation for protection against cisplatin-induced peripheral neuropathy: final results. *Support Care Cancer.* 2006;14:1134-1140.

10 Neuro-ophthalmology

"Cloud-like Enhancement" Is a Magnetic Resonance Imaging Abnormality Specific to Neuromyelitis Optica

Ito S, Mori M, Makino T, et al (Chiba Univ, Japan)

Ann Neurol 66:425-428, 2009

Neuromyelitis optica (NMO) is presumably mediated by an autoantibody against aquaporin-4 densely expressed at the blood-brain barrier. In 18 patients with NMO, brain magnetic resonance imaging (MRI) findings were systematically reviewed. Brain MRI abnormalities were found for 89% of the patients, and the most prominent feature was "cloud-like enhancement," multiple patchy enhancing lesions with blurred margin, found in 90% of the patients with positive contrast enhancement. In NMO, brain MRI abnormalities are frequent, and cloud-like enhancement appears to be an MRI finding specific to NMO, possibly caused by primary involvement of the blood-brain barrier by the autoantibodies.

▶ This article looked at MRI findings in 18 patients who met the 2006 Wingerchuk[1] diagnostic criteria for neuromyelitis optica (NMO) and compared them with 39 patients with multiple sclerosis (MS) who were negative for the anti-aquaporin-4 (AQP4) antibody. Each group of patients had had their disease for similar lengths of time (12 years NMO group, 11 years MS group), and the mean age at onset was 37.6 for the NMO group and 29.7 for the MS group.

They compared MRI findings between "initial" and "final" brain MRIs, but the definition of these terms was not included in the article. Initial MRIs were only performed on 5 NMO patients, 2 of which had abnormal contrast enhancing lesions and 1 of the 2 had "cloud-like enhancement." In the MS group with initial brain MRIs, 3 of 4 had contrast enhancement that was termed "isolated." They defined "cloud-like enhancement" as multiple patchy enhancement with blurred margin in adjacent regions, in comparison with isolated enhancing lesions. Follow-up MRIs were done on all the patients in the study with 16 of 18 NMO MRIs and 38 of 39 MS MRIs with any abnormality. Apparently contrast was not given in all MRI studies. Contrast enhancement was of the "cloud-like" variety in 9 of 10 NMO and 1 of 13 MS patients, whereas 12 of 13 MS patients had isolated enhancement and only 1 of 10 NMO patients.

This study is confusing in that the definition of timing for initial MRIs and follow-up MRIs was not given. Treatment and clinical findings were also not given in relationship to the follow-up MRI (mention is made of 7 of 8 patients getting intravenous steroids before MRI scans but which patients and which

MRIs was not detailed). There may be a possible difference in the contrast enhancement characteristics of brain MRI lesions in NMO versus MS. Further corroborating studies should be carried out.

J. Leavitt, MD

Reference

1. Wingerchuk DM, Lennon VA, Pittock SJ, Lucchinetti CF, Weinshenker BG. Revised diagnostic criteria for neuromyelitis optica. *Neurology.* 2006;66: 1485-1489.

Early MRI in optic neuritis: The risk for disability

Swanton JK, Fernando KT, Dalton CM, et al (Inst of Neurology, London, UK)
Neurology 72:542-550, 2009

Background.—MRI findings influence the risk of patients with optic neuritis (ON) developing clinically definite (CD) multiple sclerosis (MS) but their influence on future disability is less clear.

Objective.—To investigate in patients with ON the influence of lesion number, location and activity, and non-lesion MRI measures obtained on early scans on disability.

Methods.—A total of 106 of 143 prospectively recruited patients with ON had reached a scheduled 5-year follow-up, of whom 100 were evaluated clinically. Lesion number, location, and activity measures were analyzed at baseline (within 3 months of onset) and lesion activity measures were studied at 3-month follow-up. Brain atrophy, magnetization transfer ratio, and spectroscopy measures were also analyzed. Ordinal logistic regression assessed the association between early MRI findings and subsequent disability.

Results.—At median 6 years follow-up, 48% had converted to CDMS and 52% remained with clinically isolated syndrome (median Expanded Disability Status Scale 2 and 1). In the final models, both the presence and the number of spinal cord lesions at baseline (odds ratios [OR] 3.30, 1.94) and new T2 lesions at follow-up (OR 7.12, 2.06) were significant independent predictors of higher disability. Disability was also predicted by the presence at baseline of gadolinium-enhancing lesions (OR 2.78) and number of infratentorial lesions (OR 1.82). Only spinal cord lesions predicted disability in patients converting to CDMS.

Conclusion.—Spinal cord, infratentorial, and gadolinium lesions within 3 months of optic neuritis onset and new T2 lesions after 3 months predicted disability after 6 years; only spinal cord lesions were predictive of disability in those developing clinically definite multiple sclerosis.

▶ One hundred patients with clinically isolated optic neuritis were prospectively recruited over 10 years and followed for at least 5 years. All patients had baseline brain and spinal cord MRI as well as MR spectroscopy (MRS) and magnetization transfer imaging (MTI) done within 3 months of onset of optic neuritis and at 3 months follow-up.

The neurology exam and Expanded Disability Status Scale (EDSS) score at the 5-year follow-up were all performed by a single physician (although the EDSS score was obtained by phone in 25 patients). Poser criteria[1] were used to determine clinically definite multiple sclerosis (CDMS). At last follow-up (median 6 years), 48% had converted to CDMS whereas 52% remained as clinically isolated syndromes.

They analyzed early MRIs with regard to lesion number, features, location, and activity to try to determine if there were any factors that could predict eventual disability. Initial MRIs correlated with EDSS with regard to spinal cord lesions (number and presence). The 3-month follow-up MRIs with new T2 lesions were significantly associated with EDSS score. The MRS and MTI at 3 months did not show any significant measurable changes. For the 48% who converted to CDMS, the only significant predictor on early MRI was baseline cord lesions. Their findings with regard to the initial brain MRI not correlating with disability agree with the latest report of the Optic Neuritis Treatment Trial.[2] This is an interesting study in that MRI of the spine is not often done in clinically isolated optic neuritis cases and perhaps should be considered more often.

J. Leavitt, MD

References

1. Poser CM, Paty DW, Scheinberg L, et al. New diagnostic criteria for multiple sclerosis: guidelines for research protocols. *Ann Neurolog.* 1983;13:227-231.
2. Optic Neuritis Study Group. Multiple sclerosis risk after optic neuritis. Final optic neuritis treatment trial follow-up. *Arch Neurol.* 2008;65:727-732.

Functional Visual Loss in Idiopathic Intracranial Hypertension

Ney JJ, Volpe NJ, Liu GT, et al (Univ of Pennsylvania School of Medicine, Philadelphia; et al)

Ophthalmology 116:1808-1813, 2009

Objective.—To identify and describe patients with idiopathic intracranial hypertension (IIH) with concurrent functional visual loss (FVL).

Design.—Observational, retrospective case series.

Participants.—Seventeen patients with IIH and FVL.

Methods.—Clinical features were collected retrospectively. Data from 281 cases of IIH were analyzed for concurrence of FVL.

Main Outcome Measures.—Occurrence of FVL diagnosed at presentation or on subsequent follow-up.

Results.—Seventeen patients had FVL and IIH. Of the 17 patients with FVL and IIH, 11 (65%) had FVL on presentation, with the remaining 6 patients developing FVL after initial presentation. Two patients in this cohort had documented recurrence of their IIH. There were several common patterns of FVL. All 17 patients had functional visual fields, with 82% having tubular fields and 71% exhibiting nonphysiologic constriction on perimetry testing. Seventy-six percent of patients had nerve/field mismatch showing no atrophic disc changes. Eighty-eight percent of patients had significant psychiatric, psychosocial, or other medical comorbidities. The majority of patients were managed surgically at some point in their clinical history, with 53% having nerve decompression, shunt, or both. Three patients had optic nerve sheath fenestrations after the diagnosis of FVL.

Conclusions.—Results suggest a high prevalence of FVL in IIH with a potential association with psychiatric illness and psychosocial stressors requiring careful consideration before surgical intervention.

▶ Retrospective review of 281 cases of idiopathic intracranial hypertension (IIH) revealed 17 that also had functional visual loss. This article reports the types of functional abnormalities in this group. Of the cases of patients with functional field loss, there were 82% with tubular fields, 71% with nonphysiologic constriction, 12% with spiraling on a Goldmann field, and 12% with crossed isopters on a Goldmann field. The majority (76%) had a nerve/field mismatch which they defined as no optic atrophy or gliosis in 13 and some optic atrophy but not consistent with field loss in 4. More than half (53%) had vision/behavior mismatch, 35% had fluctuating inconsistent vision, 29% had a functional neurologic exam, and 18% had monocular diplopia.

Their cases had significant concomitant psychiatric and/or psychosocial stressors in 88%, including chronic disease (fibromyalgia, systemic lupus erythematosus [SLE], hyperthyroidism, morbid obesity, malignant hypertension [HTN], diabetes mellitus [DM], stroke, multiple sclerosis [MS], sleep apnea, Crohn's disease, and asthma) in 59%; 24% each with mood disorder, substance abuse, or malingering; 6% each with borderline personality, motor vehicle accident (MVA), periodic homelessness, and 47% with multiple factors.

They correctly point out that real aspects of IIH on the vision system have to be addressed. The decision to treat medically versus surgically is normally based on progressive visual decline, which needs to be tempered when there are elements of functional vision loss. They suggest that functional patients may be more willing to undergo surgical treatment, which may reinforce the notion that the vision loss is real. Like previous studies of functional vision loss[1] the functional loss was persistent in the majority of their cases with only 2 showing improvement.

J. Leavitt, MD

Reference

1. Kathol RG, Cox TA, Corbett JJ, Thompson HS, et al. Functional visual loss: follow-up of 42 cases. *Arch Ophthalmol.* 1983;101:729-735.

High-sensitivity C-reactive protein measurements in patients with non-arteritic anterior ischaemic optic neuropathy: a clue to the presence of a microinflammatory response

Kesler A, Irge D, Rogowski O, et al (Tel Aviv Univ, Israel)

Acta Ophthalmol 87:216-221, 2009

Purpose.—To explore the possibility that individuals with non-arteritic anterior ischaemic optic neuropathy (NA-AION) harbour a heightened microinflammatory response compared to carefully matched controls.

Methods.—Diagnosis and follow-up were performed by a senior neuro-ophthalmologist (A.K.). The inflammatory biomarkers included white blood cell count, Westergren erythrocyte sedimentation rate (ESR), quantitative fibrinogen as well as high-sensitivity C-reactive protein (hs-CRP). The values of the inflammatory biomarkers of four and five matched controls were compared to patients with NA-AION.

Results.—We examined 33 NA-AION patients and 151 controls matched for age, gender, body mass index, oral temperature, smoking status and atherothrombotic risk factors. A significantly elevated concentration was noted for hs-CRP ($P = 0.021$): 3.3 mg/l for NA-AION patients and 2.1 mg/l for controls. Accelerated ESR (18.8 versus 13.5 mm/hr, $P = 0.025$) was noted in the NA-AION patients.

Conclusion.—Following appropriate matching to apparently healthy controls, patients with NA-AION presented a microinflammatory response, revealed by the presence of increased hs-CRP concentrations and accelerated ESR. The finding, if confirmed in future studies, might shed more light on the eventual pathophysiological processes involved in the disease and pave the way for new therapeutic approaches.

▶ The premise of this article is that patients with nonarteritic anterior ischemic optic neuropathy (NA-AION) may have a microinflammatory condition that predisposes them to develop the disease. They measured sedimentation rate (ESR) and high-sensitivity C-reactive protein (hs-CRP) in 33 patients with NA-AION compared with 151 controls. They used 4 to 5 controls per NA-AION patient and matched for a number of criteria (age, sex, body mass index, oral temperature, smoking status, and atherothrombotic risk factors). One limit of this study is that the blood work was collected up to 2 months after the onset of NA-AION.

They analyzed medication use in the 2 groups (medications included anticoagulant, hormone replacement, antihypertensive, cholesterol lowering medications, oral hypoglycemic, antiarrhythmic, and thyroid medications), and the only statistically significant difference was that the NA-AION group took more aspirin (63.6% vs 30.5%). This would indicate that the NA-AION patients were seen and started on aspirin before they were referred to the study center.

Comparing the ESR and hs-CRP between the 2 groups they found that the *P*-value for hs-CRP was .021 with the estimated marginal mean of 3.3 in the NA-AION group and 2.1 in the controls. Ten of the NA-AION patients had ESR > 30 and the corresponding hs-CRP was not included. They eliminated the diagnosis of A-AION because with long-term (1-3 years) follow-up there were no manifestations/clinical signs for AION or giant cell arteritis. The 2 patients with ESR > 60 had temporal artery biopsies, which were negative.

Previous studies have compared ESR and CRP in A-AION and NA-AION patients and found that the A-AION patients had significantly higher ESR and CRP ($P < .0001$).

This is an interesting preliminary study. The pathogenesis of NA-AION is controversial. A very recent review of ischemic optic neuropathy[1] did not discuss the contribution of ESR or CRP in the diagnosis of NA-AION.

J. Leavitt, MD

Reference

1. Hayreh SS. Ischemic optic neuropathy. *Prog Retin Eye Res.* 2009;28:34-62.

Neuromyelitis Optica IgG Serostatus in Fulminant Central Nervous System Inflammatory Demyelinating Disease

Magaña SM, Pittock SJ, Lennon VA, et al (Mayo Clinic College of Medicine, Rochester, MN)
Arch Neurol 66:964-966, 2009

Background.—The aquaporin-4–specific serum autoantibody neuromyelitis optica (NMO) IgG is a validated biomarker distinguishing NMO spectrum disorders from multiple sclerosis (MS). Because fulminant attacks are more common in NMO spectrum disorders than in MS, some investigators suggest that NMO IgG may be a marker of destructive demyelination rather than a disease-specific biomarker. To our knowledge, this study is the first to compare NMO IgG serostatus among patients with fulminant central nervous system inflammatory demyelinating disease (CNS IDD).

Objective.—To determine whether NMO IgG distinguishes patients with NMO spectrum disorders from those with other fulminant corticosteroid-refractory CNS IDD.

Design.—Descriptive historical cohort.

Setting.—Neuroimmunology laboratory and neurology practice, Mayo Clinic College of Medicine, Rochester, Minnesota.

Patients.—Serum samples from 74 patients who underwent plasmapheresis between February 24, 1993, and November 22, 2007, for a corticosteroid-refractory CNS IDD were tested for NMO IgG by indirect immunofluorescence assay.

Main Outcome Measures.—Two blinded observers scored serum samples tested at 1:120 dilution. Clinical data were obtained by medical record review.

Results.—Preplasmapheresis serum samples were available from 74 patients (ratio of women to men, 2:5); the mean interval between blood draw and plasmapheresis was 13 days. At the time of plasmapheresis, the mean age of patients was 46 years (age range, 7-80 years); the mean

Expanded Disability Status Scale score was 7.0 (score range, 3.5-9.5 [10.0 is death]). Diagnoses included MS (18 patients with definite and 11 patients with probable), longitudinally extensive transverse myelitis involving at least 3 vertebral segments (20 patients), NMO(14 patients), transverse myelitis involving fewer than 3 vertebral segments (8 patients), optic neuritis (2 patients), and acute disseminated encephalomyelitis (1 patient). Neuromyelitis optica IgG was detected in 20 patients (27%) (10 with longitudinally extensive transverse myelitis, 9 with NMO, and 1 with recurrent optic neuritis) and was not detected in any patient with MS, short transverse myelitis, monophasic optic neuritis, or acute disseminated encephalomyelitis.

Conclusion.—Neuromyelitis optica IgG is a specific biomarker for NMO spectrum disorders and is not simply a marker of destructive CNS IDD.

▶ Seventy-four patients with steroid refractory central nervous system (CNS) inflammatory demyelinating disease (IDD) underwent plasmapheresis at Mayo Clinic Rochester between February 24, 1993 and November 22, 2007. Their stored preplasmapheresis serum (taken 0-3 months before plasmapheresis) was analyzed in a masked fashion for the aquaporin-4-specific autoantibody neuromyelitis optica (NMO) IgG to see if there was any way to distinguish fulminating demyelinating disease from NMO. Diagnoses at the time of plasmapheresis included multiple sclerosis (MS) (29 patients), longitudinally extensive transverse myelitis (LETM) (20 patients), NMO (14 patients), short transverse myelitis (TM) (8 patients), optic neuritis (ON) (2 patients) and acute disseminated encephalomyelitis (ADEM) (1 patient). NMO IgG was found in 20 patients (27%)—10 with LETM, 9 with NMO, and 1 with recurrent ON. None of the patients with MS, ADEM, short TM or monophasic ON had a positive NMO IgG. Fifty percent of the NMO IgG positive patients had a relapse at the last follow-up, including 5 LETM patients who progressed to NMO.

They concluded that the absence of the NMO IgG in even the worst MS patients (requiring plasmapheresis) was another indicator that NMO and MS are distinct clinical entities. Also, the presence of the NMO IgG only in the NMO or NMO spectrum patients corroborates that the NMO IgG is not just a marker for severe CNS IDD but a biomarker specifically for NMO. NMO has a more fulminant course than MS with a different natural history and response to therapies so the distinction between the diseases should be determined early in the course of the disease.

J. Leavitt, MD

NMO-IgG detected in CSF in seronegative neuromyelitis optica

Klawiter EC, Alvarez E III, Xu J, et al (Washington Univ, St Louis, MO)

Neurology 72:1101-1103, 2009

Neuromyelitis optica (NMO) is an inflammatory and demyelinating disease characterized by recurrent attacks of optic neuritis (ON) and longitudinally extensive transverse myelitis (LETM). NMO is associated with antibodies against the aquaporin-4 (AQP4) water channel. NMO–immunoglobulin G (IgG) predicts a relapsing course and is a supportive criterion for NMO. The high risk of relapse, sometimes with devastating effects, makes early diagnosis important. Early identification permits counseling and consideration for immunosuppressive therapy. The serum NMO-IgG assay, using indirect immunofluorescence, is 73% sensitive and 91% specific for clinically defined NMO. While helpful when positive, the sensitivity is insufficient to exclude the diagnosis. We describe 3 of 26 patients with NMO at our institution with NMO-IgG positivity restricted to CSF.

▶ The authors report 3 cases with recurring numbness and/or weakness of extremities with resolution of the events after treatment with steroids alone, steroids with rituximab or azathioprine. None of their cases meet the diagnostic criteria for neuromyelitis (NMO) but would fit into the category of NMO spectrum disorder (eg, idiopathic single or recurrent events of longitudinally extensive myelitis [> 3 vertebral segment spinal cord lesion seen on MRI]).[1] All 3 had negative serum NMO Abs but positive spinal fluid NMO Abs.

Serum NMO Abs have become a distinguishing factor in differentiating NMO from multiple sclerosis (MS). Serum is fairly routinely stored and NMO Abs can be tested on stored serum retrospectively as was recently published.[2] NMO Abs in clinically definite NMO patients have similar titers of NMO Ab in serum and cerebrospinal fluid[3] suggesting that the NMO Ab is made peripherally. A more recent article also looked at cerebrospinal fluid and determined that NMO Ab is produced intrathecally and specifically targets aquaporin-4[4] early in the disease course. These articles suggest that NMO Abs in cerebrospinal fluid may become more important in our knowledge of the disease process and help refine the diagnosis of NMO versus NMO spectrum disorder in distinction from MS.

J. Leavitt, MD

References

1. Wingerchuk SM, Lennon VA, Lucchinetti CF, Pittock SJ, Weinshenker BG. The spectrum of neuromyelitis optica. *Lancet.* 2007;6:805-815.
2. Nishiyama S, Ito T, Misu T, et al. A case of NMO seropositive for aquaporin-4 antibody more than 10 years before onset. *Neurology.* 2009;72:1960-1961.
3. Takahashi T, Fujihara K, Nakashima I, et al. Anti-aquaporin-4 antibody is involved in the pathogenesis of NMO: a study on antibody titre. *Brain.* 2007; 130:1235-1243.
4. Bennett JL, Lam C, Kalluri SR, et al. Intrathecal pathogenic anti-aquaporin-4 antibodies in early neuromyelitis optica. *Ann Neurol.* http://www3.interscience.wiley.com. Published July 13, 2009. Accessed November 19, 2009.

Optical coherence tomography differs in neuromyelitis optica compared with multiple sclerosis

Naismith RT, Tutlam NT, Xu J, et al (Washington Univ, St Louis, MO)

Neurology 72:1077-1082, 2009

Background.—Neuromyelitis optica (NMO) is associated with destructive inflammatory lesions, resulting in necrosis and axonal injury. Disability from multiple sclerosis (MS) is due to a combination of demyelination and varying axonal involvement. Optical coherence tomography (OCT), by measuring retinal nerve fiber layer (RNFL) as a surrogate of axonal injury, has potential to discriminate between these two conditions.

Methods.—Included were 22 subjects with NMO or NMO spectrum disorders and 47 with MS. Seventeen subjects with NMO and all with MS had a remote history of optic neuritis (ON) in at least one eye, at least 6 months before OCT. Linear mixed modeling was used to compare the two diagnoses for a given level of vision loss, while controlling for age, disease duration, and number of episodes of ON.

Results.—After ON, NMO was associated with a thinner mean RNFL compared to MS. This was found when controlling for visual acuity (56.7 vs 66.6 μm, $p = 0.01$) or for contrast sensitivity (61.2 vs 70.3 μm, $p = 0.02$). The superior and inferior quadrants were more severely affected in NMO than MS.

Conclusions.—Optic neuritis (ON) within neuromyelitis optica (NMO) is associated with a thinner overall average retinal nerve fiber layer compared to multiple sclerosis, with particular involvement of the superior and inferior quadrants. This suggests that NMO is associated with more widespread axonal injury in the affected optic nerves. Optical coherence tomography can help distinguish the etiology of these two causes of ON, and may be useful as a surrogate marker of axonal involvement in demyelinating disease.

▶ Optical coherence tomography (OCT) was performed on 22 neuromyelitis optica (NMO) or NMO spectrum disorder patients and 47 multiple sclerosis (MS) patients. All the MS patients and 17 of 22 NMO patients had a history of optic neuritis in the remote past, in at least one eye. During acute optic neuritis the retinal nerve fiber layer may be increased in thickness. Their NMO subjects had more episodes of optic neuritis, worse vision and contrast sensitivity, and a higher Expanded Disability Status Scale (EDSS) score than the MS cohort. The OCT showed a thinner retinal nerve fiber layer in the NMO patients compared with the MS group. The data were not different enough to distinguish NMO optic neuritis from MS cases of optic neuritis. This study correlates with past literature and clinical experience in which NMO optic neuritis had a poorer prognosis than MS optic neuritis.[1]

J. Leavitt, MD

Reference

1. Papais-Alvarenga RM, Carellos SC, Alvarenga MP, Holander C, Bichara RP, Thuler LC. Clinical course of optic neuritis in patients with relapsing neuromyelitis optica. *Arch Opthahlmol.* 2008;126:12-16.

Optical coherence tomography helps differentiate neuromyelitis optica and MS optic neuropathies

Ratchford JN, Quigg ME, Conger A, et al (Johns Hopkins Univ School of Medicine, Baltimore, MD; Univ of Texas Southwestern Med Ctr, Dallas; et al)
Neurology 73:302-308, 2009

Objective.—To evaluate the retinal nerve fiber layer (RNFL) thickness and macular volume in neuromyelitis optica (NMO) spectrum patients using optical coherence tomography (OCT).

Background.—OCT can quantify damage to retinal ganglion cell axons and can identify abnormalities in multiple sclerosis and optic neuritis (ON) eyes. OCT may also be useful in the evaluation of patients with NMO.

Methods.—OCT and visual function testing were performed in 26 NMO spectrum patients with a history of ON, 17 patients with isolated longitudinally extensive transverse myelitis (LETM) without ON, 378 patients with relapsing-remitting multiple sclerosis (RRMS), and 77 healthy controls at 2 centers.

Results.—Substantial RNFL thinning was seen in NMO ON eyes (63.6 μm) relative to both RRMS ON eyes (88.3 μm, $p < 0.0001$) and control eyes (102.4 μm, $p < 0.0001$). A first episode of ON was estimated to cause 24 μm more loss of RNFL thickness in NMO than RRMS. Similar results were seen for macular volume. ON also was associated with more severe visual impairment in NMO spectrum patients than in RRMS patients. Eyes in the LETM group and unaffected NMO eyes were not significantly different from controls, though conclusions about these subgroups were limited by small sample sizes.

Conclusions.—Optical coherence tomography (OCT) shows more severe retinal damage after optic neuritis (ON) episodes in neuromyelitis optica (NMO) than in relapsing-remitting multiple sclerosis. Identification of substantial retinal nerve fiber layer loss (>15 μm) after ON in a non-multiple sclerosis patient should prompt consideration of an NMO spectrum condition. OCT may be a useful tool for the evaluation of patients with NMO.

► This is another study of optical coherence tomography (OCT) in neuromyelitis optica (NMO) patients (26 NMO spectrum disorder with a history of optic neuritis) compared with multiple sclerosis (MS) patients (378 of which 41% had a history of optic neuritis). Other groups measured with OCT included a control group of 77 subjects and 17 patients with isolated longitudinally extensive transverse myelitis. OCT was not possible to obtain in 8 blind eyes in the NMO group. OCT documented more retinal nerve fiber layer (RNFL) thinning in the NMO group compared with the control group with an absolute difference of 38%. The NMO eyes had a statistically significant thinner RNFL than MS subjects who had had optic neuritis, although the NMO subjects had had more episodes of optic neuritis. A subanalysis of the subjects who had only 1 episode of optic neuritis found greater thinning after the first episode than in subsequent events whether the patient had NMO or MS.

They conclude that there are a few situations in which OCT might be helpful in distinguishing NMO from MS. More severe thinning of the RNFL with a history of optic neuritis would be more consistent with NMO. They don't define severe, but suggest that a RNFL thickness at or below 60 μm corresponds to poor vision. More severe vision loss is consistent with the typical natural history of optic neuritis in NMO. The other situation in which OCT may be helpful is if there is greater than 15 μm difference in RNFL thickness between a patient's 2 eyes. This finding was more consistent with NMO (75%) than relapsing-remitting multiple sclerosis (RRMS) (24%). OCT is 1 element of the total evaluation of a patient with optic neuritis. Clinical history and examination, brain MRI, spinal fluid, and NMO-immunoglobulin G (IgG) antibody must be looked at in conjunction with OCT to determine the etiology in optic neuritis patients.

J. Leavitt, MD

11 Neuroradiology

Acute Toxic Leukoencephalopathy: Potential for Reversibility Clinically and on MRI With Diffusion-Weighted and FLAIR Imaging

McKinney AM, Kieffer SA, Paylor RT, et al (Univ of Minnesota Med Ctr and Hennepin County Med Ctr, Minneapolis; et al)

AJR Am J Roentgenol 193:192-206, 2009

Objective.—Toxic leukoencephalopathy may present acutely or subacutely with symmetrically reduced diffusion in the periventricular and supraventricular white matter, hereafter referred to as periventricular white matter. This entity may reverse both on imaging and clinically. However, a gathering together of the heterogeneous causes of this disorder as seen on MRI with diffusion-weighted imaging (DWI) and an analysis of their likelihood to reverse has not yet been performed. Our goals were to gather causes of acute or subacute toxic leukoencephalopathy that can present with reduced diffusion of periventricular white matter in order to promote recognition of this entity, to evaluate whether DWI with apparent diffusion coefficient (ADC) values can predict the extent of chronic FLAIR abnormality (imaging reversibility), and to evaluate whether DWI can predict the clinical outcome (clinical reversibility).

Materials and Methods.—Two neuroradiologists retrospectively reviewed the MRI examinations of 39 patients with acute symptoms and reduced diffusion of periventricular white matter. The reviewers then scored the extent of abnormality on DWI and FLAIR. ADC ratios of affected white matter versus the unaffected periventricular white matter were obtained. Each patient's clinical records were reviewed to determine the cause and clinical outcome. Histology findings were available in three patients. Correlations were calculated between the initial MRI markers and both the clinical course and the follow-up extent on FLAIR using Spearman's correlation coefficient.

Results.—Of the initial 39 patients, seven were excluded because of a nontoxic cause (hypoxic–ischemic encephalopathy [HIE] or congenital genetic disorders) or because of technical errors. In the remaining 32 patients, no correlation was noted between any of the initial MRI markers (percentage of ADC reduction, DWI extent, or FLAIR extent) with the clinical outcome. Three patients had histologic correlation. However, moderate correlation was seen between the extent of abnormality on initial FLAIR and the extent on follow-up FLAIR ($r = 0.441$, $p = 0.047$). Of the 13 patients who underwent repeat MRI at 21 days or longer, the reduced diffusion resolved in all but one. Significant differences were noted between ADC values in affected white matter versus unaffected periventricular white matter on initial ($p < 0.0001$) but not on follow-up MRI ($p = 0.13$), and in affected white matter on initial versus follow-up ($p = 0.0014$) in those individuals who underwent repeat imaging on the same magnet ($n = 9$), confirming resolution of the DWI abnormalities.

Conclusion.—Acute toxic leukoencephalopathy with reduced diffusion may be clinically reversible and radiologically reversible on DWI, and may also be reversible, but to a lesser degree, on FLAIR MRI. None of the imaging markers measured in this study appears to correlate with clinical outcome, which underscores the necessity for prompt recognition of this entity. Alerting the clinician to this potentially reversible syndrome can facilitate treatment and removal of the offending agent in the early stages.

▶ The common and shared appearance of the multitude of disorders and insults that may lead to acute toxic leukoencephalopathy (ATL) has not yet been well defined based on diffusion-weighted imaging (DWI) or fluid attenuated inversion recovery (FLAIR) imaging. There are a number of case reports or small studies describing diffuse white matter insults on FLAIR and/or DWI in a myriad of causes that include, but are not limited to, chemotherapy, carbon monoxide poisoning, toxic drug ingestions/inhalations, hepatic disease/hyperammonemia, and a number of medications. This author and his colleagues set out to define a common appearance of these disorders based on a retrospective review and to demonstrate that this appearance can range from being rather subtle to profound but is a potentially reversible condition if this characteristic imaging appearance is noted on DWI or FLAIR MRI. However, some patients had severe outcomes, and factors that precipitated those poor outcomes were not identified. An incomplete list of disorders is provided that may cause this diffuse symmetric white matter involvement on FLAIR or DWI MRI, although this should be an adequate foundation for classifying the imaging appearances and grading the severity for future studies evaluating ATL.

The disorder that most commonly can simulate this appearance is the subacute phase of hypoxic-ischemic encephalopathy (HIE), where cortical insults and resultant axonal degeneration are probably the factors that lead to subacute phase white matter abnormalities on FLAIR and DWI. However, these cases, typically, have a much poorer outcome than ATL. Notably, none of the measured imaging markers correlated with the clinical outcome, which would seem to underscore the potential reversibility of the disease even in severely involved cases based on MRI.

A. M. McKinney IV, MD

Aging of the Cervical Spine in Healthy Volunteers: A 10-Year Longitudinal Magnetic Resonance Imaging Study

Okada E, Matsumoto M, Ichihara D, et al (Keio Univ, Tokyo, Japan; et al)

Spine 34:706-712, 2009

Study Design.—Prospective longitudinal study, mean follow-up period; 11.7 ± 0.8 years was conducted from 1995 to 2007.

Objective.—To clarify normal aging process of cervical spine and correlation between progression of disc degeneration and development of clinical symptoms.

Summary of Background Data.—Aging of the cervical spine can inevitably occur in anyone. Long-term longitudinal studies following the same individuals are necessary to elucidate the accurate aging processes of the cervical spine.

Methods.—Two hundred twenty-three subjects of 497 original cohorts (123 men, 100 women, mean age: 39.0 ± 15.0, follow-up rate: 44.9%). Subjects, who underwent MRI 10 years ago, underwent another MRI, neurologic examination, and questionnaire survey regarding symptoms related to cervical spine and life style. Following 5 MR findings representing intervertebral disc degeneration were evaluated: (1) decrease in signal intensity of disc, (2) anterior compression of dura and spinal cord, (3) posterior disc protrusion (PDP), (4) disc space narrowing (DSN), and (5) foraminal stenosis (FS).

Results.—Progression of degenerative findings was observed in 189 subjects (81.1%). Progression of decrease in signal intensity of disc was observed in 59.6%, anterior compression of dura and spinal cord in 61.4%, PDP in 70.0%, DSN in 26.9%, and FS in 9.0%. Logistic regression analysis revealed that incidence of progression of PDP, DSN, FS was higher in elderly subjects. There were no correlations between any degenerative MR findings and sex, smoking, alcohol, sport, or body mass index. Neck pain, shoulder stiffness, and numbness in upper extremities were recognized in 9.9%, 30.0%, and 4.0% of subjects, and 1 or more clinical symptoms have developed in 34.1% during 10 years.

Conclusion.—Progression of degeneration of cervical spine on MRI was frequently observed during 10-year period, with development of symptoms in 34% of subjects. No factor related to progression of degeneration of cervical spine was identified except for age.

► The authors provide this study as an approximately 10-year follow-up to their previous MRI study, which demonstrated that incidence of cervical spine findings increased with age and that 17% and 12% of male and female teenagers and 86% and 89% of male and female subjects older than 60 years have degenerative findings to some degree.[1] In this study, the 10-year follow-up MRIs of volunteers demonstrated that progression of degenerative findings in previously asymptomatic subjects closely correlated with increasing age and that none of the measured factors (gender, smoking, alcohol, sports, and body mass index) correlated with a progression in degenerative findings.

Although the increase with age is at first glance intuitive, the lack of other associated factors combined with the fact that these patients were initially asymptomatic raises the question in this author's mind that genetics probably plays a major role in the susceptibility toward degenerative findings, although this susceptibility increases in all patients with age. The presence of mild degenerative findings in the teenage population, albeit a minority, would lend some support to this concept.

A. M. McKinney IV, MD

Reference

1. Matsumoto M, Fujimura Y, Suzuki N, et al. MRI of cervical intervertebral discs in asymptomatic subjects. *J Bone Joint Surg Br.* 1998;80:19-24.

Automated MRI measures identify individuals with mild cognitive impairment and Alzheimer's disease

Desikan RS, Alzheimer's Disease Neuroimaging Initiative (Massachusetts General Hosp, Charlestown; et al)
Brain 132:2048-2057, 2009

Mild cognitive impairment can represent a transitional state between normal ageing and Alzheimer's disease. Non-invasive diagnostic methods are needed to identify mild cognitive impairment individuals for early therapeutic interventions. Our objective was to determine whether automated magnetic resonance imaging-based measures could identify mild cognitive impairment individuals with a high degree of accuracy. Baseline volumetric T_1-weighted magnetic resonance imaging scans of 313 individuals from two independent cohorts were examined using automated software tools to identify the volume and mean thickness of 34 neuroanatomic regions. The first cohort included 49 older controls and 48 individuals with mild cognitive impairment, while the second cohort included 94 older controls and 57 mild cognitive impairment individuals. Sixty-five patients with probable Alzheimer's disease were also included for comparison. For the discrimination of mild cognitive impairment, entorhinal cortex thickness, hippocampal volume and supramarginal gyrus thickness demonstrated an area under the curve of 0.91 (specificity 94%, sensitivity 74%, positive likelihood ratio 12.12, negative likelihood ratio 0.29) for the first cohort and an area under the curve of 0.95 (specificity 91%, sensitivity 90%, positive likelihood ratio 10.0, negative likelihood ratio 0.11) for the second cohort. For the discrimination of Alzheimer's disease, these three measures demonstrated an area under the curve of 1.0. The three magnetic resonance imaging measures demonstrated significant correlations with clinical and neuropsychological assessments as well as with cerebrospinal fluid levels of tau, hyperphosphorylated tau and abeta 42 proteins. These results demonstrate that automated magnetic resonance imaging measures can serve as an *in vivo* surrogate for disease severity, underlying neuropathology and as a non-invasive diagnostic method for mild cognitive impairment and Alzheimer's disease.

▶ As there would be great clinical utility in being able to separate mild cognitive impairment (MCI) from early Alzheimer disease (AD) based on imaging, an automated or computer-aided detection (CAD) approach could facilitate early detection. CAD has been used previously in a number of other brain and non-cerebral disorders. However, often CAD is similar to or does not add much additional information (and actually may lead to unnecessary work up) relative to neuroradiologists experienced in a particular disorder.

However, in this report the authors used a CAD algorithm with coregistration to measure cortical thickness and volume in various regions of interest, obtained neuropsychological testing, and calculated/correlated which measures best separated MCI from controls using online patient databases. Significant differences were obtained for numerous regions, while the sensitivity (73%-90%) and specificity (91%-94%) were relatively high. The correlation between the various cerebrospinal fluid markers and MRI measures of entorhinal cortex, supramarginal gyrus thickness, and hippocampal volumes would seem to validate these findings.

The importance of such findings is that even an experienced neuroradiologist will have difficulty in separating these disorders, even with the aid of 3-dimensional (3D) imaging, etc. The authors do point out a potential significant limitation that this was not used in a clinical setting where other subtypes of dementia and various other clinical disorders that may cause cognitive impairment would need to be ruled out. Hence, while evaluation by a neuroradiologist is critical in excluding other disorders, the CAD technique that the authors describe could be invaluable in distinguishing these 2 disorders.

A. M. McKinney IV, MD

CT Angiography for Brain Death Diagnosis

Frampas E, Videcoq M, de Kerviler E, et al (CHU Nantes Hôtel-Dieu, Nantes, France; Hôpital Mére et Enfants, Nantes, France; Hôpital Saint-Louis, Paris, France; et al)

AJNR Am J Neuroradiol 30:1566-1570, 2009

Background and Purpose.—Lack of cerebral circulation is an important confirmatory test for brain death (BD). Conventional angiography remains the standard imaging method, but CT angiography (CTA) is emerging as an alternative. France accepts BD diagnoses relying on a score based on lack of opacification of 7 intracerebral vessels in CTA images. The purpose of this study was to validate the efficiency of this score and to evaluate the sensitivity of a novel 4-point CTA score in confirming BD.

Materials and Methods.—A prospective multicentric study was conducted during 12 months with 105 patients referred for CTA to confirm a clinical diagnosis of BD. Clinical data were recorded. CTA images were interpreted first by local radiologists at the referent center, resulting in a 7-point score based on lack of opacification of the pericallosal and cortical segments of the middle cerebral arteries (MCAs), internal cerebral veins (ICVs), and 1 great cerebral vein per patient and, second, by a consensus panel of 3 expert radiologists, blinded to the initial scores, resulting in novel 4-point scores based on the lack of opacification of the cortical segments of the MCAs and ICVs.

Results.—Injection of contrast medium did not alter renal function. With the initial 7-point score, sensitivity was 62.8%. With the simplified 4-point score, sensitivity was 85.7% and specificity was 100%. Opacification of ICVs was absent in 98.1% of patients.

Conclusions.—Lack of opacification in the cortical segments of the MCAs and internal veins in CTA is efficient and reliable for confirming BD.

▶ Frampas et al address an interesting and yet critical scenario that most neuroradiologists have become embroiled in at some point regarding CT angiography (CTA): What are the significant intracranial vascular findings in surveillance for brain death? They did not approach it from the standpoint that the diagnosis of brain death was not yet suspected or in the hyperacute phase (< 12 hours onset of coma), which may occur in emergent scans immediately postsevere traumatic brain injury where CTA may be ordered immediately following the unenhanced CT showing severe hemorrhage, herniation, and fractures (I have personally encountered this a number of times). However, their prospective evaluation of CTA in brain death (BD) is no less important in 105 patients with clinical suspicion of BD, where the mean time from initial coma and absence of brain stem reflexes were 67 hours, and the mean time of apnea test was 87 hours. A previous 7-point CTA scoring by Dupas et al included the pericallosal arteries, middle cerebral arteries (MCA), internal cerebral veins (ICV), and great cerebral vein.[1] In this article, Frampas et al modified that scoring system to a more select and novel system of both MCAs and ICVs, which was 85.7% sensitive (when all 4 vessels do not opacify by 60 seconds after contrast medium injection). They did conduct the 7-point scoring system as well, which was only 62.7% sensitive (when all 7 vessels do not opacify). They maintain that the examination was 100% specific based on 10 catheter angiograms and 12 EEGs performed for confirmation when the CTA score was < 7. One should note that given that several days were present between the onset of coma and absence of brain stem reflexes and positive apnea test, along with the scoring of patients known to clinically have brain death, there is an expectation bias. In this author's opinion, prospective studies of CTAs in patients presenting with severe traumatic brain injury and herniation with CTA within the first 24 to 48 hours of admission could be of further importance, because in those patients it would be helpful to know the status of these arteries as well as potentially also evaluate the internal carotid artery, dural sinuses, and possibly even the external carotid to internal carotid ratio in density/contrast concentration.

A. M. McKinney IV, MD

Reference

1. Dupas B, Gayet-Delacroix M, Villers D, Antonioli D, Vecchierini MF, Soulillou JP. Diagnosis of brain death using two-phase spiral CT. *AJNR Am J Neuroradiol.* 1998;19:641-647.

Differences in CT Perfusion Maps Generated by Different Commercial Software: Quantitative Analysis by Using Identical Source Data of Acute Stroke Patients

Kudo K, Sasaki M, Yamada K, et al (Iwate Med Univ, Morioka, Japan; Kyoto Prefectural Univ of Medicine, Japan; et al)

Radiology 254:200-209, 2010

Purpose.—To examine the variability in the qualitative and quantitative results of computed tomographic (CT) perfusion imaging generated from identical source data of stroke patients by using commercially available software programs provided by various CT manufacturers.

Materials and Methods.—Institutional review board approval and informed consent were obtained. CT perfusion imaging data of 10 stroke patients were postprocessed by using five commercial software packages, each of which had a different algorithm: singular-value decomposition (SVD), maximum slope (MS), inverse filter (IF), box modulation transfer function (bMTF), and by using custom-made original software with standard (sSVD) and block-circulant (bSVD) SVD methods. Areas showing abnormalities in cerebral blood flow (CBF), mean transit time (MTT), and cerebral blood volume (CBV) were compared with each other and with the final infarct areas. Differences among the ratios of quantitative values in the final infarct areas and those in the unaffected side were also examined.

Results.—The areas with CBF or MTT abnormalities and the ratios of these values significantly varied among software, while those of CBV were stable. The areas with CBF or MTT abnormalities analyzed by using SVD or bMTF corresponded to those obtained with delay-sensitive sSVD, but overestimated the final infarct area. The values obtained from software by using MS or IF corresponded well with those obtained from the delay-insensitive bSVD and the final infarct area. Given the similarities between CBF and MTT, all software were separated in two groups (ie, sSVD and bSVD). The ratios of CBF or MTTs correlated well within both groups, but not across them.

Conclusion.—CT perfusion imaging maps were significantly different among commercial software even when using identical source data, presumably because of differences in tracer-delay sensitivity.

► The negative results of the phase III Desmoteplase in Acute Ischemic Stroke (DIAS-2) trial[1] in the 3- to 9-hour window postsymptom onset have led to a resurgence in evaluating and discussing the technical differences in various CT perfusion (CTP) and MR perfusion (MRP) techniques regarding scan parameters, postprocessing algorithms, and software, as these differences may have led to suboptimal patient selection in that study. The lack of standardization among CTP and MRP postprocessing vendors arises from the fact that most of the original studies validating CTP were based on deconvolution algorithms, while most of these seminal validation studies between the 1990s to early 2000s used deconvolution algorithms that were typically in normal humans or animals. Hence, there was a delay in recognizing the shortcomings of the available CTP algorithms.

This article is part of a new process of revisiting CTP algorithms by comparison between several of the major CTP postprocessing vendors. This article compares the results in 10 patients with acute stroke with final infarct size as well as with what can be termed delay-invariant algorithms. The authors noted a significant overestimation of the ischemic regions on cerebral blood flow (CBF) and mean transit time (MTT) maps with the standard delay-sensitive singular value decomposition (SVD) algorithms versus the delay-invariant SVD (dSVD) and block-circulant decomposition algorithms. The reason that SVD algorithms (the most commonly used and initially validated software) may overestimate these parameters is that the SVD algorithm assumes that the signal intensity in the tissue of interest (cerebrum) does not arrive before the measured arterial input (a chosen artery), which may be an incorrect assumption in the setting of blocked vessels and other scenarios. Hence, delay-invariant SVD and block-circulant methods were shown to be more accurate with final infarct size. Notably, the cerebral blood volume (CBV), considered the best marker of infarct, did not change significantly between vendors. These phenomenons have already been demonstrated on MRP as well. An excellent discussion and overview of these concepts and the significance of this article are provided by Konstas and Lev in an editorial in the January issue of *Radiology*.[2]

Although SVD algorithms may overestimate the at-risk penumbra, it should be noted that CBV did not change significantly between these algorithms and that it has not yet been evaluated whether the penumbra overestimation (by way of overestimating MTT and underestimating CBF) is a bad thing (ie, this has not been shown yet to change therapy or outcome). Could it be that these algorithms are more sensitive even though the early data would lead one to think that SVD is not as specific as dSVD? Hence, prospective studies are forthcoming, but in the meantime this author would recommend that those with available SVD software as well as dSVD or block-circulant software should review both delay-sensitive (SVD) and delay-invariant (dSVD) deconvolutional maps in concert until these questions of postprocessing algorithm/software standardization are settled. This author's preliminary experience is that dSVD is more specific in predicting the final infarct size, while SVD appears more sensitive but more prone to artifacts and surreptitious conditions or inappropriate vascular (arterial and venous input) selection that can lead to simulated infarcts.

A. M. McKinney IV, MD

References

1. Liebeskind DS. Reversing stroke in the 2010s: lessons from Desmoteplase In Acute ischemic Stroke-2 (DIAS-2). *Stroke*. 2009;40:3156-3158.
2. Konstas AA, Lev MH. CT perfusion imaging of acute stroke: the need for arrival time, delay insensitive, and standardized postprocessing algorithms? *Radiology*. 2010;254:22-25.

Differentiation of Recurrent Glioblastoma Multiforme from Radiation Necrosis after External Beam Radiation Therapy with Dynamic Susceptibility-weighted Contrast-enhanced Perfusion MR Imaging

Barajas RF Jr, Chang JS, Segal MR, et al (Univ of California, San Francisco)
Radiology 253:486-496, 2009

Purpose.—To investigate whether cerebral blood volume (CBV), peak height (PH), and percentage of signal intensity recovery (PSR) measurements derived from the results of T2*-weighted dynamic susceptibility-weighted contrast material–enhanced (DSC) magnetic resonance (MR) imaging performed after external beam radiation therapy (EBRT) can be used to distinguish recurrent glioblastoma multiforme (GBM) from radiation necrosis.

Materials and Methods.—Fifty-seven patients were enrolled in this HIPAA-compliant institutional review board–approved retrospective study after they received a diagnosis of GBM, underwent EBRT, and were examined with DSC MR imaging, which revealed progressive contrast enhancement within the radiation field. A definitive diagnosis was established at subsequent surgical resection or clinicoradiologic follow-up. Regions of interest were retrospectively drawn around the entire contrast-enhanced region. This created T2*-weighted signal intensity–time curves that produced three cerebral hemodynamic MR imaging measurements: CBV, PH, and PSR. Welch *t* tests were used to compare measurements between groups.

Results.—Mean, maximum, and minimum relative PH and relative CBV were significantly higher ($P < .01$) in patients with recurrent GBM than in patients with radiation necrosis. Mean, maximum, and minimum relative PSR values were significantly lower ($P < .05$) in patients with recurrent GBM than in patients with radiation necrosis.

Conclusion.—These findings suggest that DSC perfusion MR imaging may be used to differentiate recurrent GBM from EBRT-induced radiation necrosis.

▶ Building on previous studies[1] that have demonstrated differences in various MR perfusion (MRP) values between recurrent glioblastoma multiforme (GBM) and radiation necrosis, the authors set out to evaluate whether recurrent tumor could be discriminated from radiation necrosis based on selecting the contrast enhancing portion as the region of interest (ROI). This mode of generating the ROI is important, as there has been dispute among neuroradiologists as to which ROI to select (whether the area that enhances the most, is the most solid, or gets the darkest on dynamic perfusion images) and as to which MRP values are the most sensitive for tumor (many parameters have been suggested). One nice factor in this study is the reproducibility; it is rather quite simple for most neuroradiologists, neurosurgeons, or neurologists to select the enhancing portion and encircle it as a ROI.

Based on that relatively reproducible method, the authors found that relative peak height (rPH) analysis of the dynamic first-pass contrast curve and relative cerebral blood volume (rCBV) were elevated compared with the visually non-affected white matter (NAWM); an rPH threshold of >2.17 was seen only in recurrent tumor. While rPH and rCBV had sensitivities of only 89% and 79%, respectively, with less specificity, and also, the sensitivities and specificities are lower than when MRP is used in the initial diagnosis,[2] one must keep in mind that there are no set standards or thresholds and that MRP is a work in progress not to be interpreted in an information void. In other words, there are other imaging characteristics and sequences such as diffusion-weighted imaging (DWI), MR spectroscopy, susceptibility-weighted imaging (SWI), and subtraction techniques that can tilt the scale of diagnosis in 1 direction or another. Personally, I have found this article quite helpful in providing additional reproducible measurements to the neuroradiologist's armamentarium in diagnosing recurrent high-grade primary brain tumors. In particular, it seems that a combination of calculating MRP-based rCBV and rPH along with the postcontrast findings on T1-weighted imaging (T1WI), DWI, and, recently, SWI may act in synergy to augment our diagnosis rates of recurrent tumor. At this point what is necessary is a prospective study using the mentioned techniques to develop a diagnosis diagram of some sort. The benefit of MRP, DWI, and SWI is the feasibility with which such images can be obtained in the same sitting as the routine brain MRI sequences with the addition of less than 5 to 10 minutes of total scanning time for these 3 techniques, depending on the technical abilities of a given MR scanner.

A. M. McKinney IV, MD

References

1. Barajas RF, Chang JS, Sneed PK, Segal MR, McDermott MW, Cha S. Distinguishing recurrent intra-axial metastatic tumor from radiation necrosis following gamma knife radiosurgery using dynamic susceptibility-weighted contrast-enhanced perfusion MR imaging. *AJNR Am J Neuroradiol.* 2009;30:367-372.
2. Arvinda HR, Kesavadas C, Sarma PS, et al. Glioma grading: sensitivity, specificity, positive and negative predictive values of diffusion and perfusion imaging. *J Neurooncol.* 2009;94:87-96.

Motor Homunculus: Passive Mapping in Healthy Volunteers by Using Functional MR Imaging—Initial Results

Kocak M, Ulmer JL, Ugurel MS, et al (The Med College of Wisconsin, Milwaukee; et al)

Radiology 251:485-492, 2009

Purpose.—To determine the concurrence of activation in the primary motor cortex, induced by paradigms of active and passive movement of extremities, by using blood oxygen level–dependent functional magnetic resonance (MR) imaging.

Materials and Methods.—The HIPAA-compliant study was approved by the institutional review board, and written informed consent was obtained from the participating volunteers. Functional MR imaging data were collected from 11 healthy volunteers (four women, seven men; age range, 24–42 years) during active and passive movements of hand, elbow, shoulder, ankle, knee, and hip. These data were then mapped onto three-dimensional anatomic images. Volumes of activation were determined by using cross-correlation analysis at a coefficient threshold of 0.4 ($P < .01$). Regions of interest were drawn in pre- and postcentral gyri based on anatomic criteria. The mean number of activated voxels in the pre- and postcentral gyri induced by active and passive movements was compared by using Wilcoxon analysis. Concurrence ratios and proportional ratios of activation between active and passive movements were calculated for each somatotopic location.

Results.—Primary motor cortex activation tended to increase with active compared with passive movements, although in the precentral gyrus, hand, elbow, and shoulder movements showed no statistically significant difference in mean number of activated voxels. In the postcentral gyrus, only the shoulder revealed a significant difference ($P < .05$). Concurrence ratios (activation volume overlap of two tasks/ combined activation area of both tasks) ranged from 0.44 to 0.57. Proportional ratios (activation volume overlap of passive task with active task/total activation volume of passive task) ranged from 0.64 to 0.82.

Conclusion.—Passive movement paradigms may be an alternative to or complement to active movement tasks in patient populations.

► In this quite interesting study, the authors used functional MRI (fMRI) to demonstrate that motor cortex activation occurs to some degree use passive movements. The study used 6 joints (hand, elbow, shoulder, ankle, knee, and hip) in 11 volunteers, whereby the differences between active and passive motion of these joints were measured using blood oxygen level dependent (BOLD) measurements in the precentral and postcentral gyri at various anatomic landmarks. A statistical analysis was then applied comparing these landmarks in the active versus the passive states. As expected, there was somewhat greater activation overall in the active versus the passive state with most movements; however, surprisingly there were no significant differences specifically for the ankle, knee, and hip in the precentral gyri between active versus passive states. The authors point out an anatomic basis for this activation based on previous research describing how afferent inputs may modulate efferent outputs from the primary motor cortex.

These results may significantly further the abilities of fMRI research by enabling passive studies of the primary motor homunculus in the precentral gyrus. One of the greatest potential uses in this author's opinion is in early pediatric patients and in developmental delay, although this has yet to be proven facile and validated in the sedated population. Research in animals or in patients with dementia, Parkinson's, or other neurologic conditions preventing voluntary motor control are other possibilities that come immediately to mind. Hence, this preliminary study points to a significant alternative method of evaluating motor cortex activation via passive movement paradigms, which will require further studies in various populations to determine the reproducibility of these results.

A. M. McKinney IV, MD

Somatostatin Receptor Scintigraphy for Optic Nerve Sheath Meningiomas

Saeed P, Tanck MWT, Freling N, et al (Univ of Amsterdam, The Netherlands)
Ophthalmology 116:1581-1586, 2009

Objective.—To investigate the value of somatostatin receptor scintigraphy (SSRS) in the diagnosis of optic nerve sheath meningiomas (ONSMs).

Design.—Prospective, comparative case series.

Participants.—SSRS was used to investigate 68 orbits in 61 patients diagnosed with an orbital tumor.

Methods.—Patients were injected intravenously with 200 MBq of indium-111 (^{111}In)-octreotide. SSRS with single photon emission computed tomography (SPECT) was performed 24 hours after injection.

Main Outcome Measures.—The ^{111}In-octreotide uptake in orbital lesions was determined by semiquantitative uptake-ratio analysis (lesion/brain) on attenuation-corrected transverse SPECT slices.

Results.—All orbital meningiomas, including 14 ONSMs and 12 spheno-orbital meningiomas, showed high median ^{111}In-octreotide uptake ratios of 7.2 (range, 4.6–15.4) and 16.3 (range, 4.6–15.4), respectively. In 7 patients with a diagnosis of ONSM, the SSRS uptake ratio was significantly decreased 2.7 (1–6.8) after treatment with 54 Gy of radiotherapy. Median uptake ratios of other tumors were vascular anomalies/vascular tumors, 1.2 (range, 0.5–3.3); non-Hodgkin lymphomas, 2.9 (range, 0.9–4.2); optic nerve gliomas, 1.5 (range, 0.2–3.3); and idiopathic orbital inflammation, 1.6 (range, 1.4–1.9). By using a threshold uptake ratio of 5.9, the sensitivity of SSRS with ^{111}In-octreotide for ONSM was 100%, with a specificity of 97.2%.

Conclusions.—SSRS is a useful additional tool in diagnosing ONSM and has 100% sensitivity and 97% specificity at a threshold uptake ratio of 5.9.

▶ This was a nonrandomized collection of patients ("Patients" section in Materials and Methods identifies "Sixty-one patients" and the listing of tumor types in Table 1 in the original article adds up to 61, but the "Results" section includes "16 male and 46 female patients") diagnosed with an orbital tumor who were referred to an orbit clinic. Of these, 14 were diagnosed with an optic nerve sheath meningioma (ONSM) and 12 with sphenoid wing meningioma (the other cases had other primary orbital tumors or inflammation). Half of the ONSM cases had histopathological confirmation of the diagnosis. Meningiomas have been found to be rich in somatostatin receptors (SSR). Scintigraphy for SSR can be performed using indium-111 (^{111}In)-diethylenetriamine pentaacetic acid-octreotide uptake to help distinguish meningioma from other entities. The uptake ratios (comparing the involved orbit to noninvolved brain) for all forms of meningioma were statistically significant when compared with nonmeningioma orbital tumors ($P < .001$). Median uptake ratios were 16.3 for sphenoid wing meningiomas and 7.2 for ONSM. For the 7 histologically proven cases of ONSM, they calculated a sensitivity of 100% with a specificity of 97.2% using a score of 5.9 as the cutoff. This distinguished ONSM from vascular lesions, non-Hodgkin's lymphoma, and optic nerve glioma. The 1 ONSM case shown in the figure in the original article was not a classic ONSM and may be the type of case in which this test would be most useful—a large nondescript tumor. For lesions less than 1-cm size, scintigraphy may not be helpful. On a cautionary note, melanoma can have SSRs as well, so a metastatic melanoma should be in the differential. Most cases of ONSM have classic features on neuroimaging (tram tracking and contrast enhancement) and can be radiated without histopathology once vision loss occurs. In those cases that are not classic, SSR scintigraphy may be a useful nonsurgical diagnostic tool. Limitations of the technique may occur if the tumor size is too small.

J. Leavitt, MD

The Accuracy of [^{18}F]Fluorodeoxyglucose Positron Emission Tomography as Confirmed by Biopsy in the Diagnosis of Spine Metastases in a Cancer Population

Laufer I, Lis E, Pisinski L, et al (Memorial Sloan-Kettering Cancer Ctr, NY; Harlem Hosp, NY)

Neurosurgery 64:107-114, 2009

Objective.—To determine the accuracy of [^{18}F]fluorodeoxyglucose (FDG) positron emission tomography (PET) in the diagnosis of vertebral metastases in patients with cancer using needle-biopsy results and patient follow-up data.

Methods.—A retrospective chart review of all patients who underwent a needle biopsy of a spinal lesion and underwent FDG-PET within

6 weeks of the biopsy was performed. Biopsy results and magnetic resonance imaging and computed tomographic appearance of the biopsied lesion, as well as long-term clinical follow-up data, were recorded for each patient. A total of 82 patients with solid tumors and hematological spine metastases were included in this study.

Results.—The mean standardized uptake values of lesions with active cancer were 7.1 and 2.1 in benign lesions ($P < 0.02$). In patients with metastatic solid tumors, the mean standardized uptake value was 7.3. Stratification of solid tumor lesions according to whether they had a sclerotic appearance on computed tomographic scans showed that FDG-PET was a significantly better predictor of cancer status in lytic or mixed lesions. In patients with a history of solid tumors, there was 100% concordance between the FDG-PET and needle-biopsy diagnoses in nonsclerotic lesions, when the standardized uptake value cutoff of 2 was used.

Conclusion.—FDG-PET is an accurate screening test for vertebral metastases in cancer patients. It is especially accurate in patients with nonsclerotic vertebral lesions and a history of solid malignancy.

▶ As [^{18}F]fluorodeoxyglucose (FDG)-PET is increasingly used in the initial work up to evaluate for metastatic disease of the lungs, mediastinum, neck, abdomen/pelvis, and lymph nodes, there is a need to determine the accuracy of FDG-PET in regard to the vertebral lesions visualized. As the authors state, up to 10% of all metastases are found in the vertebral column[1] and hence, there are many malignancies that may present with metastastic disease to the bone first. Thus, although FDG-PET is not yet indicated as the primary examination to evaluate for metastatic bone disease, it would be extremely helpful to figure out the chance that hot or elevated metabolic activity bone lesion is a metastasis. The authors retrospectively reviewed CT-guided biopsy results to determine the status of FDG-PET lesions.

The authors demonstrate that nonsclerotic (ie lytic) vertebral lesions with elevated standardized uptake value (SUV) >2.0 had a 100% sensitivity and specificity for being metastases. The sensitivity (98%) was similar, but the specificity was (50%) much lower for lesions that were mixed density or sclerotic with that SUV threshold. However, the mean SUV in malignant lesions was 7.1 and in benign lesions was 2.1. Notably, the sensitivity of MRI or CT as compared with FDG-PET or a prospective analysis of FDG-PET-positive lesions was not performed.

Therefore, their results suggest that a cutoff SUV of 2.0 is excellent for determining a nonsclerotic lesion to be a metastasis, but one should exercise care in the setting of a sclerotic lesion (such as commonly occurs with prostate or breast metastases) or mixed lytic-sclerotic lesions, as many benign sclerotic lesions can have slightly elevated metabolic uptake. Again, this study was based on a retrospective review of CT-guided biopsy results, where benign-appearing lesions would not usually be accepted for biopsy, thus possibly leading to some expectation bias in this study. A prospective analysis of FDG-PET-positive lesions is necessary. Hence, a slightly more cautious SUV threshold between 2.5 and 3.0 for predicting a metastatic lesion would be this author's suggestion based on experience in FDG-PET interpretation for 7 years and previous literature.[2]

A. M. McKinney IV, MD

References

1. Bilsky MH, Shannon FJ, Sheppard S, Prabhu V, Boland PJ. Diagnosis and management of a metastatic tumor in the atlantoaxial spine. *Spine*. 2002;27:1062-1069.
2. Tian R, Su M, Tian Y, et al. Dual-time point PET/CT with F-18 FDG for the differentiation of malignant and benign bone lesions. *Skeletal Radiol*. 2009;38:451-458.

Usefulness of Contrast-Enhanced T1-Weighted Sampling Perfection with Application-Optimized Contrasts by Using Different Flip Angle Evolutions in Detection of Small Brain Metastasis at 3T MR Imaging: Comparison with Magnetization-Prepared Rapid Acquisition of Gradient Echo Imaging

Kato Y, Higano S, Tamura H, et al (Tohoku Univ Graduate School of Medicine, Sendai, Japan)

AJNR Am J Neuroradiol 30:923-929, 2009

Background and Purpose.—Early accurate diagnosis of brain metastases is crucial for a patient's prognosis. This study aimed to compare the conspicuity and detectability of small brain metastases between contrast-enhanced 3D fast spin-echo (sampling perfection with application-optimized contrasts by using different flip angle evolutions [SPACE]) and 3D gradient-echo (GE) T1-weighted (magnetization-prepared rapid acquisition of GE [MPRAGE]) images at 3T.

Materials and Methods.—Sixty-nine consecutive patients with suspected brain metastases were evaluated prospectively by using SPACE and MPRAGE on a 3T MR imaging system. After careful evaluation by 2 experienced neuroradiologists, 92 lesions from 16 patients were selected as brain metastases. We compared the shorter diameter, contrast rate (CR), and contrast-to-noise ratio (CNR) of each lesion. Diagnostic ability was compared by using receiver operating characteristic (ROC) analysis. Ten radiologists (5 neuroradiologists and 5 residents) participated in the reading.

Results.—The mean diameter was significantly larger by using SPACE than MPRAGE (mean, 4.5 ± 3.7 versus 4.3 ± 3.7 mm, $P = .0014$). The CR and CNR of SPACE (mean, 57.3 ± 47.4%, 3.0 ± 1.9, respectively) were significantly higher than those of MPRAGE (mean, 37.9 ± 41.2%, 2.6 ± 2.2; $P < .0001$, $P = .04$). The mean area under the ROC curve was significantly larger with SPACE than with MPRAGE (neuroradiologists, 0.99 versus 0.88, $P = .013$; residents, 0.99 versus 0.78, $P = .0001$).

Conclusions.—Lesion detectability was significantly higher on SPACE than on MPRAGE, irrespective of the experience of the reader in neuroradiology. SPACE should be a promising diagnostic technique for assessing brain metastases.

▶ With the advent of routine clinical availability of 3 T MR imaging several years ago, there has been an ongoing debate in neuroradiologic literature as to which sequences are optimal for detecting metastases using a standard intravenous gadolinium bolus. This basically pits T1-weighted 3-dimensional rapid gradient echo (T1-3DRGE) sequences and T1-weighted fluid attenuation inversion recovery (T1-FLAIR) versus standard T1-weighted spin echo sequences (T1-SE). Some initial studies utilizing various sequences at 3 T had determined that the detection of metastatic lesions was slightly higher using T1-3DRGE, but notably that sequence used thinner slice thicknesses (via a 3D acquisition) than the other 2 sequences.[1]

Although there are other recent studies comparing these sequences, in this study by Kato et al a similar thickness and plane with 3D acquisition for both T1-3DRGE and for T1-SE was used, which elevates the relevance of this article due to the fairness in comparison. The authors showed that T1-SE using a 3D acquisition had a significantly higher sensitivity than T1-3DRGE (95.7% vs 50.4%) for lesions < 5-mm size. This is in accordance with other recent articles and with evidence that there is a higher contrast-to-noise ratio with T1-SE images at 3 T.[2,3] Notably, readers must be aware that although T1-SE images are likely superior in demonstrating contrast enhancement, the gray-white matter differentiation is less than that for T1-3DRGE at 3 T because for T1-SE the difference in T1 times for gray and white matter is closer at 3 T than at 1.5 T. Hence, some still advocate T1-3DRGE acquisitions at 3 T after contrast administration for surgical planning MRI or for superior depiction of anatomy.

A. M. McKinney IV, MD

References

1. Kakeda S, Korogi Y, Hiai Y, et al. Detection of brain metastasis at 3T: comparison among SE, IR-FSE and 3D-GRE sequences. *Eur Radiol.* 2007;17:2345-2351.
2. Furutani K, Harada M, Mawlan M, Nishitani H. Difference in enhancement between spin echo and 3-dimensional fast spoiled gradient recalled acquisition in steady state magnetic resonance imaging of brain metastasis at 3-T magnetic resonance imaging. *J Comput Assist Tomogr.* 2008;32:313-319.
3. Komada T, Naganawa S, Ogawa H, et al. Contrast-enhanced MR imaging of metastatic brain tumor at 3 tesla: utility of T(1)-weighted SPACE compared with 2D spin echo and 3D gradient echo sequence. *Magn Reson Med Sci.* 2008; 7:13-21.

12 Pediatric Neurology

Brain Tumor Signs and Symptoms: Analysis of Primary Health Care Records from the UKCCS

Ansell P, Johnston T, Simpson J, et al (Univ of York, UK; et al)

Pediatrics 125:112-119, 2010

Objective.—To compare the frequency of brain tumor signs and symptoms in children with and without brain tumors.

Methods.—This was a UK population-based retrospective analysis of primary care records. Participants were 195 children (1–14 years) newly diagnosed with brain tumors and 285 controls matched by age, gender, and region. Comparisons included total number of prediagnosis consultations, number with ≥1 symptom suggestive of a brain tumor, total number of symptoms, number of different symptoms, and number of visits with specific combinations of symptoms.

Results.—On average, cases consulted more often than controls between birth and diagnosis/pseudodiagnosis with brain tumor signs and symptoms. Their consultation rate with ≥1 suggestive symptom escalated in the 2 years before diagnosis. Symptom prevalence was higher among cases than controls, a relative difference of 3.29 times as many consultations with ≥1 suggestive symptom (95% confidence interval [CI]: 2.82–3.83) and 7.01 as many with more than 1 (95% CI: 5.38–9.13). In each 6-month period in the 4 years before diagnosis, cases had at least twice as many consultations with ≥1 suggestive symptom (20.81 times as many in the 6 months before diagnosis [95% CI: 14.29–30.30]) and 2–3 times more records of suggestive symptoms (28.35 times more in the 6 months before diagnosis [95% CI: 19.05–42.19]). Symptoms rarely or not observed among control children included head tilt, odd head movements, odd posture, back or neck stiffness, and unsteadiness without obvious cause.

Conclusion.—Key to identifying the 1 child among many who merits prompt investigation is recognition of unusual symptoms, or specific symptom patterns.

▶ This retrospective analysis of primary care records from children in the United Kingdom establishes the sign and symptom patterns present in children with brain tumors. Remarkably, this report states that a general practitioner in the United Kingdom will see only 1 child younger than 15 years presenting with cancer in 20 years of practice; brain tumors comprise 18% of these. Twenty-one relevant signs and symptoms were sought in the records. Seven times more cases than controls presented with more than 1 of these symptoms. Vomiting, headache, visual problems, unsteadiness, and anorexia were the frequent symptoms. Headache combined with vomiting, visual problems or disequilibrium, and vomiting with disequilibrium were the most frequent symptom combinations. The authors state, "There was little evidence of findings from neurological examination in our data." In the 6 months before diagnosis, cases had 28 times more records of suggestive symptoms; in each 6-month interval in the 4 years before diagnosis, cases had 2 to 3 times more. Sensitivity to unusual symptoms or symptom patterns should facilitate recognition of these patients.

G. N. Breningstall, MD

Hair-Grooming Syncope in Children

Evans WN, Acherman R, Kip K, et al (Children's Heart Ctr, Las Vegas, NV)
Clin Pediatr 48:834-836, 2009

Objectives.—This report describes children undergoing pediatric cardiology evaluation for syncope in which a hair-grooming trigger was determined as the stimulus.

Methods.—A review of our database revealed 1525 patients with syncope seen by our program of whom 111 had a hair-grooming trigger determined as a cause.

Results.—Of the 111 patients, 78% were girls. We found characteristic difference between boys and girls with boys experiencing syncope more during hair cutting whereas girls experienced syncope more during hair combing and brushing. Electrocardiograms and echocardiograms were performed as part of syncope evaluation and no significant abnormalities were found in either test in this patient group.

Conclusions.—This is the largest reported group of children presenting with syncope that had a hair-grooming trigger. Our data also include the first series of boys with the condition. The hair-grooming trigger appears to stimulate a benign form of neurocardiogenic reflex syncope.

► A common form of reflex syncope in children is hair-grooming syncope, predominantly affecting girls. This is a review of 111 patients with hair-grooming syncope, with 22% of these boys. Previous reports have focused on girls only. Hair cutting was the common trigger in boys versus hair combing or grooming in girls. Seventy-six percent were standing at the time of syncope and 34% were sitting or kneeling. Electrocardiograms and echocardiograms were unrevealing. What is not discussed is the common occurrence of brief myoclonic or convulsive movements with syncope of whatever sort and the common misperception of such events as possibly epileptic. Sitting while hair grooming is being performed and hydration before hair grooming are suggested as the preventive measures.

G. N. Breningstall, MD

Intellectual, Adaptive, and Behavioral Functioning in Children With Urea Cycle Disorders

Krivitzky L, Babikian T, Lee H-S, et al (George Washington Univ School of Medicine and Health Sciences; UCLA School of Medicine, Los Angeles, CA; Univ of South Florida, Tampa; et al)

Pediatr Res 66:96-101, 2009

Inborn errors of urea synthesis lead to an accumulation of ammonia in blood and brain and result in high rates of mortality and neurodevelopmental disability. This study seeks to characterize the cognitive, adaptive, and emotional/behavioral functioning of children with urea cycle disorders (UCDs). These domains were measured through testing and parent questionnaires in 92 children with UCDs [33 neonatal onset (NO), 59 late onset (LO)]. Results indicate that children who present with NO have poorer outcome than those who present later in childhood. Approximately half of the children with NO performed in the range of intellectual disability (ID), including a substantial number (~30%) who were severely impaired. In comparison, only a quarter of the LO group was in the range of ID. There is also evidence that the UCD group has difficulties in aspects of emotional/behavioral and executive skills domains. In conclusion, children with UCDs present with a wide spectrum of cognitive outcomes. Children with NO disease have a much higher likelihood of having an ID, which becomes even more evident with increasing age. However, even children with LO UCDs demonstrate evidence of neurocognitive and behavioral impairment, particularly in aspects of attention and executive functioning.

▶ Urea cycle disorders (UCDs) have neurological, specifically cognitive morbidity. This has diminished with the advent of improved recognition and more effective therapy. In the severe cases with neonatal onset, 50% have intellectual disability (ID), with 31% moderate to severe. In late onset, the ID percentage is 25%. Distal UCDs, autosomal recessive disorders, especially citrullinemia, with 50% ID and 33% moderate to severe, carry greater cognitive morbidity than ornithine transcarbamylase deficiency (OTC), 2:1 female heterozygotes, with 20% ID and 6% moderate to severe. Patients with distal UCDs more frequently had neonatal onset, but less frequently had hyperammonemic episodes than patients with OTC. There may be additional mechanisms contributing to the cognitive morbidity of distal defects. The cognitive impairment of UCDs is more difficult to identify before 3 years of age, with only 8% (all neonatal onset) showing impairment, although the composite scores on developmental testing were below average. Older children demonstrated below average scores in social difficulties, attention problems, and metacognitive skills (initiation, planning/organization, working memory, and self-monitoring).

G. N. Breningstall, MD

Moderate Hypothermia to Treat Perinatal Asphyxial Encephalopathy

Azzopardi DV, for the TOBY Study Group (Hammersmith Hosp, London, UK; et al)

N Engl J Med 361:1349-1358, 2009

Background.—Whether hypothermic therapy improves neurodevelopmental outcomes in newborn infants with asphyxial encephalopathy is uncertain.

Methods.—We performed a randomized trial of infants who were less than 6 hours of age and had a gestational age of at least 36 weeks and perinatal asphyxial encephalopathy. We compared intensive care plus cooling of the body to 33.5°C for 72 hours and intensive care alone. The primary outcome was death or severe disability at 18 months of age. Prespecified secondary outcomes included 12 neurologic outcomes and 14 other adverse outcomes.

Results.—Of 325 infants enrolled, 163 underwent intensive care with cooling, and 162 underwent intensive care alone. In the cooled group, 42 infants died and 32 survived but had severe neurodevelopmental disability, whereas in the noncooled group, 44 infants died and 42 had severe disability (relative risk for either outcome, 0.86; 95% confidence interval [CI], 0.68 to 1.07; $P = 0.17$). Infants in the cooled group had an increased rate of survival without neurologic abnormality (relative risk, 1.57; 95% CI, 1.16 to 2.12; $P = 0.003$). Among survivors, cooling resulted in reduced risks of cerebral palsy (relative risk, 0.67; 95% CI, 0.47 to 0.96; $P = 0.03$) and improved scores on the Mental Developmental Index and Psychomotor Developmental Index of the Bayley Scales of Infant Development II ($P = 0.03$ for each) and the Gross Motor Function Classification System ($P = 0.01$). Improvements in other neurologic outcomes in the cooled group were not significant. Adverse events were mostly minor and not associated with cooling.

Conclusions.—Induction of moderate hypothermia for 72 hours in infants who had perinatal asphyxia did not significantly reduce the combined rate of death or severe disability but resulted in improved neurologic outcomes in survivors. (Current Controlled Trials number, ISRCTN89547571.)

▶ Two randomized controlled trials of hypothermia treatment for perinatal asphyxial encephalopathy preceding this one did not have sufficient power to detect significant differences in important individual neurological outcomes.

Unlike one of these previous trials, this large trial showed no significant reduction in death or severe disability in the treated neonates (45% cooled vs 53% noncooled). However, the cooled neonates in this study had increased survival without neurological abnormality (44% vs 28%), a lower incidence of cerebral palsy (28% vs 41%), and better developmental outcomes. The effect of cooling did not vary according to the severity of abnormality on amplitude-integrated electroencephalography at study entry. Also, randomization at less than 4 hours versus 4 to 6 hours did not affect the outcome of cooling. Outcome assessments were performed at 18 months of age.

G. N. Breningstall, MD

Neurodevelopmental outcome at 2 years in children born preterm treated by amnioreduction or fetoscopic laser surgery for twin-to-twin transfusion syndrome: comparison with dichorionic twins

Lenclen R, Ciarlo G, Paupe A, et al (Unité de Réanimation Néonatale, Centre Hospitalier Poissy-Saint-Germain, Poissy, France; et al)

Am J Obstet Gynecol 201:291.e1-291.e5, 2009

Objective.—We sought to assess long-term neurodevelopment of children born prematurely treated for twin-to-twin transfusion syndrome and dichorionic (DC) twins.

Study Design.—In all, 21 and 88 children treated with amnioreduction (AR) and fetoscopic laser surgery (FLS), respectively, and 222 DC twins matched for gestational age at delivery were assessed with Ages and Stages Questionnaire and standardized examination at 2 years of age.

Results.—Normal development was noted in 81% in the AR group, 88.6% in the FLS group, and 93.1% in the DC twins. Minor and major neurologic impairment was found in 9.5% and 9.5% following AR, in 6.8% and 4.6% of FLS children, and in 3.4% and 3.4% in DC twins, respectively. Ages and Stages Questionnaire assessment was similar in FLS and DC children but scores were lower ($P = .01$) and domains were more often abnormal (60% vs 27%; $P = .005$) following AR.

Conclusion.—Neurodevelopmental outcome is similar in twin-to-twin transfusion syndrome survivors treated by FLS and in DC control subjects; but survivors treated with AR have an increased risk of neurodevelopmental delay at 2 years of age.

► Having recent experience with 2 twin-to-twin transfusion syndrome (TTTS) twins treated with fetoscopic laser surgery (FLS), each resulting in one fetal demise and major sequelae in the survivor twin, I was interested in what the broader experience with this intervention might be. A previous article by the same group had demonstrated a 77% survivorship of treated TTTS twins, contrasting with an 88% survivorship of dichorionic twin controls. This article shows impressively favorable outcome, with the neurodevelopmental status of

TTTS survivors treated by FLS being similar to that of dichorionic twin controls. The outcomes of TTTS survivors treated with amnioreduction were less favorable. This is a large study, with 88 TTTS and 21 amnioreduction survivors and 203 dichorionic twin controls. An Ages and Stages Questionnaire, comparable with the Bayley Scales of Infant Development, and neurologic assessment were used.

G. N. Breningstall, MD

Noninvasive testing, early surgery, and seizure freedom in tuberous sclerosis complex

Wu JY, Salamon N, Kirsch HE, et al (Mattel Children's Hosp at UCLA, Los Angeles, CA; Univ of California, Los Angeles; Univ of California, San Francisco; et al)

Neurology 74:392-398, 2010

Background.—The unambiguous identification of the epileptogenic tubers in individuals with tuberous sclerosis complex (TSC) can be challenging. We assessed whether magnetic source imaging (MSI) and coregistration of ^{18}fluorodeoxyglucose PET (FDG-PET) with MRI could improve the identification of the epileptogenic regions noninvasively in children with TSC.

Methods.—In addition to standard presurgical evaluation, 28 children with intractable epilepsy from TSC referred from 2000 to 2007 had MSI and FDG-PET/MRI coregistration without extraoperative intracranial EEG.

Results.—Based on the concordance of test results, 18 patients with TSC (64%) underwent surgical resection, with the final resection zone confirmed by intraoperative electrocorticography. Twelve patients are seizure free postoperatively (67%), with an average follow-up of 4.1 years. Younger age at surgery and shorter seizure duration were associated with postoperative seizure freedom. Conversely, older age and longer seizure duration were linked with continued seizures postoperatively or prevented surgery because of nonlateralizing or bilateral independent epileptogenic zones. Complete removal of presurgery MSI dipole clusters correlated with postoperative seizure freedom.

Conclusions.—Magnetic source imaging and ^{18}fluorodeoxyglucose PET/MRI coregistration noninvasively localized the epileptogenic zones in many children with intractable epilepsy from tuberous sclerosis complex (TSC), with 67% seizure free postoperatively. Seizure freedom after surgery correlated with younger age and shorter seizure duration. These findings support the concept that early epilepsy surgery is associated with seizure freedom in children with TSC and intractable epilepsy.

► In patients with tuberous sclerosis and intractable epilepsy, a tuber is generally the seizure focus. However, these patients may have more than 20 tubers.

This article describes success with noninvasive determination of which of the tubers might ameliorate the epilepsy by surgical resection. Twenty-eight patients were assessed; 18 patients underwent surgery, all of whom had FDG-PET/MRI coregistration and 10 of whom had magnetic source imaging (MSI). FDG-PET/MRI coregistration provided further localization over ictal EEG in 35% and MSI in 80%. Twelve of 18 patients were seizure-free postoperatively. Seizure-free patients were younger and their duration of seizures was shorter. All 7 patients with complete removal of the dipole clusters and 2/5 with partial removal were seizure-free. Six of 7 patients with colocalizing MSI and FDG-PET/MRI coregistration were seizure-free. The 67% overall seizure-free outcome was comparable with that obtained after invasive EEG recording of ictal onsets.

G. N. Breningstall, MD

Subtle hemorrhagic brain injury is associated with neurodevelopmental impairment in infants with repaired congenital heart disease

Soul JS, Robertson RL, Wypij D, et al (Children's Hosp Boston, MA; et al)

J Thorac Cardiovasc Surg 138:374-381, 2009

Objective.—Perioperative stroke and periventricular leukomalacia have been reported to occur commonly in infants with congenital heart disease. We aimed to determine the incidence and type of brain injury in infants undergoing 2-ventricle repair in infancy and to determine risk factors associated with such injury.

Methods.—Forty-eight infants enrolled in a trial comparing 2 different hematocrits during surgical repair of congenital heart disease underwent brain magnetic resonance imaging scans and neurodevelopmental testing at 1 year of age.

Results.—Eighteen (38%) of our subjects had tiny foci of hemosiderin by susceptibility imaging, without evidence of abnormalities in corresponding regions on conventional magnetic resonance imaging sequences. Subjects with foci of hemosiderin had a significantly lower Psychomotor Developmental Index at 1 year of age (79.6 ± 16.5, mean ± standard deviation) compared with subjects without these foci (89.5 ± 15.3; $P = .04$). Older age at surgery and diagnostic group were significantly associated with the presence of hemosiderin foci. Only 1 subject had a small stroke (2%), and 2 subjects had periventricular leukomalacia (4%).

Conclusion.—Foci of hemosiderin without radiologic evidence of ischemic brain injury are an abnormality associated with adverse neurodevelopmental outcome not previously described in magnetic resonance imaging studies of children with surgically repaired congenital heart disease. The association of hemosiderin foci with older age at surgery and cardiac diagnosis, and not with risk factors associated with brain injury, in previous studies suggests that the cause and pathogenesis of this abnormality are different from ischemic brain lesions reported previously.

▶ There are a number of interesting features in this study of brain MRI and neurodevelopmental outcome in 48 infants who underwent surgical repair of congenital cardiac disease. Abnormal neurological examination results were least frequent in the infants who had transposition of the great arteries (TGA), which, in contrast to ventricular septal defect (VSD) and tetralogy of Fallot (TOF), had the highest perioperative morbidity. Eighteen of 23 infants with an MRI abnormality had tiny foci of signal abnormality on the MPGR sequence consistent with hemosiderin. Only 1 patient had a focal stroke. The occurrence of hemosiderin foci was notably greater in infants with VSD and TOF, than in the infants with TGA. Infants with TGA underwent surgery at a younger age. Infants with hemosiderin foci had a 10-point lower Psychomotor Developmental Index score, but similar Mental Developmental Index scores.

G. N. Breningstall, MD

13 Sleep Disorders

Brain Activation Changes Before and After PAP Treatment in Obstructive Sleep Apnea

Castronovo V, Canessa N, Strambi LF, et al (Vita-Salute San Raffaele Univ and San Raffaele Scientific Inst, Milan, Italy; et al)

Sleep 32:1161-1172, 2009

Study Objectives.—Obstructive sleep apnea syndrome (OSAS) is associated with cognitive and functional deficits, most of which are corrected after positive airway pressure (PAP) treatment. Previous studies investigating the neural underpinnings of OSAS failed to provide consistent results both on the cerebral substrates underlying cognitive deficits and on the effect of treatment on these anomalies. The aims of the study were a) to investigate whether never-treated OSA patients demonstrated differences in brain activation compared to healthy controls during a cognitive task; and b) to investigate whether any improvements in cognitive functioning found in OSA patients after treatment reflected a change in the underlying cerebral activity.

Design.—OSA patients and healthy controls underwent functional magnetic resonance imaging (fMRI) scanning. They were compared on performance and brain activation during a 2-back working-memory task. Patients were also re-evaluated after 3 months treatment with PAP. Cognitive functions were evaluated using neurocognitive tests. Sleepiness (ESS), mood (Beck Depression Inventory) and, quality-of-life (SF-36) were also assessed.

Setting.—The Sleep Disorders Center and CERMAC at the Vita-Salute San Raffaele University.

Patients or Participants.—17 OSA patients and 15 age- and education-matched healthy controls.

Interventions.—PAP treatment for 3 months.

Measurements and Results.—Compared to controls, never-treated OSA patients showed increased activations in the left frontal cortex, medial precuneus, and hippocampus, and decreased activations in the caudal pons. OSA patients showed decreases in activation with treatment in the left inferior frontal gyrus and anterior cingulate cortex, and bilaterally in the hippocampus. Most neurocognitive domains, impaired at baseline, showed significant improvement after treatment.

Conclusions.—OSA patients showed an overrecruitment of brain regions compared to controls, in the presence of the same level of performance on a working-memory task. Decreases of activation in prefrontal and hippocampal structures were observed after treatment in comparison to baseline. These findings may reflect a neural compensation mechanism in never-treated patients, which is reduced by effective treatment.

▶ Many providers are concerned that once sleep apnea is diagnosed and positive airway pressure (PAP) is prescribed people will not use the device. Another objection to aggressively pursuing treatment for sleep apnea sufferers is that treatment benefit is not always obvious. Both of these concerns are often the case with milder degrees of the disorder. As the authors have described, sleep apnea sufferers have measurable impairments of brain function including memory. Sleep apnea subjects in this study were typically in the severe range, with apnea/hypopnea index (AHI) above 30/hr. They also had significant time spent while sleeping below 90% SpO_2. There is abundant evidence that higher levels of available circulating O_2 promote better brain functioning in many ways. PAP-treated subjects in this study did use the device on the average of greater than 5 hours per night, which is certainly not uncommon in compliant users. For those who are in the majority of patients who are using PAP and believe they do feel better and function better, the authors have shown significant improvements in memory function.

B. Nolan, MD

Effect of Acute and Chronic Physical Exercise on Patients with Periodic Leg Movements

Esteves AM, De Mello MT, Pradella-Hallinan M, et al (Federal Univ of São Paulo-UNIFESP, Brazil)

Med Sci Sports Exerc 41:237-242, 2009

Purpose.—Nonpharmacological interventions may lead to an improvement in sleep quality. The objective of our study was to evaluate the effects of acute intensive exercise and chronic exercise on sleep patterns in patients with periodic leg movements (PLM).

Methods.—The study involved acute and chronic exercise. The acute intensive exercise group consisted of 22 volunteers who underwent a maximum effort test and a polysomnography (PSG) on the same night. The chronic exercise group included 11 patients who performed 72 physical training sessions undergoing three PSG studies on the night of sessions 1, 36, and 72. Blood samples were collected from both acute and chronic groups for β-endorphin dosage.

Results.—Our results showed that both forms of physical exercise lowered PLM levels. The acute physical exercise increased sleep efficiency, rapid eye movement (REM) sleep, and reduced wake after sleep onset, whereas the chronic physical exercise increased sleep efficiency, REM. sleep, and reduced sleep latency. We also found a significant negative correlation between β-endorphin release after acute intensive exercise and PLM levels ($r = -0.63$).

TABLE 2.—Sleep Pattern Variables—Baseline and Acute Intensive Physical Exercise Using a PLM Severity Classification (Mild, Moderate, and Severe)

	Mild		Moderate		Severe	
	Baseline	Acute Physical Exercise	Baseline	Acute Physical Exercise	Baseline	Acute Physical Exercise
WASO (min)	104.95 ± 53.51	66.10 ± 33.58*	58.50 ± 26.67	55.28 ± 41.01	141.75 ± 86.61	110.30 ± 52.63
REM sleep (%)	16.95 ± 5.47	21.76 ± 4.13*	18.10 ± 9.81	18.75 ± 8.41	14.46 ± 10.46	18.20 ± 8.57
PLM index	15.55 ± 4.60	11.68 ± 6.78*	32.44 ± 4.57	30.00 ± 12.06	59.91 ± 7.04	41.43 ± 26.27

Values are presented as mean ± SD; results from Student's *t*-test ($P < 0.05$).
*Differing from baseline values.

TABLE 3.—Sleep Pattern Variables, Baseline and After Physical Training Sessions 1, 36, and 72

	Baseline	1	36	72	*F*	*P*
TST (h)	5.08 ± 0.60	5.71 ± 0.56	5.69 ± 0.42	6.06 ± 0.51*	$F_{(3, 27)} = 3.4$	0.03
Sleep efficiency (%)	65.03 ± 7.77	73.00 ± 7.24*	75.30 ± 4.74*	74.84 ± 5.81*	$F_{(3, 27)} = 4.4$	0.01
Stage changes	75.51 ± 16.13	74.66 ± 8.90	78.22 ± 13.93	71.77 ± 7.84	$F_{(3, 27)} = 0.1$	0.94
Sleep latency (min)	39.4 ± 9.50	23.25 ± 6.87*	23.65 ± 4.83*	28.90 ± 8.09	$F_{(3, 27)} = 3.5$	0.02
REM sleep latency (min)	143.22 ± 25.19	124.50 ± 32.29	75.61 ± 9.81*	102.22 ± 29.25	$F_{(3, 24)} = 2.0$	0.04
WASO (min)	109.22 ± 25.23	98.72 ± 37.42	59.83 ± 11.72	79.11 ± 27.72	$F_{(3, 24)} = 0.1$	0.94
Wake index (h)	10.45 ± 2.06	13.15 ± 2.88	9.88 ± 2.34	11.16 ± 1.94	$F_{(3, 27)} = 0.5$	0.64
Stage 1 (%)	5.21 ± 1.78	3.74 ± 1.28	3.54 ± 0.85	3.66 ± 0.84	$F_{(3, 27)} = 0.4$	0.78
Stage 2 (%)	72.21 ± 3.42	66.20 ± 3.09	65.12 ± 2.57*	68.79 ± 2.10	$F_{(3, 27)} = 2.3$	0.02
Stage 3 (%)	1.90 ± 0.63	2.97 ± 0.90	1.93 ± 0.78	1.05 ± 0.24	$F_{(3, 27)} = 1.9$	0.14
Stage 4 (%)	5.17 ± 2.07	6.55 ± 1.61	6.78 ± 2.11	4.00 ± 1.17	$F_{(3, 27)} = 0.7$	0.51
REM sleep (%)	15.50 ± 2.82	20.50 ± 1.85*	22.60 ± 2.16*	22.48 ± 1.64*	$F_{(3, 27)} = 6.8$	<0.01
Apnea index	3.68 ± 1.93	3.32 ± 1.62	2.42 ± 1.14	3.01 ± 0.95	$F_{(3, 27)} = 0.2$	0.86
PLM index	27.21 ± 4.73	18.69 ± 5.34	25.05 ± 7.43	14.79 ± 3.69*	$F_{(3, 27)} = 2.3$	0.05

Values are presented as mean ± SD; results from repeated-measures ANOVA, *post hoc* Duncan ($P < 0.05$).
*Differing from baseline.

Conclusion.—Physical exercise may improve sleep patterns and reduce PLM levels. The correlation between β-endorphin release after acute intensive exercise and PLM levels might be associated with the impact physical exercise has on the opiodergic system. We suggest that physical exercise may be a useful nonpharmacological treatment for PLM (Tables 2 and 3).

▶ Over the years, there have been other reports that physical exercise may provide symptomatic relief to sufferers from periodic limb movements in sleep and restless legs syndrome. This study used polysomnographic measures to demonstrate measurable differences with both acute and long-term interventions with exercise. Improvement in sleep efficiency, percentage of random eye movement (REM) sleep, and reduction in indices for periodic limb movements would be expected to provide a better quality of sleep in these individuals. Supplementation of iron, when needed, and increased physical exercise would appear to provide more physiologically attractive alternatives to dopaminergic agents, benzodiazepines, and oral narcotics.

B. Nolan, MD

Effect of Retirement on Sleep Disturbances: the GAZEL Prospective Cohort Study

Vahtera J, Westerlund H, Hall M, et al (Univ of Turku and Turku Univ Hospital, Finland; Stockholm Univ, Sweden; Univ of Pittsburgh School of Medicine, PA; et al)

Sleep 32:1459-1466, 2009

Objectives.—Changes in health following retirement are poorly understood. We used serial measurements to assess the effect of retirement on sleep disturbances.

Design.—Prospective cohort study.

Setting.—The French national gas and electricity company.

Participants.—Fourteen thousand seven hundred fourteen retired employees (79% men).

Measurements and Results.—Annual survey measurements of sleep disturbances ranging from 7 years before to 7 years after retirement (a mean of 12 measurements). Before retirement 22.2% to 24.6% of participants reported having disturbed sleep. According to repeated-measures logistic-regression analysis with generalized estimating equations estimation, the odds ratio (OR) for having a sleep disturbance in the postretirement period was 0.74 (95% confidence interval 0.71-0.77), compared with having a sleep disturbance in the preretirement period. The postretirement improvement in sleep was more pronounced in men (OR 0.66 [0.63-0.69]) than in women (OR 0.89 [0.84-0.95]) and in higher-grade workers than lower-grade workers. Postretirement sleep improvement was explained by the combination of preretirement risk factors suggesting removal of work-related exposures as a mechanism. The only exception to the general improvement in sleep after retirement was related to retirement on health grounds. In this group of participants, there was an increase in sleep disturbances following retirement.

Conclusions.—Repeated measurements provide strong evidence for a substantial and sustained decrease in sleep disturbances following retirement. The possibility that the health and well-being of individuals are significantly worse when in employment than following retirement

TABLE 2.—Changes in Sleep Disturbances Following Retirement[a]

Covariate	Interaction with Time	Sleep Disturbances[b] OR	95% CI
Sex	$P < 0.0001$		
Men		0.66	0.63-0.69
Women		0.89	0.84-0.95
Age at retirement, y	$P = 0.008$		
≤ 53		0.77	0.72-0.81
54-56		0.71	0.67-0.75
≥ 57		0.72	0.67-0.78
Grade	$P < 0.0001$		
Higher		0.63	0.59-0.67
Intermediate		0.74	0.70-0.77
Lower		0.85	0.78-0.92
Marital status	$P = 0.823$		
Type of retirement	$P < 0.0001$		
Statutory		0.69	0.66-0.72
Early		1.46	1.27-1.69
Night work	$P = 0.002$		
No		0.75	0.72-0.78
Yes		0.66	0.62-0.70
Job demands			
Psychological	$P < 0.0001$		
Low		0.91	0.86-0.97
Moderate		0.72	0.68-0.76
High		0.59	0.56-0.63
Physical	$P = 0.784$		
Job satisfaction	$P = 0.952$		
Body mass index, kg/m^2	$P = 0.006$		
≤ 24.9		0.77	0.73-0.81
25.0- 29.9		0.66	0.62-0.70
≥ 30.0		0.74	0.67-0.82
Alcohol consumption, units/d	$P = 0.140$		
Suboptimal self-rated health	$P = 0.019$		
No		0.74	0.71-0.78
Yes		0.68	0.64-0.72
Mental fatigue	$P < 0.0001$		
No		0.86	0.82-0.90
Yes		0.56	0.53-0.60
Physical fatigue	$P = 0.007$		
No		0.74	0.70-0.78
Yes		0.68	0.64-0.72
Physical illness	$P = 0.378$		
Depression	$P < 0.0001$		
No		0.76	0.73-0.80
Yes		0.55	0.52-0.59

[a]Overall odds ratio (OR) for sleep disturbances and their 95% confidence interval (CI) in the 7 years after retirement, compared with the 7 years prior to retirement, are derived from repeated-measures logistic regression generalized estimating equations analyses adjusted for sex, age at retirement, year and time of data collection (1989-99 or 2000-07).

[b]In year +1 to +7 compared with the years −1 to −7.

presents a great challenge to improve the quality of work life in Western societies in which the cost of the aging population can only be met through an increase in average retirement age (Table 2).

► There is a common notion that older adults do not sleep as well as younger adults. This large population study supports the important conclusion that healthy, retired older adults appear to sleep better than their preretirement counterparts. Also of note is that, unhealthy, older individuals, on the other hand, do not sleep as well either. The authors do point out in the text that the population studied may not represent the average working circumstances of most people and that the assessments were limited and subjective. Retirement age for over 80% of those studied was less than 57 years. With the present global economic stresses, it seems unlikely that potentially beneficial improvements in the workplace will occur in the near future. Those who do decide to retire may at least have the prospect of improved sleep.

B. Nolan, MD

Efficacy of an Internet-Based Behavioral Intervention for Adults With Insomnia

Ritterband LM, Thorndike FP, Gonder-Frederick LA, et al (Univ of Virginia Health System, Charlottesville; et al)
Arch Gen Psychiatry 66:692-698, 2009

Context.—Insomnia is a major health problem with significant psychological, health, and economic consequences. However, availability of one of the most effective insomnia treatments, cognitive behavioral therapy, is significantly limited. The Internet may be a key conduit for delivering this intervention.

Objective.—To evaluate the efficacy of a structured behavioral Internet intervention for adults with insomnia.

Design, Setting, and Participants.—Forty-five adults were randomly assigned to an Internet intervention (n = 22) or wait-list control group (n = 23). Forty-four eligible participants (mean [SD] age, 44.86 [11.03] years; 34 women) who had a history of sleep difficulties longer than 10 years on average (mean [SD], 10.59 [8.89] years) were included in the analyses.

Intervention.—The Internet intervention is based on well-established face-to-face cognitive behavioral therapy incorporating the primary components of sleep restriction, stimulus control, sleep hygiene, cognitive restructuring, and relapse prevention.

Main Outcome Measures.—The Insomnia Severity Index and daily sleep diary data were used to determine changes in insomnia severity and the main sleep variables, including wake after sleep onset and sleep efficiency.

Results.—Intention-to-treat analyses showed that scores on the Insomnia Severity Index significantly improved from 15.73 (95% confidence interval [CI], 14.07 to 17.39) to 6.59 (95% CI, 4.73 to 8.45) for the Internet group but did not change for the control group (16.27 [95% CI, 14.61 to 17.94] to 15.50 [95% CI, 13.64 to 17.36]) ($F_{1,42} = 29.64$; $P < .001$). The Internet group maintained their gains at the 6-month follow-up. Internet participants also achieved significant decreases in wake after sleep onset (55% [95% CI, 34% to 76%]) and increases in sleep efficiency (16% [95% CI, 9% to 22%]) compared with the nonsignificant control group changes of wake after sleep onset (8% [95% CI, −17% to 33%) and sleep efficiency (3%; 95% CI, −4% to 9%).

Conclusions.—Participants who received the Internet intervention for insomnia significantly improved their sleep, whereas the control group did not have a significant change. The Internet appears to have considerable potential in delivering a structured behavioral program for insomnia.

Trial Registration.—clinicaltrials.gov Identifier:NCT00328250 (Table 2).

▶ In a telethon conducted last year at our own center, we were overwhelmed but not surprised by the number of callers reporting night-to-night difficulty

TABLE 2.—Sleep Diary Data Changes by Treatment Condition

Sleep Variable and Period	Internet Participants (n = 22) Mean (SD)	Internet Participants (n = 22) Improvement, %	Control Participants (n = 22) Mean (SD)	Control Participants (n = 22) Improvement, %	$F_{1,42}$	P Value
Primary variable						
WASO, min						
Preassessment	66.74 (40.81)		56.43 (19.38)		10.80	.002
Postassessment	29.89 (19.83)[a]	55	51.81 (26.58)	8		
SOL, min						
Preassessment	31.84 (27.90)		35.43 (21.43)		2.74	.11
Postassessment	18.12 (12.84)	43	32.75 (16.49)	8		
Secondary variable						
Sleep efficiency, %						
Preassessment	77.3 (14.7)		79.6 (7.7)		8.29	.006
Postassessment	89.3 (5.0)[a]	16	81.6 (7.3)	3		
Total sleep time, min						
Preassessment	349.92 (88.00)		365.65 (61.46)		2.95	.09
Postassessment	404.92 (61.46)	16	380.04 (59.82)	4		
Awakenings, No.						
Preassessment	2.38 (1.48)		2.38 (1.02)		6.80	.01
Postassessment	1.52 (1.07)[b]	36	2.40 (1.39)	1		
Time in bed, min						
Preassessment	448.70 (61.66)		457.50 (53.41)		0.01	.92
Postassessment	453.55 (67.38)	1	464.59 (51.90)	2		
Restored, scale score[c]						
Preassessment	2.69 (0.65)		2.71 (0.62)		5.69	.02
Postassessment	3.21 (0.70)	19	2.88 (0.66)	6		
Soundness of sleep, scale score[d]						
Preassessment	2.83 (0.59)		2.83 (0.64)		3.12	.09
Postassessment	3.23 (0.61)	14	2.94 (0.74)	4		

Abbreviations: SOL, sleep-onset latency; WASO, wake after sleep onset.
[a] $P \leq .001$ based on paired-samples t tests to examine time effects within each treatment condition.
[b] $P = .005$ based on paired-samples t tests to examine time effects within each treatment condition.
[c] Scored on a scale from 1 to 5, with 1 indicating exhausted and 5 indicating very refreshed.
[d] Scored on a scale from 1 to 5, with 1 indicating very restless and 5 indicating very sound.

with insomnia. That was around the time of a severe downturn in the local and world economy. Even before the current economic woes, chronic insomnia was found to affect more than 10% of adults. Although behavioral interventions have been found to be quite effective for most insomnia sufferers, they are not widely available. This study has limitations in sample size and using wait-listed controls for comparison. Nonetheless, these results should provide some encouragement for the millions of insomnia sufferers still waiting for a better remedy. Larger numbers of study subjects and better refined confirmation of these findings may lead to greater availability of effective needed interventions for chronic insomnia sufferers.

B. Nolan, MD

Elevated Anti-Streptococcal Antibodies in Patients with Recent Narcolepsy Onset

Aran A, Lin L, Nevsimalova S, et al (Stanford Univ School of Medicine, Palo Alto, CA; Charles Univ in Prague, Czech Republic; et al)
Sleep 32:979-983, 2009

Study Objectives.—Narcolepsy-cataplexy has long been thought to have an autoimmune origin. Although susceptibility to narcolepsy, like many autoimmune conditions, is largely genetically determined, environmental factors are involved based on the high discordance rate (~75%) of monozygotic twins. This study evaluated whether *Streptococcus pyogenes* and *Helicobacter pylori* infections are triggers for narcolepsy.

Design.—Retrospective, case-control.

Setting.—Sleep centers of general hospitals.

Participants.—200 patients with narcolepsy/hypocretin deficiency, with a primary focus on recent onset cases and 200 age-matched healthy controls. All patients were DQB1*0602 positive with low CSF hypocretin-1 or had clear-cut cataplexy.

Measurements and Results.—Participants were tested for markers of immune response to β hemolytic streptococcus (anti-streptolysin O [ASO]; anti DNAse B [ADB]) and *Helicobacter pylori* [Anti Hp IgG], two bacterial infections known to trigger autoimmunity. A general inflammatory marker, C-reactive protein (CRP), was also studied. When compared to controls, ASO and ADB titers were highest close to narcolepsy onset, and decreased with disease duration. For example, ASO ≥ 200 IU (ADB ≥ 480 IU) were found in 51% (45%) of 67 patients within 3 years of onset, compared to 19% (17%) of 67 age matched controls (OR = 4.3 [OR = 4.1], P < 0.0005) or 20% (15%) of 69 patients with long-standing disease (OR = 4.0 [OR = 4.8], P < 0.0005]. CRP (mean values) and Anti Hp IgG (% positive) did not differ from controls.

TABLE 1.—Combination of Anti-Streptolysin O (ASO) ≥ 200 IU and Anti DNAse B (ADB) ≥ 480 IU in Patients with Narcolepsy and Age-Matched Controls

Interval from Disease Onset	ASO and ADB	ASO or ADB
Up to 1 year (n = 23)	43% [1,2]	65% [1,2]
Controls	4.5%	26%
1-3 years (n = 42)	33% [3,4]	57% [3,4]
Controls	9.5%	30%
3-10 years (n = 64)	16%	40%
Controls	11%	28%
≥ 10 years (n = 65)	6%	29%
Controls	3%	25%

[1]OR = 16.1 (ASO and ADB); 5.3 (ASO or ADB), P < 0.01 versus age matched controls
[2]OR = 11.7 (ASO and ADB); 4.5 (ASO or ADB), P < 0.01 versus patients > 10 years from onset
[3]OR = 4.8 (ASO and ADB); 3.2 (ASO or ADB), P < 0.05 versus age matched controls
[4]OR = 7.6 (ASO and ADB); 4.5 (ASO or ADB), P < 0.01 versus patients > 10 years from onset

Conclusions.—Streptococcal infections are probably a significant environmental trigger for narcolepsy (Table 1).

► Clinical symptoms and findings in narcolepsy appear to be the result of the relatively selective loss of a population of hypocretin (orexin) producing cells in the hypothalamus.[1] The work presented here provides additional evidence for a possible link to an environmental trigger in narcolepsy. The study improves our understanding of another potential connection between the likely hereditary predisposition and possible environmental role in narcolepsy. If narcolepsy is in fact another autoimmune manifestation of antecedent group A streptococcal infection, one might expect the prevalence of the disorder to be higher in areas where antibiotic treatment for these infections is less frequent. Additional environmental triggers have been postulated and are not necessarily excluded by the present work. Further study of these associations should help to better elucidate the role of such mechanisms.

B. Nolan, MD

Reference

1. Peterson PC, Husain AM. Pediatric narcolepsy. *Brain Dev.* 2008;30:609-623 [published online ahead of print March 28 2008].

Insomnia and Sleep Duration as Mediators of the Relationship Between Depression and Hypertension Incidence

Gangwisch JE, Malaspina D, Posner K, et al (Columbia Univ, NY; New York Univ; et al)
Am J Hypertens 23:62-69, 2010

Background.—Depression has been found to predict the incidence of hypertension and other adverse cardiovascular events in prospective studies. Insomnia and short sleep duration, which are typical symptoms of depression, have also been shown to increase the risk for hypertension incidence. Insomnia is associated with increased activation of the hypothalamic–pituitary–adrenal axis, and short sleep duration raises average 24-h blood pressure, which over time could lead to structural adaptations that gradually reset the entire cardiovascular system to operate at an elevated pressure equilibrium. No previous published population studies have examined whether insomnia and sleep duration mediate the relationship between depression and hypertension incidence.

Methods.—We conducted multivariate longitudinal (1982–1992) analyses stratified by age of the First National Health and Nutrition Examination Survey (NHANES I) ($n = 4{,}913$) using Cox proportional hazards models.

Results.—Middle-aged subjects who suffered from depression at baseline were 44% more likely to be diagnosed with hypertension over the follow-up period after controlling for covariates (hazard ratio (HR) = 1.44, 95% confidence interval (CI) 1.15–1.80). Both short sleep duration and insomnia were also significantly associated with hypertension incidence. Consistent with insomnia and sleep duration acting as mediators of the relationship between depression and hypertension incidence, the inclusion of these variables in the multivariate models appreciably attenuated the association (HR = 1.27, 95% CI 1.00–1.61). Depression, sleep duration, and insomnia were not significantly associated with hypertension incidence in elderly subjects.

Conclusions.—These results suggest the hypothesis that treatment of sleep problems in middle-aged individuals suffering from depression could reduce their risk for developing hypertension, and its vascular and cardiac complications (Fig 1, Table 3).

▶ The question of whether hypertension is "essential" has been a troubling conundrum for decades. Establishing and reducing risk factors for hypertension

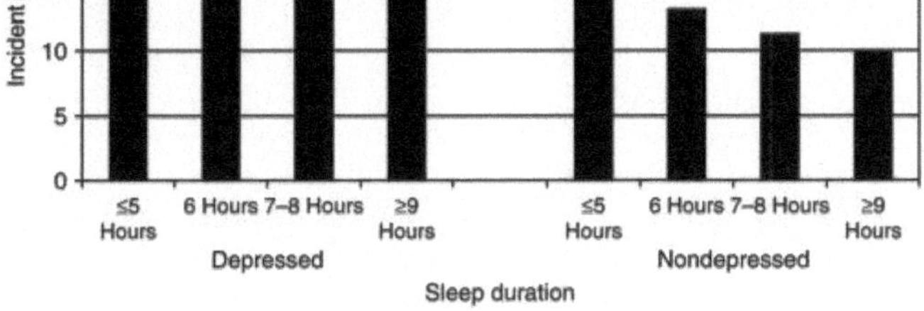

FIGURE 1.—Relationship between sleep duration and hypertension incidence in both depressed and nondepressed middle-aged subjects. (Reprinted from Gangwisch JE, Malaspina D, Posner K, et al. Insomnia and sleep duration as mediators of the relationship between depression and hypertension incidence. *Am J Hypertens*. 2010;23:62-69, with permission from American Journal of Hypertension, Ltd.)

TABLE 3.—Hazards Ratios (95% CI) as Computed with Cox Proportional Hazards Models for Hypertension Incidence Over the Follow-Up Period by Depression, Sleep Duration, and Insomnia at Baseline

	Model 1[a]	Model 2[b]	Model 3[c]	Model 4[d]	Model 5[e]
Ages 32–86					
Depression	1.61 (1.34–1.94)	1.41 (1.16–1.71)	1.37 (1.13–1.67)	1.32 (1.08–1.62)	1.31 (1.07–1.60)
Sleep duration					
≤5 h			1.34 (1.04–1.73)		1.25 (0.96–1.63)
6 h			1.02 (0.84–1.24)		0.99 (0.81–1.21)
7–8 h			1.00		1.00
≥9 h			1.15 (0.87–1.53)		1.17 (0.88–1.56)
Insomnia				1.04 (1.01–1.07)	1.03 (1.00–1.07)
Ages 32–59					
Depression	1.65 (1.33–2.05)	1.44 (1.15–1.80)	1.39 (1.10–1.74)	1.28 (1.01–1.62)	1.27 (1.00–1.61)
Sleep duration					
≤5 h			1.66 (1.25–2.22)		1.50 (1.11–2.02)
6 h			1.07 (0.86–1.34)		1.03 (0.82–1.30)
7–8 h			1.00		1.00
≥9 h			0.97 (0.64–1.47)		0.99 (0.65–1.50)
Insomnia				1.07 (1.03–1.11)	1.05 (1.01–1.09)
Ages 60–86					
Depression	1.45 (1.02–2.07)	1.29 (0.89–1.87)	1.32 (0.91–1.93)	1.34 (0.92–1.97)	1.33 (0.91–1.96)
Sleep duration					
≤5 h			0.80 (0.46–1.38)		0.81 (0.46–1.44)
6 h			0.83 (0.54–1.29)		0.84 (0.54–1.31)
7–8 h			1.00		1.00
≥ 9 h			1.29 (0.85–1.94)		1.28 (0.85–1.94)
Insomnia				0.98 (0.92–1.03)	0.99 (0.93–1.06)

CI, confidence interval.
[a]Model 1, unadjusted.
[b]Model 2, adjusted for age, sex, race/ethnicity, education, body weight, diabetes, alcohol consumption, cigarette smoking, physical activity, and pulse rate.
[c]Model 3, adjusted for variables in Model 2 plus sleep duration.
[d]Model 4, adjusted for variables in Model 2 plus insomnia.
[e]Model 5, adjusted for variables in Model 2 plus sleep duration and insomnia.

have important potential for reducing the associated collectively immense health care costs of individuals and society. Depression and insomnia are 2 prevalent and modifiable disorders that are associated with hypertension. Health care providers generally are aware of the importance of identifying and treating hypertension, but greater awareness of the importance and potential health implications of insomnia is needed. Studies consistently show that greater than 10% of the population is affected by chronic insomnia, but few health care settings inquire about such symptoms. Even fewer providers actively address the assessment and treatment of such sleep difficulties. Nonetheless, effective treatment interventions are available for insomnia as they are also for depression and hypertension. Greater awareness of these important associations and more widespread use of effective interventions can greatly reduce health-related costs and suffering.

B. Nolan, MD

Obstructive Sleep Apnea Syndrome Is Associated with Overactive Bladder and Urgency Incontinence in Men

Kemmer H, Mathes AM, Dilk O, et al (Erasmus MC, Rotterdam, The Netherlands; Saarland Univ Hosp, Germany)

Sleep 32:271-275, 2009

Study Objective.—To investigate the incidence of overactive bladder (OAB) and urgency incontinence (Ul) in men with obstructive sleep apnea syndrome (OSAS).

Design.—Prospective questionnaire study.

Setting.—Saarland University Hospital.

Patients.—All male patients who underwent full-night in-laboratory polysomnography between November 2006 and April 2007.

Interventions.—Overactive bladder symptom score (OABSS) and International Consultation on Incontinence Questionnaire, Short-Form (ICIQ-SF).

Measurements and Results.—OSAS severity was assessed according to the apnea-hypopnea-index (AHI). Return rate of questionnaires was 100% (n = 100). Patients with upper airway resistance syndrome (UARS) served as controls. Evaluation of OABSS revealed that patients with moderate and severe OSAS presented with a significantly higher incidence of symptoms of OAB than patients with mild OSAS and UARS ($P < 0.05$). Further, the ICIQ-SF revealed a higher occurrence of UI in patients with severe OSAS than in those with mild OSAS and UARS ($P < 0.05$).

Conclusions.—Increasing severity of OSAS appears to be associated with an increasing occurrence of overactive bladder and urgency incontinence in men. This relationship may have clinical implications for the treatment of affected patients.

▶ Sleep professionals frequently encounter symptoms of nocturia in patients with sleep disorders. The association of nocturia and incontinence with sleep-related breathing disorders does not seem to be widely appreciated outside of the sleep community, however. This study shows that the urinary symptoms were directly related to the severity of the sleep apnea in their subjects. In addition to loud snoring, the symptoms of urinary frequency, urgency, and nocturia should alert clinicians to the increased likelihood of significant sleep apnea. Effective interventions including nasal positive airway pressure are available that may substantially improve overall health and quality of life for individuals, including those with neurological disorders who are experiencing these comorbidities.

B. Nolan, MD

Obstructive sleep apnoea and its association with gestational hypertension

Champagne K, Schwartzman K, Opatrny L, et al (McGill Univ, Montreal, Quebec, Canada; et al)

Eur Respir J 33:559-565, 2009

Hypertension develops in 10% of pregnancies. Snoring, a marker of obstructive sleep apnoea, is a newly identified risk factor for gestational hypertension. Moreover, obstructive sleep apnoea is an independent risk factor for incident hypertension in the non-pregnant population. The aim of the present study was to test the hypothesis that obstructive sleep apnoea is associated with new onset of hypertension among pregnant females.

A case–control study was performed involving 17 pregnant females with gestational hypertension and 33 pregnant females without hypertension. Subjects were frequency-matched for gestational age and recruited in a tertiary obstetrical centre. Obstructive sleep apnoea was ascertained by polysomnography and defined by an apnoea/hypopnoea index (AHI) of ≥15 events$\cdot h^{-1}$, without requirement for desaturation.

The mean ± SD AHI for normotensive pregnant females was 18.2 ± 12.2 events$\cdot h^{-1}$ compared with 38.6 ± 36.7 events$\cdot h^{-1}$ for females with hypertensive pregnancies. The crude odds ratio for the presence of obstructive sleep apnoea given the presence of gestational hypertension was 5.6. The odds ratio was 7.5 (95% confidence interval 3.5–16.2), based on a logistic regression model with adjustment for maternal age, gestational age, pre-pregnancy body mass index, prior pregnancies, and previous live births.

TABLE 4.—Adjusted Odds Ratio (OR) for Each Variable and its Association with Gestational Hypertension

Variables	Adjusted OR (95% CI)	p-Values
Sleep apnoea# versus no sleep apnoea	7.5 (3.5–16.2)	<0.0001
BMI per 1 kg$\cdot m^{-2}$ increase	1.2 (1.1–1.4)	0.001
Maternal age per 1-yr increase	1.2 (0.95–1.4)	0.14
Pregnancy status		
Previous pregnancy but no live birth	12.8 (3.5–46.0)	<0.0001
First pregnancy	3.4 (0.25–45.5)	0.35
Previous live birth¶	1	
Gestational age		
20–27 weeks	1.1 (0.4–3.2)	0.80
27–34 weeks	0.8 (0.5–1.2)	0.32
>34 weeks¶	1	

CI: confidence interval; BMI: body mass index.
#sleep apnoea was defined by an apnoea/hypopnoea index ≥15$\cdot h^{-1}$;
¶this category served as the reference group.

In conclusion, gestational hypertension appears to be strongly associated with the presence of obstructive sleep apnoea (Table 4).

▶ Hypertension has long been known to be associated with snoring and sleep related breathing disorders (SRBD). Correction of SRBD has also been shown to improve hypertension. Other symptoms of sleep apnea, including excessive daytime sleepiness increase as pregnancy progresses. This study shows a strong association with sleep apnea and hypertension in pregnancy. The degree of desaturation reported in this study appears mild in comparison with typical nonpregnant individuals with moderate to severe sleep apnea. Even mild desaturation, though, may be poorly tolerated by subjects who are not accustomed to experiencing lower levels of oxygen. Poor quality sleep usually results. Fortunately, sleep symptoms typically improve following parturition. However, the health of the mother as well as the unborn child should raise concern about the ill effects of hypertension and hypoxemia, even if mild, during pregnancy. Improved oxygenation, correction of blood pressure, and better quality sleep would appear to be a desirable goal even for the limited period of time later in pregnancy. I would echo the authors' suggestion that further studies using best management of sleep apnea, including nasal positive airway pressure are warranted for suspected sleep apnea in pregnancy.

B. Nolan, MD

Perceived Insufficient Rest or Sleep Among Adults - United States, 2008

Centers for Disease Control and Prevention (CDC)

MMWR Morb Mortal Wkly Rep 58:1175-1179, 2009

The importance of chronic sleep insufficiency is under-recognized as a public health problem, despite being associated with numerous physical and mental health problems, injury, loss of productivity, and mortality (*1*,*2*). Approximately 29% of U.S. adults report sleeping <7 hours per night (*3*) and 50–70 million have chronic sleep and wakefulness disorders (*1*). A CDC analysis of 2006 data from the Behavioral Risk Factor Surveillance System (BRFSS) in four states showed that an estimated 10.1% of adults reported receiving insufficient rest or sleep on all days during the preceding 30 days (*4*). To examine the prevalence of insufficient rest or sleep in all states, CDC analyzed BRFSS data for all 50 states, the District of Columbia (DC), and three U.S. territories (Guam, Puerto Rico, and U.S. Virgin Islands) in 2008. This report summarizes the results, which showed that among 403,981 respondents, 30.7% reported no days of insufficient rest or sleep and 11.1% reported insufficient rest or sleep every day during the preceding 30 days. Females (12.4%) were more likely than males (9.9%) and non-Hispanic blacks (13.3%) were more likely than other racial/ethnic groups to report insufficient rest or sleep. State estimates of 30 days of insufficient rest or sleep ranged from 7.4% in North Dakota to 19.3% in West Virginia. Health-care providers should consider adding an assessment of chronic rest or sleep insufficiency to routine office visits

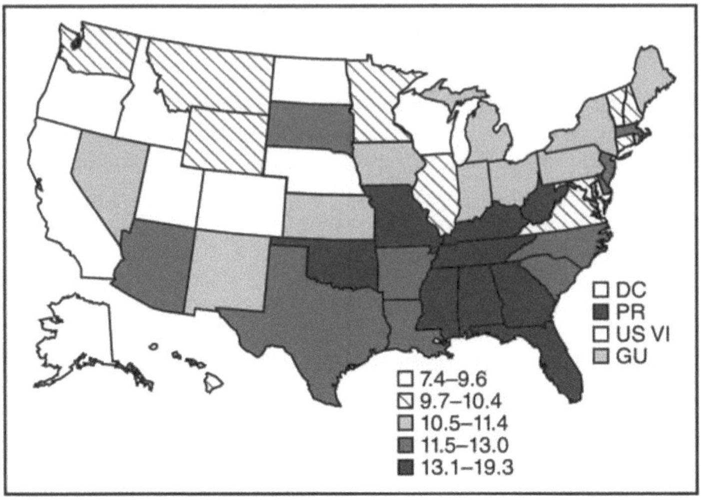

FIGURE 1.—Age-adjusted* percentage of adults who reported 30 days of insufficient rest or sleep† during the preceding 30 days—Behavioral Risk Factor Surveillance System, United States,§ 2008. * Age adjusted to 2000 projected U.S. population. † Determined by response to the question, "During the past 30 days, for about how many days have you felt you did not get enough rest or sleep?" § Includes the 50 states, District of Columbia, Guam, Puerto Rico, and U.S. Virgin Islands. (Courtesy of Centers for Disease Control and Prevention (CDC). Perceived insufficient rest or sleep among adults – United States, 2008. *MMWR Morb Mortal Wkly Rep*. 2009;58:1175-1179.)

so they can make needed interventions or referrals to sleep specialists (Fig 1).

▶ This is a statistically powerful study that provides important data on rest and sleep. Less than 1 person in 3 reported getting sufficient amounts every day. Over 10% reported getting insufficient amounts on any day. Despite similar requirements, women are getting significantly less rest and sleep than their male counterparts. Whether these data are a holdover from the outdated but still prevalent notion that sleep is a waste of time is difficult to say. There are undoubtedly many underlying contributing factors resulting in these findings. There is little doubt, however, that health care providers should be asking about sleep symptoms more systematically because sleep derangements are so frequently associated with a variety of health risks.[1] Individuals who are getting insufficient rest or sleep need to consider pursuing active interventions with their health care provider or consult a sleep specialist.

B. Nolan, MD

Reference

1. Centers for Disease Control and Prevention (CDC). Perceived insufficient rest or sleep among adults — United States, 2008. *MMWR Morb Mortal Wkly Rep*. 2009;58:1175-1179.

REM, not incubation, improves creativity by priming associative networks

Cai DJ, Mednick SA, Harrison EM, et al (Univ of California at San Diego, La Jolla; Univ of Southern California, Los Angeles)

Proc Natl Acad Sci U S A 106:10130-10134, 2009

The hypothesized role of rapid eye movement (REM) sleep, which is rich in dreams, in the formation of new associations, has remained anecdotal. We examined the role of REM on creative problem solving, with the Remote Associates Test (RAT). Using a nap paradigm, we manipulated various conditions of prior exposure to elements of a creative problem. Compared with quiet rest and non-REM sleep, REM enhanced the formation of associative networks and the integration of unassociated information. Furthermore, these REM sleep benefits were not the result of an improved memory for the primed items. This study shows that compared with quiet rest and non-REM sleep, REM enhances the integration of unassociated information for creative problem solving, a process, we hypothesize, that is facilitated by cholinergic and noradrenergic neuromodulation during REM sleep (Fig 3).

▶ There exist clear physiological differences in the characteristics of wake, nonrandom eye movement (REM) sleep, and REM sleep. The functions of sleep and more specifically the function of REM sleep has been a long-standing matter of conjecture. This study provides further insights into these essential processes. Despite use of the "remote associates test (RAT)," the reader can appreciate that the subjects in this study were polysomnographically-monitored humans who were given the opportunity to either nap or "incubate" while remaining awake. As more research is completed, we can gain greater

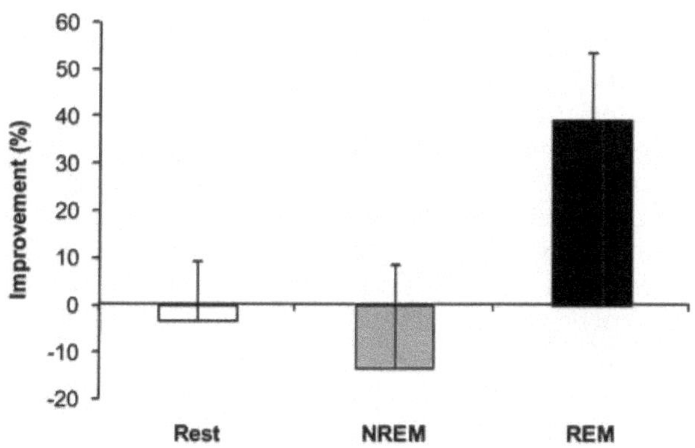

FIGURE 3.—REM sleep facilitates the use of prior information for creative problem solving. Subjects who had REM sleep displayed a significant improvement above NREM and quiet rest groups ($P = 0.047$, 1-way ANOVA and post hoc analysis). Strikingly, although the quiet rest and NREM nap groups received the same priming, they displayed no improvement on the primed RAT items, whereas the REM group improved by almost 40% above the morning performance. (Reprinted from Cai DJ, Mednick SA, Harrison EM, et al. REM, not incubation, improves creativity by priming associative networks. *Proc Natl Acad Sci U S A*. 2009;106:10130-10134. Copyright 2009 National Academy of Sciences, U S A.)

understanding of how the brain processes information, which increasingly appears to be one of the important functions of sleep.

B. Nolan, MD

Sleep-related breathing and sleep-wake disturbances in ischemic stroke

Hermann DM, Bassetti CL (Univ Hosp Essen, Germany; Univ Hosp Zurich, Switzerland)

Neurology 73:1313-1322, 2009

Background.—Sleep-related breathing disturbances (SDB) and sleep-wake disturbances (SWD) are often neglected in stroke patients. Recent studies suggest that they are frequent and have an impact on stroke outcome.

Methods.—We review current knowledge about frequency, clinical presentation, and consequences of poststroke SDB and SWD, and discuss treatment options.

Results.—SDB, presenting with obstructive, central, or mixed apneas, is present in 50%–70% of stroke patients. We recommend screening for SDB in all stroke patients by respirography. Continuous positive airway pressure (CPAP) is the treatment of choice for obstructive SDB, which reverses the vascular risk of the patients. In the absence of controlled trials, CPAP treatment should be reserved for patients with severe obstructive SDB, daytime symptoms (e.g., sleepiness), or high cardiovascular risk profile. Oxygen and adaptive servoventilation may be used for central SDB. SWD including insomnia, disturbances of wakefulness (hypersomnia, excessive daytime sleepiness, fatigue), sleep-related movement disorders (restless legs syndrome, periodic limb movements during sleep), and parasomnias (REM sleep behavior disorder) are found in 10%–50% of patients. SWD are associated with cognitive disturbances and may compromise neurologic recovery. Hypnotics and sedative antidepressants may aggravate SDB and neurologic recovery and should be used with caution. For disturbances of wakefulness, dopaminergic drugs, modafinil, or activating antidepressants may be considered. Poststroke sleep-related movement disorders can be treated with dopaminergic drugs; REM sleep behavior disorder with clonazepam.

Conclusions.—Sleep-related breathing disturbances and sleep-wake disturbances are frequent conditions that affect stroke outcome. In view of existing treatment options, these conditions deserve the neurologist's awareness (Table 2).

▶ Sleep-disordered breathing is still widely overlooked by neurologists and other providers caring for stroke patients in typical clinical settings. Nonetheless, there is compelling evidence that sleep apnea and other sleep disturbances are highly prevalent in stroke patients. The authors have brought together important data from a variety of sources that provide clear information on how to identify, evaluate, and treat these conditions. While future studies

TABLE 2.—Effect of CPAP After Stroke

Study	Patients	Age, y	Body mass index (BMI), kg/m²	Findings
Wessendorf et al. (2001)[51]	105 stroke patients (ischemic and hemorrhagic) with SDB, defined by respiratory disturbance index ≥15/h (80 men, 25 women); patients were recruited in a rehabilitation unit 60 days poststroke and followed up over 10 days	61 ± 19	27 ± 4	70% of patients tolerated CPAP during hospital stay (mean CPAP pressure: 9 ± 2 cm H_2O) and remained on treatment after discharge; in these patients, CPAP reduced respiratory events by 82% and increased minimal SaO_2 from 76 ± 10 to 89 ± 45%; nonacceptance of CPAP was associated with poor Barthel index and presence of aphasia; subjective well-being was significantly improved in compliant vs noncompliant patients; in a sample of 16 subjects, mean nocturnal blood pressure decreased in compliant, but not in noncompliant patients (−8 ± 7 mm Hg vs 1 ± 8mm Hg)
Sandberg et al. (2002)[55]	63 patients with ischemic stroke; SDB defined by respiratory disturbance index ≥15/h; Patients were recruited in a rehabilitation unit 2–4 weeks poststroke and followed up over 28 days	77 ± 8 (no CPAP) and 78 ± 6 (CPAP)	25 ± 5 (no CPAP) and 24 ± 4 (CPAP)	In this randomized trial, CPAP was used by 31 out of 33 patients for 4 weeks; compared to the control group (no treatment), depressive symptoms improved in patients randomized to CPAP; no significant treatment effect was found with regard to Mini-Mental State Examination (MMSE) or Barthel-Activities of Daily Living (ADL) index; low cognitive level (MMSE score) explained poor use (mean 4.1 ± 3.6 hours/night) with CPAP
Hui et al. (2002)[13]	34 patients with ischemic stroke with an AHI ≥10/h; patients were recruited 4 days poststroke and followed up over up to 3 months	64 ± 13	24 ± 4	CPAP titration successfully performed in 47% of patients (mean CPAP pressure: 11 ± 1 cm H_2O); however, only 12% with long-term compliance (average CPAP use: 2.5 ± 0.6 h/night), 100% of which were snorers and 75% of which suffered from daytime sleepiness
Martinez-Garcia et al. (2005)[54]	51 patients with ischemic stroke with an AHI ≥20/h, recruited 2 months poststroke and followed up over 18 months	73 ± 9	27 ± 4	15 of 51 patients (29%) tolerated CPAP and continued therapy over at least 1 month (mean CPAP pressure: 8 ± 4 cm H_2O; mean CPAP use: 6.4 ± 2.2 h/night); patients on CPAP exhibited an AHI decrease from 41 ± 14 to 4 ± 3/h; incidence of new vascular events (stroke, angina, myocardiac infarcts) was significantly lower in compliant compared with noncompliant patients (7% vs 36%); treatment tolerance reduced vascular risk by fivefold, when adjusted for other vascular risk factors, Canadian Stroke Scale, and Barthel index (1 new vascular event less for every 4 patients treated)

(Continued)

Table 2. Effect of CPAP After Stroke

Study	Patients	Age, y	Body mass index (BMI), kg/m^2	Findings
Hsu et al. (2006)[56]	30 patients with stroke with an AHI ≥30/h, for which 658 patients had to be screened; randomization to CPAP therapy over 8 weeks or no treatment; treatment initiated 21–25 days after the stroke, patients followed up over up to 6 months; patients balanced for NIH Stroke Scale (NIHSS) score and Epworth Sleepiness Scale score	Mean 73 (no CPAP) and 74 (CPAP)	Mean 25 (no CPAP) and 27 (CPAP)	In this randomized trial, objective CPAP use was poor, averaging to 1.4 h/night; the study was prematurely stopped due to poor recruitment; CPAP treatment resulting in no significant improvements in neurologic outcome, anxiety, depression, as well as quality of life; no significant difference in 24 h daytime and nighttime systolic blood pressure, diastolic blood pressure, and mean arterial blood pressure between groups; only 7 of 15 patients (47%) kept using the CPAP device over more than 4 weeks; treatment discontinued in 8 patients because of problems with mask or machine, stroke-related confusional states, or upper airway symptoms; CPAP use positively correlated with better Barthel index and better language capabilities
Bassetti et al. (2006)[3]	70 acute ischemic stroke patients with AHI ≥15/h or AHI >10/h plus excessive daytime sleepiness (EDS); patients were recruited within 1 week poststroke and followed up over up to 5 years	56 ± 13	26 ± 4	CPAP treatment successfully initiated in 69% of patients, with compliance until patient discharge in 51% and longterm compliance in only 15%; CPAP users did not differ from nonusers with respect to age, gender, BMI, history of hypertension, diabetes, or coronary disease; no difference in EDS, initial NIHSS, and initial AHI
Palombini and Guilleminault (2006)[52]	32 patients with stroke evaluated for CPAP study; 11 patients refused to participate, 21 patients assessed by respirography; 14 patients with AHI ≥10/h enrolled during acute hospital stay; patients followed up over 8 weeks	62 ± 13	23 ± 3	12 out of 14 patients agreed to initiate CPAP at home (mean pressure 8 ± 4 cmH_2O), 7 of which (50%) continued CPAP usage over the whole observation period; treatment stopped because of problems with cognition and orientation, inability to apply headgear, mask, and hose, and to readjust equipment
Broadley et al. (2007)[18]	16 stroke patients with AHI ≥15/h enrolled during first poststroke days and followed up over 6 weeks	Mean 71	27 ± 4	13 out of 16 patients agreed to initiate CPAP therapy, which was tolerated by 8 patients; control respirography in the end of the observation period confirmed persistence of obstructive sleep apnea in the whole sample (AHI in all patients ≥10/h)

Scala et al. (2009)[53]	12 patients (4 men, 8 women) recruited within 48 h after stroke and studied over a single night	75 ± 5	27 ± 5	90%, 60%, and 50% of patients exhibiting respiratory disturbance index ≥5/h, ≥10/h, and ≥15/h; CPAP acceptance was 84%, 42% using CPAP >6 h and 42% between 1 and 3 h per night (mean 5.2 ± 4.0 h)
Martinez-Garcia et al. (2009)[57]	166 patients with ischemic stroke, 96 of them with AHI ≥20/h were offered CPAP; patients were recruited 2 months poststroke and followed up over 5 years	Mean 76 (no CPAP) and 71 (CPAP)	Mean 28 (no CPAP) and 27 (CPAP)	In this prospective observational study, a lower mortality (50%) was found in 28 out of 96 patients with AHI ≥20/h and long-term CPAP use, compared with patients with AHI ≥20/h not using CPAP (68%)

Data are mean ± SD.
CPAP = continuous positive airway pressure; SDB = sleep-related breathing disturbances; AHI = apnea-hypopnea index.
Editor's Note: Please refer to original journal article for full references.

may help to establish better guidelines for patient selection for specific interventions, it should be apparent from the current evidence that continuing to ignore sleep disorders in stroke patients is not likely to serve the patients' best interests. Increased clinical awareness and recognition of sleep disorders in patients with cerebrovascular disease along with proper diagnosis and appropriate treatment in selected patients may be expected to lead to reduction in patient risks and improvement in overall outcomes.

B. Nolan, MD

Triggering of Nocturnal Arrhythmias by Sleep-Disordered Breathing Events

Monahan K, Storfer-Isser A, Mehra R, et al (Vanderbilt Univ Med Ctr, Nashville, TN; Case School of Medicine, Cleveland, OH; et al)

J Am Coll Cardiol 54:1797-1804, 2009

Objectives.—This study sought to evaluate respiratory disturbances as potential triggers for arrhythmia in patients with sleep-disordered breathing (SDB).

Background.—SDB is associated with an increased risk of atrial fibrillation and nonsustained ventricular tachycardia (NSVT) as well as a predilection for sudden cardiac death during nocturnal sleeping hours. However, prior research has not established whether respiratory disturbances operate as triggers for nocturnal arrhythmias.

Methods.—Overnight polysomnograms from the Sleep Heart Health Study (n = 2,816) were screened for paroxysmal atrial fibrillation and NSVT. We used the case-crossover design to determine whether apneas and/or hypopneas are temporally associated with episodes of paroxysmal atrial fibrillation or NSVT. For each arrhythmia, 3 periods of sinus rhythm were identified as control intervals. Polysomnograms were examined for the presence of respiratory disturbances, oxygen desaturations, and cortical arousals within a 90-s hazard period preceding each arrhythmia or control period.

Results.—Fifty-seven participants with a wide range of SDB contributed 62 arrhythmias (76% NSVT). The odds of an arrhythmia after a respiratory disturbance were nearly 18 times (odds ratio: 17.5; 95% confidence interval: 5.3 to 58.4) the odds of an arrhythmia occurring after normal breathing. The absolute rate of arrhythmia associated with respiratory disturbances was low (1 excess arrhythmia per 40,000 respiratory disturbances). Neither hypoxia nor electroencephalogram-defined arousals alone increased arrhythmia risk.

Conclusions.—Although the absolute arrhythmia rate is low, the relative risk of paroxysmal atrial fibrillation and NSVT during sleep is markedly increased shortly after a respiratory disturbance. These results

TABLE 4.—Risk of Arrhythmia After Respiratory Disturbance Compared With Risk of Arrhythmia During Normal Nocturnal Breathing

	Arrhythmias Included in Each Analysis	Odds Ratio (95% CI)
Primary overall analysis	62	17.5 (5.3–58.4)
Subanalysis by arrhythmia type		
PAF	15	17.9 (2.2–144.2)
NSVT	47	17.4 (4.0–75.7)
Subanalysis by sleep stage		
NREM	42	14.2 (4.2–48.0)
REM	20	*
Subanalysis by respiratory disturbance subtype		
No respiratory disturbance	18	Reference
Respiratory disturbance without hypoxia (nadir $SpO_2 \leq 92\%$) or arousal	14	24.1 (5.4–106.6)
Respiratory disturbance with hypoxia	20	13.6 (3.7–50.6)
Respiratory disturbance with arousal	10	21.8 (4.5–106.3)

CI = confidence interval; other abbreviations as in Tables 1 and 2.
*Unable to be calculated.

support a direct temporal link between SDB events and the development of these arrhythmias (Table 4).

▶ Time-honored techniques of 24-hour cardiac monitoring may identify arrhythmias but not necessarily the underlying cause. A variety of cardiac arrhythmias may be associated with sleep-disordered breathing (SDB). On overnight sleep recordings, relative slowing and speeding of heart rate with apneas is commonplace. This study shows the statistically greatly increased risk for individuals with SDB to manifest 2 serious forms of cardiac arrhythmia. Overnight sleep recording frequently identifies patients with hundreds of apneas per night. One excess arrhythmia per 40 000 abnormal respiratory events may not seem like a lot but, as the authors indicate, individuals with sleep apnea may have that many events in less than 6 months. There is evidence already indicating that treatment of SDB with nasal positive airway pressure reduces overall risk for those with moderate to severe SDB. Further study of the subgroup with cardiac arrhythmias is, in my estimation, likely to provide additional support for earlier identification and treatment of SDB.

B. Nolan, MD

NEUROSURGERY

PAUL KLIMO, JR, MD, MPH

14 Brain Tumors

ABC Surgical Risk Scale for skull base meningioma: a new scoring system for predicting the extent of tumor removal and neurological outcome: Clinical article

Adachi K, Kawase T, Yoshida K, et al (Keio Univ, Tokyo, Japan)

J Neurosurg 111:1053-1061, 2009

Object.—Surgery for skull base meningiomas (SBMs) can lead to complications because these lesions are difficult to approach and can involve cranial nerves and arteries. The authors propose a scoring system to evaluate the relative risks and benefits of surgical treatment of SBMs.

Methods.—The authors used a 2-step process to construct their scale. First, they derived significant predictive variables from retrospective data on 132 SBM cases treated surgically (primary surgeries only) between May 2000 and December 2005. Next, they validated the predictive accuracy of their scoring system in 60 consecutive cases treated surgically between January 1995 and April 2000, including both primary and repeated surgeries. Finally, they investigated the effect of the surgery on the patients' preoperative symptoms for consecutive cases treated surgically between January 1995 and December 2005, including both primary surgeries and retreatments.

Results.—Five items that predicted surgical risk were identified: 1) tumor attachment size; 2) arterial involvement; 3) brainstem contact; 4) central cavity location; and 5) cranial nerve group involvement. The authors named their scoring system the ABC Surgical Risk Scale, after the initial letters of these items. Each factor was assigned a score of 0–2 points, and an additional point was added for previous surgical treatment or for radiation, giving a possible total score of 12 points. On average, the scoring system allocated 2 points for gross-total resections, 6.1 points for near-total resections, and 9 points for subtotal resections, with significant differences between groups. For cases scoring ≥ 8 points, the percentage of cases showing neurological deterioration postoperatively exceeded the percentage showing improvement.

Conclusions.—The authors conclude that this scoring system can be used to predict the extent of tumor removal and that the scores reflect the surgical risk.

▶ The authors of this article describe a simple scoring system for risk assessment of surgical removal of skull base meningiomas. It is based primarily on the following factors that can increase the risk of surgery: attachment size, arterial involvement, brainstem contact, central cavity location, cranial nerve involvement, and prior radiation or surgery. The scoring system is also useful in predicting the likelihood of gross total removal. Those that are at lower risk for surgery are more likely to be amenable to gross total or near total removal. Those that are at higher risk of neurological deterioration after complete removal may be more suitable for subtotal resection and possible radiosurgery of the residual tumor. Although the authors have validated this scoring system in their practice, this system should be validated by other high-volume skull base meningioma centers.

J. K. Liu, MD

Alterations of *BRAF* and *HIPK2* loci predominate in sporadic pilocytic astrocytoma

Yu J, Deshmukh H, Gutmann RJ, et al (Washington Univ School of Medicine, St Louis, MO; et al)

Neurology 73:1526-1531, 2009

Objective.—Independent studies have previously demonstrated that both the *HIPK2* and *BRAF* genes are amplified and rearranged, respectively, in pilocytic astrocytomas (PAs). The purpose of this study was to further investigate the frequency of *BRAF* and *HIPK2* alterations in PAs, the concordance of these events, and their relationship to clinical phenotype.

Methods.—We performed extensive characterization by array-based copy number assessment (aCGH), *HIPK2* copy number analysis, and *BRAF* rearrangement and mutation analysis in a set of 79 PAs, including 9 tumors from patients with neurofibromatosis type 1 (NF1).

Results.—We identified 1 of 3 previously identified *BRAF* rearrangements in 42/70 sporadic PAs. An additional 2 tumors with no rearrangement also exhibited *BRAF* mutation, including a novel 3-base insertion. As predicted from the genomic organization at this locus, 22/36 tumors with *BRAF* rearrangement also exhibited corresponding *HIPK2* amplification. However, 14/36 tumors with *BRAF* rearrangement had no detectable *HIPK2* gene amplification and 6/20 tumors demonstrated *HIPK2* amplification without apparent *BRAF* rearrangement or mutation. Only 12/70 PAs lacked detectable *BRAF* or *HIPK2* alterations. Importantly, none of the 9 PA tumors from NF1 patients exhibited *BRAF* rearrangement or mutation.

Conclusions.—*BRAF* rearrangement represents the most common genetic alteration in sporadic, but not neurofibromatosis type 1-associated, pilocytic astrocytomas (PAs). These findings implicate BRAF in the pathogenesis of these common low-grade astrocytomas in children, and suggest that PAs arise either from *NF1* inactivation or *BRAF* gain of function.

▶ This study of the molecular basis of pilocytic astrocytomas (PAs) from one of the leading laboratories in the world studying neurofibromatosis sheds new light on the etiology of PAs. Recent evidence has shown that *BRAF* is linked to numerous cancers. It is frequently mutated in low-grade gliomas, but is rarely disturbed in high-grade gliomas. This study finds that *BRAF* is mutated (rearranged) in a majority of sporadic PA cases. However, PAs arising in *NF1* patients do not exhibit alterations of the *BRAF* gene. This study suggests that *BRAF* is critical to the genesis of PAs and further differentiates the etiology of sporadic and *NF1*-associated PAs.

G. Rao, MD

Complications of Particle Embolization of Meningiomas: Frequency, Risk Factors, and Outcome

Carli DFM, Sluzewski M, Beute GN, et al (St Elisabeth Ziekenhuis, Tilburg, the Netherlands)

Am J Neuroradiol 31:152-154, 2010

Background and Purpose.—Particle embolization is widely used in the treatment of meningiomas. We assessed the frequency and outcome of complications of embolization of meningiomas and tried to identify risk factors.

Materials and Methods.—Between 1994 and 2009, a total of 198 patients with 201 meningiomas underwent embolization. Indication for embolization was preoperative in 165 meningiomas and adjunctive to radiosurgery in 8. In the remaining 28 meningiomas, embolization was initially offered as a sole therapy. There were 128 women and 70 men with a mean age of 54.4 years (median age, 54 years; range, 15–90 years). Complications were defined as any neurologic deficit or death that occurred during or after embolization. Logistic regression was used to identify the following possible risk factors: age above median, female sex, tumor size above median, meningioma location in 5 categories, use of small particle size (45–150 μm), the presence of major peritumoral edema, and arterial supply in 3 categories.

Results.—Complications occurred in 11 patients (5.6%; 95% confidence interval [CI], 3.0%–9.8%). Ten complications were hemorrhagic, and 1 was ischemic. Six of 10 patients with hemorrhagic complications underwent emergency surgery with removal of the hematoma and meningioma. Complications of embolization resulted in death in 2 and dependency in 5 patients (7/198, 3.5%; 95% CI, 1.6%–2.0%). The use of small particles (45–150 μm) was the only risk factor for complications (odds ratio [OR], 10.21; CI, 1.3–80.7; P =.028).

Conclusions.—In this series, particle embolization of meningiomas had a complication rate of 5.6%. We believe that the use of small polyvinyl alcohol (PVA) particles (45–150 μm) should be discouraged.

▶ Particle embolization as an adjunct to surgery or radiosurgery is a common practice. This report details the complications associated with the procedure when used either as an adjunct to definitive treatment or as a sole therapy. This large retrospective series indicates that complications are probably more common than most surgeons suspect at almost 6% of cases. Surprisingly, a majority of cases required surgical intervention to evacuate a hematoma. The authors find that small particles (45-150 μm) are a significant risk for complications and have adjusted their practice accordingly.

G. Rao, MD

Identification and Functional Characterization of microRNAs Involved in the Malignant Progression of Gliomas

Malzkorn B, Wolter M, Liesenberg F, et al (Heinrich-Heine-Univ, Düsseldorf, Germany; et al)
Brain Pathol 20:539-550, 2010

Diffuse astrocytoma of World Health Organization (WHO) grade II has an inherent tendency to spontaneously progress to anaplastic astrocytoma WHO grade III or secondary glioblastoma WHO grade IV. We explored the role of microRNAs (miRNAs) in glioma progression by investigating the expression profiles of 157 miRNAs in four patients with primary WHO grade II gliomas that spontaneously progressed to WHO grade IV secondary glioblastomas. Thereby, we identified 12 miRNAs (miR-9, miR-15a, miR-16, miR-17, miR-19a, miR-20a, miR-21, miR-25, miR-28, miR-130b, miR-140 and miR-210) showing increased expression, and two miRNAs (miR-184 and miR-328) showing reduced expression upon progression. Validation experiments on independent series of primary low-grade and secondary high-grade astrocytomas confirmed miR-17 and miR-184 as promising candidates, which were selected for functional analyses. These studies revealed miRNA-specific influences on the viability, proliferation, apoptosis and invasive growth properties of A172 and T98G glioma cells *in vitro*. Using mRNA and protein expression profiling, we identified distinct sets of transcripts and proteins that were differentially expressed after inhibition of miR-17 or overexpression of miR-184 in glioma cells. Taken together, our results support an important role of altered miRNA expression in gliomas, and suggest miR-17 and miR-184 as interesting candidates contributing to glioma progression.

▶ MicroRNAs (miRNAs) are noncoding RNA molecules that posttranscriptionally regulate gene expression by modulating mRNA transcripts. miRNA-mediated regulation of gene expression is very complex, and a single miRNA may affect multiple gene targets. The authors studied glioblastoma multiforme samples to identify miRNAs that are upregulated in the malignant transformation of grade 2 astrocytomas to grade 3 and grade 4 astrocytomas. The authors identify miRNAs that play a role in tumor progression and indicate that these may become the targets of novel therapeutic strategies.

G. Rao, MD

Impact of Morphology, MIB-1, p53 and *MGMT* on Outcome in Pilocytic Astrocytomas

Horbinski C, Hamilton RL, Lovell C, et al (Univ of Kentucky, Lexington; Univ of Pittsburgh, PA; et al)

Brain Pathol 20:581-588, 2010

Pilocytic astrocytoma (PA) is the most common glioma in the pediatric population. PAs can exhibit variable behavior that does not always correlate with location, yet at present there is no way to predict which tumors will be more aggressive. To address this problem, an institutional cohort of 147 PAs (118 with outcome data) from both cerebellar and noncerebellar locations (spine, diencephalon, midbrain, brainstem and cortex) was utilized. Parameters included quantification of characteristic morphologic variables as well as genes previously shown to be of relevance in high-grade gliomas, including MIB-1, p53 and *MGMT*. In this cohort, the classic biphasic appearance was most common in cerebellar tumors, whereas noncerebellar tumors were predominantly microcystic. Associations with outcome suggest that the presence of degenerative atypia may be a favorable factor in PAs. Oligodendroglial morphology and the absence of leptomeningeal invasion are adverse histologic factors, but only in cerebellar tumors. Conversely, MIB-1 proliferation index and p53 and *MGMT* expression do not correlate with outcome. Morphologic biomarkers thus do exist for PAs, but the utility of each biomarker varies according to location. These results suggest that PAs differ fundamentally according to location; therefore, biological behavior may not simply depend on extent of resection.

▶ Pilocytic astrocytomas (PAs), although common, receive little basic science study, primarily because of the perception that they are curable tumors. However, they can be the source of significant morbidity and for recurrent or unresectable tumors, and there are few therapeutic options. A better understanding of the biology of PAs should help develop new therapies for these tumors. The authors of this study apply multiple variables to better describe and understand this tumor type. Using a large tumor bank, they show that tumor location correlates with outcome. Further, they show that histologic features, such as degenerative atypia, were associated with a reduced risk of adverse outcomes. Unlike higher grade gliomas, p53, MIB-1, or MGMT status did not correlate with outcome. This study helps sort out some important issues of this common tumor type.

G. Rao, MD

Maternally Expressed Gene 3, an Imprinted Noncoding RNA Gene, Is Associated with Meningioma Pathogenesis and Progression

Zhang X, Gejman R, Mahta A, et al (Massachusetts General Hosp, Boston)

Cancer Res 70:2350-2358, 2010

Meningiomas are common tumors, representing 15% to 25% of all central nervous system tumors. *NF2* gene inactivation on chromosome 22 has been shown as an early event in tumorigenesis; however, few factors underlying tumor growth and progression have been identified. The chromosomal abnormalities of 14q32 are often associated with meningioma pathogenesis and progression; therefore, it has been proposed that an as yet unidentified tumor suppressor is present at this locus. *Maternally expressed gene 3 (MEG3)* is an imprinted gene located at 14q32 which encodes a noncoding RNA with an antiproliferative function. We found that MEG3 mRNA is highly expressed in normal arachnoidal cells. However, *MEG3* is not expressed in the majority of human meningiomas or the human meningioma cell lines IOMM-Lee and CH157-MN. There is a strong association between loss of *MEG3* expression and tumor grade. Allelic loss at the *MEG3* locus is also observed in meningiomas, with increasing prevalence in higher grade tumors. In addition, there is an increase in CpG methylation within the promoter and the imprinting control region of *MEG3* gene in meningiomas. Functionally, MEG3 suppresses DNA synthesis in both IOMM-Lee and CH157-MN cells by ~60% in bromodeoxyuridine incorporation assays. Colony-forming efficiency assays show that MEG3 inhibits colony formation in CH157-MN cells by ~80%. Furthermore, MEG3 stimulates p53-mediated transactivation in these cell lines. Therefore, these data are consistent with the hypothesis that *MEG3*, which encodes a noncoding RNA, may be a tumor suppressor gene at chromosome 14q32 involved in meningioma progression via a novel mechanism.

▶ The molecular contributions to meningioma formation and growth are poorly understood. Loss of chromosome 22 has long been associated with meningioma, but so is loss of chromosome 14. The authors describe a novel tumor suppressor gene, maternally expressed gene 3 (*MEG3*), as potentially relevant to meningioma pathogenesis and progression. Importantly, they show that *MEG3* is expressed in arachnoidal cells (arachnoid cap cells are the presumed cell of origin for meningiomas) but not in meningioma tissue or cell lines. They also show that transfection of *MEG3*-expressing vectors can decrease cellular proliferation in meningioma cell lines. This report describes a new discovery in meningioma biology and a promising therapeutic target.

G. Rao, MD

Postoperative nonconvulsive encephalopathic status: identification of a syndrome responsible for delayed progressive deterioration of neurological status after skull base surgery: Clinical Article

Al-Mefty O, Wrubel D, Haddad N (Univ of Arkansas for Med Sciences, Little Rock)

J Neurosurg 111:1062-1068, 2009

Object.—Over a 10-year period, the authors have observed a rare but recurring syndrome manifested by a delayed, postoperative, progressive decline in the level of consciousness to deep coma that is time-limited to several days with abrupt awakening. Extensive evaluation and workup demonstrated an abnormality on continuous electroencephalographic monitoring that implied nonconvulsive status epilepticus after the exclusion of structural, perfusion, infectious, or metabolic causes. This state has been very refractory to treatment with antiepileptic medication. In this article, the authors raise the awareness of this syndrome and its diagnosis, management, and outcome.

Methods.—The authors reviewed the medical records of a cohort of 7 patients who exemplified this syndrome who were treated during the last 5 years.

Results.—All 7 patients were women with a mean (± SD) age of 55 ± 15 years. The mean duration of surgery was 8.9 ± 1.8 hours. All patients had a stereotypical course of delayed progressive decline in their level of consciousness after surgery (average 3.3 ± 4.3 days) leading to deep coma. The unconscious state was time-limited, lasting on average 17.3 ± 13.7 days. Continuous electroencephalographic monitoring demonstrated a generalized abnormality with periodic discharges and abundant slow delta activity. A rather abrupt awakening occurred a few days after cessation of electrographic seizure activity. Structural, vascular, infectious, or metabolic causes were excluded based on an extensive workup.

Conclusions.—In this study, the authors delineate and raise the awareness of an unusual syndrome. Recognition of this syndrome is important as a cause for delayed coma after surgery. The authors stress the need for respiratory, hemodynamic, and nutritional support for these patients until recovery. The origin of this syndrome remains enigmatic and is likely to be multifactorial with a prominent pharmacological role related to anesthetic agent or medication in a setting of craniotomy that is associated with alteration of the blood-brain barrier.

▶ The authors describe a rare but important syndrome—postoperative nonconvulsive encephalopathic status—that can be seen after skull base surgery, characterized by a delayed coma after surgery that is followed by abrupt awakening after several days. I have encountered this phenomenon on a few occasions in my practice and have attributed this to postoperative encephalopathy of some sort. Making the diagnosis can be difficult since it is a diagnosis of exclusion after an extensive workup to rule out other structural, infectious, or metabolic causes. EEG monitoring should be initiated early; however, the findings may be nonspecific. Skull base and cerebrovascular surgeons should be aware of this possible postoperative condition and continue to optimize the milieu for brain recovery with supportive care during the encephalopathic comatose period. Despite the grim appearing clinical picture, there is good chance that the patient can wake up and have an excellent recovery.

J. K. Liu, MD

Preclinical Evaluation of Radiation and Perifosine in a Genetically and Histologically Accurate Model of Brainstem Glioma

Becher OJ, Hambardzumyan D, Walker TR, et al (Memorial Sloan-Kettering Cancer Ctr, NY; et al)

Cancer Res 70:2548-2557, 2010

Brainstem gliomas (BSG) are a rare group of central nervous system tumors that arise mostly in children and usually portend a particularly poor prognosis. We report the development of a genetically engineered mouse model of BSG using the RCAS/tv-a system and its implementation in preclinical trials. Using immunohistochemistry, we found that platelet-derived growth factor (PDGF) receptor α is overexpressed in 67% of pediatric BSGs. Based on this observation, we induced low-grade BSGs by overexpressing PDGF-B in the posterior fossa of neonatal nestin tv-a mice. To generate high-grade BSGs, we overexpressed PDGF-B in combination with Ink4a-ARF loss, given that this locus is commonly lost in high-grade pediatric BSGs. We show that the likely cells of origin for these mouse BSGs exist on the floor of the fourth ventricle and cerebral aqueduct. Irradiation of these high-grade BSGs shows that although single doses of 2, 6, and 10 Gy significantly increased the percent of terminal deoxynucleotidyl transferase–mediated dUTP nick end labeling (TUNEL)–positive nuclei, only 6 and 10 Gy significantly induce cell cycle arrest. Perifosine, an inhibitor of AKT signaling, significantly induced TUNEL-positive nuclei in this high-grade BSG model, but in combination with 10 Gy, it did not significantly increase the percent of TUNEL-positive nuclei relative to 10 Gy alone at 6, 24, and 72 hours. Survival analysis showed that a single dose of 10 Gy significantly prolonged survival by 27% ($P = 0.0002$) but perifosine did not ($P = 0.92$). Perifosine + 10 Gy did not result in a significantly increased survival relative to 10 Gy alone ($P = 0.23$). This PDGF-induced BSG model can serve as a preclinical tool for the testing of novel agents.

▶ Brainstem gliomas are uniformly fatal tumors that have a predilection for children. Current treatment includes radiation and chemotherapy with a survival time of approximately 19 months. Until this report, researchers were lacking a mouse model with which to study this disease. The authors report a robust and reproducible model of brainstem glioma using the RCAS/tv-a system. This model results in tumors that recapitulate what is observed in human tumors. Importantly, they were able to use this model for preclinical testing of perifosine and radiation.

G. Rao, MD

Prognostic Significance of Molecular Markers and Extent of Resection in Primary Glioblastoma Patients

Felsberg J, Rapp M, Loeser S, et al (Heinrich-Heine-Univ, Düsseldorf, Germany)

Clin Cancer Res 15:6683-6693, 2009

Purpose.—Despite multimodal aggressive treatment glioblastoma patients still face a rather poor prognosis. Recent data indicate that certain molecular markers, in particular *MGMT* promoter hypermethylation, are associated with response to alkylating chemotherapy and longer survival. The clinical significance of other glioblastoma-associated molecular aberrations and their relationship to *MGMT* promoter hypermethylation is still poorly understood.

Experimental Design.—We conducted a translational study involving 67 newly diagnosed glioblastoma patients treated at our institution from 1998 to 2004. All patients were treated by open resection, followed by radiotherapy and adjuvant temozolomide chemotherapy. The tumors were investigated for *MGMT* promoter methylation, mRNA and protein expression, as well as presence of *MGMT* sequence polymorphisms. In addition, we screened for genetic aberrations of the *EGFR*, *TP53*, *CDK4*, *MDM2*, and *PDGFRA* genes as well as allelic losses on chromosomal arms 1p, 10q, and 19q.

Results.—Correlation of molecular findings with clinical data revealed significantly longer time to progression after onset of chemotherapy and longer overall survival of patients with *MGMT*-hypermethylated tumors. In contrast, *MGMT* protein expression, *MGMT* polymorphisms, and aberrations in any of the other genes and chromosomes were not significantly linked to patient outcome. Multivariate analysis identified *MGMT* promoter hypermethylation and near-complete tumor resection as the most important parameters associated with better prognosis.

Conclusion.—Our study provides novel insights into the significance of molecular and clinical markers in predicting the prognosis of glioblastoma patients, which may improve stratification of patients into distinct prognostic subgroups.

▶ This is an interesting study evaluating the potential benefits for the treatment of glioblastoma of MGMT status and maximal surgical resection. Not surprisingly, the authors find that MGMT promoter hypermethylation was associated with a longer time to progression. Other markers, including amplification of EGFR, CDK4, MDM2, PDGFR, or TP53 mutation were not associated with patient survival. A near complete resection (NCR) defined by volumetric MRI comparing the tumor preoperatively and postoperatively conferred a survival advantage to patients. The authors then combined the variables of MGMT methylation status and extent of resection to divide patients into 4 groups: group 1, MGMT methylated and NCR; group 2, MGMT methylated and >5 cc residual tumor; group 3, MGMT unmethylated and NCR; and group 4, MGMT unmethylated and >5 cc residual tumor. Group 1 patients had a significant survival advantage compared with all other groups, but groups 2, 3, and 4 had no differences in survival. This study not only emphasizes the importance of molecular markers but also the value of surgical resection in treating glioblastoma.

G. Rao, MD

Specific Targeting of Brain Tumors with an Optical/Magnetic Resonance Imaging Nanoprobe across the Blood-Brain Barrier

Veiseh O, Sun C, Fang C, et al (Univ of Washington, Seattle; et al)

Cancer Res 69:6200-6207, 2009

Nanoparticle-based platforms have drawn considerable attention for their potential effect on oncology and other biomedical fields. However, their *in vivo* application is challenged by insufficient accumulation and retention within tumors due to limited specificity to the target, and an inability to traverse biological barriers. Here, we present a nanoprobe that shows an ability to cross the blood-brain barrier and specifically target brain tumors in a genetically engineered mouse model, as established through *in vivo* magnetic resonance and biophotonic imaging, and histologic and biodistribution analyses. The nanoprobe is comprised of an iron oxide nanoparticle coated with biocompatible polyethylene glycol–grafted chitosan copolymer, to which a tumor-targeting agent, chlorotoxin, and a near-IR fluorophore are conjugated. The nanoprobe shows an innocuous toxicity profile and sustained retention in tumors. With the versatile affinity of the targeting ligand and the flexible conjugation chemistry for alternative diagnostic and therapeutic agents, this nanoparticle platform can be potentially used for the diagnosis and treatment of a variety of tumor types.

▶ This study evaluates the applicability of nanoparticles to human brain tumors in a preclinical mouse model. A significant barrier to successful brain tumor treatment is the inability of therapy to cross the blood-brain barrier (BBB). The authors overcome this by using a nanoprobe with the capacity to cross the BBB. Using in vivo MRI, the authors demonstrate that the nanoprobe crosses into the tumor. Using bioluminescence, the authors also show that the agent specifically migrates to the tumor and not to the normal brain. This finding was confirmed histologically. This study not only proves the use of nanoparticles, but it also validates the use of the ND2:SmoA1 mouse as a useful preclinical model.

G. Rao, MD

The miR-17/92 Polycistron Is Up-regulated in Sonic Hedgehog–Driven Medulloblastomas and Induced by N-myc in Sonic Hedgehog–Treated Cerebellar Neural Precursors

Northcott PA, Fernandez-L A, Hagan JP, et al (Univ of Toronto, Ontario, Canada; Memorial Sloan-Kettering Cancer Ctr, NY; Ohio State Univ Med Ctr, Columbus; et al)

Cancer Res 69:3249-3255, 2009

Medulloblastoma is the most common malignant pediatric brain tumor, and mechanisms underlying its development are poorly understood. We identified recurrent amplification of the *miR-17/92* polycistron proto-oncogene in 6% of pediatric medulloblastomas by high-resolution single-nucleotide polymorphism genotyping arrays and subsequent interphase fluorescence *in situ* hybridization on a human medulloblastoma tissue microarray. Profiling the expression of 427 mature microRNAs (miRNA) in a series of 90 primary human medulloblastomas revealed that components of the miR-17/92 polycistron are the most highly up-regulated miRNAs in medulloblastoma. Expression of miR-17/92 was highest in the subgroup of medulloblastomas associated with activation of the sonic hedgehog (Shh) signaling pathway compared with other subgroups of medulloblastoma. Medulloblastomas in which miR-17/92 was up-regulated also had elevated levels of MYC/MYCN expression. Consistent with its regulation by Shh, we observed that Shh treatment of primary cerebellar granule neuron precursors (CGNP), proposed cells of origin for the Shh-associated medulloblastomas, resulted in increased miR-17/92 expression. In CGNPs, the Shh effector N-myc, but not Gli1, induced miR-17/92 expression. Ectopic miR-17/92 expression in CGNPs synergized with exogenous Shh to increase proliferation and also enabled them to proliferate in the absence of Shh. We conclude that miR-17/92 is a positive effector of Shh-mediated proliferation and that aberrant expression/amplification of this miR confers a growth advantage to medulloblastomas.

▶ The authors identify a microRNA (miRNA) in pediatric medulloblastoma that is associated with sonic hedgehog upregulation. miRNA are emerging as important regulators of crucial biological processes and may be critical to understanding the molecular mechanisms of cancer. The authors used high-resolution single-nucleotide polymorphism genotyping arrays and interphase fluorescence in situ hybridization on a human medulloblastoma tissue microarray. After profiling 90 human medulloblastomas, they identified a consistently up-regulated miRNA. The miRNA identified in this study, miR-17/92, is amplified and overexpressed in medulloblastoma and can drive proliferation of the granule neuron precursor (the putative cell of origin of medulloblastoma) in the absence of sonic hedgehog. Thus, miR-17/92 may be a key contributor to aberrant sonic hedgehog signaling and contribute to medulloblastoma formation.

G. Rao, MD

15 Cerebrovascular

Monitoring intracranial pressure in patients with malignant middle cerebral artery infarction: is it useful?

Poca MA, Benejam B, Sahuquillo J, et al (Autonomous Univ of Barcelona, Spain)

J Neurosurg 112:648-657, 2010

Object.—Intracranial pressure (ICP) monitoring is increasingly used in the treatment of patients with malignant middle cerebral artery (MCA) infarction. However, neurological deterioration may exist independent from intracranial hypertension. This study aimed to present the findings of continuous ICP monitoring in a cohort of patients with malignant MCA infarction and to correlate these findings with clinical and radiological features.

Methods.—The authors studied a prospective cohort of 25 patients with malignant MCA infarction consecutively admitted to the neurotrauma intensive care unit of the Vall d'Hebron University Hospital between March 2002 and September 2006. The patients were treated using a combined protocol of initial moderate hypothermia and hemicraniectomy. The latter was performed when patients showed a midline shift (MLS) ≥ 5 mm or ICP > 20 mm Hg. Six patients had an MLS ≥ 5 mm on the first CT scan and underwent surgery without prior ICP monitoring. This study focuses on the subgroup of 19 patients who underwent intraparenchymatous ICP monitoring before surgery.

Results.—Intracranial pressure readings were evaluated and correlated with pupillary abnormalities, MLS, and ischemic tissue volume. In 12 of the 19 patients, ICP values were always $\leq$ 20 mm Hg, despite a mean ($\pm$ SD) MLS of 6.7 ± 2 mm and a mean ischemic tissue volume of 241.3 ± 83 cm^3. In 2 patients with anisocoria, ICP values were also normal.

Conclusions.—In patients with a malignant MCA infarction, pupillary abnormalities and severe brainstem compression may be present despite normal ICP values. Therefore, continuous ICP monitoring cannot substitute for close clinical and radiological follow-up in the management of these patients.

▶ This is an interesting record of 19 patients with malignant middle cerebral artery infarctions who underwent intracranial pressure monitoring. The authors document significant clinical and radiographic evidence of complications associated with cerebral edema in the absence of elevated intracranial pressure recorded on the monitor.

This relatively simple study provides clear evidence that is clinically useful. Clinical judgment and close monitoring in the intensive care unit are essential in the management of these patients. Although pressure monitors are an important tool, they do not provide adequate warning of herniation in patients with large evolving infarctions.

A. S. Arthur, MD, MPH

Analysis of cerebral perfusion and metabolism assessed with positron emission tomography before and after carotid artery stenting: Clinical article

Matsubara S, Moroi J, Suzuki A, et al (Res Inst for Brain and Blood Vessels–Akita, Japan)

J Neurosurg 111:28-36, 2009

Object.—The authors analyzed cerebral perfusion and metabolism in patients with internal carotid artery stenosis before and after carotid artery stenting (CAS).

Methods.—Sixteen patients with internal carotid artery stenosis (> 70%) underwent PET scanning before CAS, 1–7 days after CAS, and 3–4 months after CAS to assess a variety of parameters related to cerebral perfusion and metabolism.

Results.—Cerebral blood flow at rest (CBF_{rest}) significantly increased in the immediate postoperative stage before returning to normal levels over the long term; this trend was also recognized on the contralateral side. In contrast, there was gradual improvement in the rate of CBF variation on acetazolamide administration (% CBF_{az}). Cerebral perfusion pressure (CBF/cerebral blood volume) increased rapidly during the acute stage and decreased in the long term, and the oxygen extraction fraction decreased slightly during the acute stage before normalizing over the long term. The cerebral metabolic rate of oxygen ($CMRO_2$) increased slightly after stenting over both the short and long term. The ratios of ipsilateral to contralateral values (asymmetry index) for CBF_{rest}, % CBF_{az}, cerebral blood volume, oxygen extraction fraction, and $CMRO_2$ tended to approach 1.0 over time.

Conclusions.—Repeated PET scanning revealed improvements in CBF, perfusion pressure, and oxygen metabolism after CAS. In particular, the vascular reserve tended to improve gradually, while CBF, cerebral perfusion pressure, and $CMRO_2$ increased rapidly and peaked soon after CAS. These results suggest that a large discrepancy between rapidly increased CBF, perfusion pressure, and a small increase in vascular reserve in the acute stage after CAS could cause hyperperfusion syndrome.

▶ While the debate continues about whether endovascular carotid artery stenting (CAS) is safer than surgical carotid endarterectomy (CEA), there needs to be further investigation into the physiologic phenomenon that occur in the acute and subacute state following CAS as there has already been some investigation into perfusion phenomena occurring post-CEA.[1] This would aid in understanding some post-CAS complications, most notably hyperperfusion syndrome. The authors describe such perfusion phenomena in 31 patients who underwent CAS after internal carotid artery (ICA) stenosis ≥70%, in whom serial positron emission tomography (PET) using radiolabeled $^{15}O_2$ within 1 month before CAS, 1 to 7 days post-CAS, and in a lesser number of patients 3 to 4 months post-CAS ($n = 8$). These studies also used acetazolamide challenge. The most notable findings, in my opinion, were (1) that in the acute stage there were significant increases in the cerebral blood flow (CBF) on the side of CAS (median of 30%, returned to normal at 3-4 months), while also increased on the contralateral side (median of 18.8%), (2) the cerebral perfusion pressure (CPP) increased significantly bilaterally in the acute phase and later decreased bilaterally at 3 to 4 months, and (3) the oxygen extraction fraction (OEF) decreased slightly in the acute phase but also later normalized. Also, the CBF at 3 to 4 months post-CAS was slightly higher than preoperatively. The cerebral metabolic rate of oxygen ($CMRO_2$) increased in the acute phase as well. These findings suggest an increased metabolic state in acutely post-CAS in previously oligemic or ischemic cerebrum.

Increased CBF immediately post-CEA has been shown by previous studies,[2] but the increase of CBF post-CAS has not yet been shown by PET, to my knowledge. The noted changes in CBF, OEF, and $CMRO_2$ are probably related to a hyperperfusion state that, in combination with the rapidly elevated CPP, may reflect an imbalance between the perfusion pressure and the cerebrovascular reserve. Notably, MR perfusion studies have also noted decreases in transit times in the treated hemisphere,[3] which would seem to corroborate these results. Hence, this study could be a window into the acute/early subacute pathophysiologic cerebrovascular response to CAS, where occasionally patients develop a hyperperfusion syndrome that can lead to significant edema or hemorrhage. Although no patients developed such a complication in this study, potentially larger studies using PET or other perfusion modalities (CT or MRI) may uncover the pre- and postprocedural perfusion values in such patients with complications. In particular, preprocedural perfusion parameters could reveal which patients are at risk for hyperperfusion syndrome, which the authors opine is a marked decrease in CPP.

A. M. McKinney IV, MD

References

1. Cikrit DF, Dalsing MC, Harting PS, et al. Cerebral vascular reactivity assessed with acetazolamide single photon emission computer tomography scans before and after carotid endarterectomy. *Am J Surg*. 1997;174:193-197.
2. Hosoda K, Kawaguchi T, Shibata Y, et al. Cerebral vasoreactivity and internal carotid artery flow help to identify patients at risk for hyperperfusion after carotid endarterectomy. *Stroke*. 2001;32:1567-1573.
3. Wilkinson ID, Griffiths PD, Hoggard N, et al. Short-term changes in cerebral microhemodynamics after carotid stenting. *AJNR Am J Neuroradiol*. 2003;24: 1501-1507.

Defining the Risk of Retreatment for Aneurysm Recurrence or Residual after Initial Treatment by Endovascular Coiling: A Multicenter Study

Ringer AJ, Rodriguez-Mercado R, Veznedaroglu E, et al (Univ of Cincinnati College of Medicine, OH; Univ of Puerto Rico Med Sciences Campus, San Juan; Thomas Jefferson Univ, Philadelphia, PA; et al)
Neurosurgery 65:311-315, 2009

Objective.—Endovascular treatment of intracranial aneurysms is less invasive than surgical repair but poses a higher risk for aneurysm recurrence, which may necessitate retreatment, thus adding to the long-term risk. Cerebrovascular neurosurgeons from 8 institutions in the United States and Puerto Rico collaborated to assess the risk of retreatment for residual or recurrent aneurysms after the initial endovascular coiling.

Methods.—Data were prospectively recorded for 311 patients with coiled intracranial aneurysms who underwent 352 retreatment procedures after angiographic or clinical recurrence (hemorrhage after initial coiling). Results analyzed included procedural complications and procedure-related morbidity. Morbidity was classified as major (modified Rankin scale score > 3) or minor, and temporary (<30 days) or permanent (>30 days).

Results.—Retreatment mortality was 0.85% per procedure and 0.96% per patient. Treatment-related rates were 0.32% per patient (0.28% per procedure) for permanent or temporary major disability; 1.29% for permanent minor disability (1.14% per procedure); and 1.61% for temporary minor disability (1.42% per procedure). Total risk for death or permanent major disability was 1.28% per patient and 1.13% per procedure.

Conclusion.—Retreatment poses a low risk for patients with recurrences of intracranial aneurysms after initial coiling; this risk is smaller than that posed by the initial endovascular therapy. The risk of disability associated with retreatment for aneurysm recurrence after coiling must be considered prospectively in the choice of treatment but with the recognition that its effects are low in the overall management risk.

► This article reviews the records of 311 patients at 8 institutions who underwent retreatment of previously coiled aneurysms. There were a total of 352 retreatments performed in these patients. From these records, the authors note a risk of death or major disability of 1.13%.

Since an increasing number of aneurysms are treated endovascularly, this issue is increasingly important in the practice of cerebrovascular neurosurgery. Although this study does not address the critical question of which aneurysms should be retreated, it provides information on the safety of endovascular retreatment procedures. It is interesting to note that endovascular aneurysm retreatment, based on these data, is actually safer than de novo aneurysm treatment, possibly due to the protective effect of the previously placed coils.

A. S. Arthur, MD, MPH

Giant Aneurysm Clipping Under Protection of an Excimer Laser–Assisted Non-occlusive Anastomosis Bypass

van Doormaal TPC, van der Zwan A, Verweij BH, et al (Univ Med Ctr Utrecht, The Netherlands)

Neurosurgery 66:439-447, 2010

Objective.—To define the safety and clinical value of giant aneurysm clipping under protection of an excimer laser–assisted non-occlusive anastomosis (ELANA) bypass.

Methods.—We report 32 patients with an uncoilable intracerebral giant aneurysm, operated on with the aid of an ELANA protective bypass between January 1, 1994, and January 1, 2008. We retrospectively collected data from patient records. Follow-up data were updated by telephone interview. We defined a favorable outcome as a successfully treated aneurysm and a better or equal postoperative modified Rankin scale (mRS) score compared with the preoperative mRS.

Results.—In total 33 bypasses were constructed, of which 31 (94%) were patent during the rest of the procedure. The first failed bypass was salvaged during a second procedure. Of the second failed bypass, the ELANA anastomosis could be reused during second bypass surgery. All 32 aneurysms could be treated. The bypasses served as protection during temporary parent vessel occlusion (n = 24, 75%), control during aneurysm rupture (n = 3, 9%), and in all patients as an indicator for recipient artery narrowing during clip placement. Four bypasses (12%) eventually had to partially (n = 3) or fully (n = 1) replace recipient artery flow at the end of surgery. Postoperatively, 3 patients (9%) had a hemorrhagic complication and 2 patients (6%) had an ischemic complication. At long-term follow-up (mean, 6.1 ± 3.4 y), 28 patients (88%) had a favorable functional outcome.

Conclusion.—The ELANA protective bypass is a safe and useful instrument for the treatment of these difficult aneurysms.

▶ This article describes the results obtained in using an excimer laser device to perform arterial bypasses useful in the treatment of giant cerebral aneurysms. It is not yet clear whether or not the excimer laser–assisted nonocclusive anastomosis (ELANA) technique will provide significant advantages to a large number of patients, but it is nonetheless an important and productive area of research. Flow replacement is essential in dealing with giant cerebral aneurysms, and the ELANA technique bears watching in this regard.

A. S. Arthur, MD, MPH

How Safe Is Arteriovenous Malformation Surgery? A Prospective, Observational Study of Surgery As First-Line Treatment for Brain Arteriovenous Malformations

Davidson AS, Morgan MK (Macquarie Univ, Sydney, Australia)

Neurosurgery 66:498-505, 2010

Objectives.—Existing studies reporting the risk of surgery for brain arteriovenous malformations (AVMs) are often biased by the exclusion of patients not offered surgery. In this study, we examine the risk of surgery, including cases excluded from surgery because of the high surgical risk.

Methods.—Data were collected on 640 consecutively enrolled AVMs in a database that included all patients not considered for surgery.

Results.—Patients with Spetzler-Martin grade 1 to 2 AVMs (n = 296) were treated with a surgical risk of 0.7% (95% confidence interval [CI], 0%-3%); patients with Spetzler-Martin grade 3 to 4 AVMs in noneloquent cortex (n = 65) were treated with a surgical risk of 17% (95% CI, 10%-28%). Patients with Spetzler-Martin grade 3 to 5 AVMs in eloquent cortex (n = 168) were treated with a surgical risk of 21% (95% CI, 15%-28%). However, because 14% of patients in this series with similar AVMs were refused surgery because of perceived surgical risk, these results are not generalizable to the population of patients with similar AVMs.

Conclusion.—The results of this series suggest that it is reasonable to offer surgery as a preferred treatment option for Spetzler-Martin grade 1 to 2 AVMs. This study also reinforces the predictive value of the Spetzler-Martin grading system, with some caveats.

▶ This is a retrospective review of a large cohort (640) of patients with arteriovenous malformations (AVMs) treated at a single institution. The analysis of the data is valid and demonstrates that surgery carries a low risk for patients with a low Spetzler-Martin grade. Higher-grade patients, with AVMs graded 3 to 5 had less predictable risks, and their treatment was less uniform in this series.

Although the Spetzler-Martin grading scale was conceived to stratify the risks of surgery for patients with AVM, much has been written about the shortcomings of the scale. In spite of these shortcomings, the scale remains both useful and widely used. This study provides excellent and clinically useful information relating this scale to surgical results at a center with significant experience in managing patients with AVM. It is a valuable addition to the literature on the surgical management of AVMs and should be required reading for neurosurgeons interested in this subject.

A. S. Arthur, MD, MPH

Intracranial Aneurysm Enlargement on Serial Magnetic Resonance Angiography: Frequency and Risk Factors

Burns JD, Huston J III, Layton KF, et al (Mayo Clinic, Rochester, MN; Baylor Univ Med Ctr, Dallas, TX)

Stroke 40:406-411, 2009

Background and Purpose.—Size of an unruptured intracranial aneurysm (UIA) may be an important risk factor for rupture. Accordingly, serial noninvasive imaging is commonly used to assess untreated UIA for enlargement. Few data exist regarding the frequency and predictors of enlargement. We obtained this information from a group of patients followed with serial MR angiography (MRA).

Methods.—We retrospectively identified 165 patients with 191 UIA followed with serial MRA. Fusiform aneurysms, UIA < 2 mm, and UIA that were surgically or endovascularly treated before the first MRA were excluded. MRA was performed using 1.5-T and 3-T MRI. Maximal diameter was determined on MRA source images. Multivariate regression analysis was used to determine independent risk factors for growth.

Results.—Twenty aneurysms (10%) grew over a median follow-up period of 47 months. Frequency of enlargement was 6.9%, 25%, and 83% for aneurysms < 8 mm, 8 to 12 mm, and > 13 mm, respectively ($P < 0.001$ for trend). Of the variables we evaluated, original aneurysm diameter (OR, 1.28 per mm;95% CI, 1.07 to 1.58) was the only independent predictor of enlargement. Aneurysms ≥8 mm in diameter were at highest risk for enlargement (OR, 7.25; 95% CI, 1.96 to 27.1). There was a trend toward increased risk of enlargement in patients with multiple aneurysms (OR, 2.50; 95% CI, 0.86 to 7.53).

Conclusions.—Over a median follow-up period of 47 months, 10% of UIA enlarged. Larger aneurysms had a significantly increased risk of enlargement. The likelihood of enlargement was highest in aneurysms with diameters ≥8 mm. However, a clinically significant proportion of small aneurysms grow, and this growth can be detected by serial MRA.

▶ As it has been estimated that there may be approximately 3 to 6 millions persons with aneurysms in the United States,[1] the question of which patients with unruptured intracranial aneurysms (UIA) to treat versus follow serially has been an ongoing controversy. The authors set out to retrospectively determine the frequency of and predictors of enlargement of conservatively treated saccular UIA using a noninvasive test, MR angiography (MRA) from both 1.5T and 3.0T magnets, with the exclusion of previously treated aneurysms as well as fusiform, mycotic, or traumatic aneurysms; tiny (< 2 mm) aneurysms were also excluded. Enlargement was defined as ≥1 mm for < 5 mm sized aneurysms and ≥2 mm for aneurysms > 5 mm in diameter over 2 separate MRA examinations at least 12 months apart (mean follow-up 56 months). They found enlargement of 10% of the 191 aneurysms (out of 165 patients included in the study), being most likely to occur in the ≥13 mm (original size) group (83% of those patients), and much less likely in the < 8 mm group (6.9%). They did not find any other statistically significant variable to predict enlargement out of age, gender, smoking history, family history of subarachnoid hemorrhage, etc.

Therefore, their data suggest that in patients with UIA < 8 mm, MRA could be used to follow these aneurysms, particular those that have not developed further or worsening symptoms. Interestingly, a smaller study from the same institution noted no aneurysm enlargement in aneurysms <9 mm over a mean of 50 months.[2] Also, in a study by Wermer et al studying <5 mm aneurysms found on screening, they did not note any growth or rupture in a subgroup of 16 patients with UIA that had a familial history of aneurysms.[3] Similarly, in a study by Matsubara et al using CTA follow-up at a mean of 17.7 months, UIA growth was detected in 2.4% of aneurysms 2 to 4 mm, and 9.1% that were 5 to 9 mm, but in 50% of lesions 10 to 20 mm.[4] Hence, in this author's opinion, as CT angiography (CTA) adequately detects aneurysms 4 to 8 mm with near 100% accuracy (while even the sensitivity and specificity in the detection of <4 mm size is above 90%), CTA (and possibly higher resolution 3T MRA) may be adequate to follow these smaller UIAs. However, given that we see so many 3 to 8 mm aneurysms that are surgically proven to have bled, this topic is still controversial, and the optimal interval of time used to follow these UIA and for how long has not been determined.[5] We await further and larger prospective studies, as the retrospective nature of these studies or the process or symptom through which these patients were obtained for may confound the study. Additionally, most studies do not follow the patients interminably or even yearly for 10 to 20 years; hence, we don't know at which point these smaller aneurysms bleed as no other risk factors other than size and familial nature have been clearly identified.

A. M. McKinney IV, MD

References

1. Menghini VV, Brown RD Jr, Sicks JD, O'Fallon WM, Wiebers DO. Clinical manifestations and survival rates among patients with saccular intracranial aneurysms: population-based study in Olmsted County, Minnesota, 1965 to 1995. *Neurosurgery.* 2001;49:251-256.
2. Phan TG, Huston J III, Brown RD Jr, Wiebers DO, Piepgras DG. Intracranial saccular aneurysm enlargement determined using serial magnetic resonance angiography. *J Neurosurg.* 2002;97:1023-1028.
3. Wermer MJ, van der Schaaf IC, Velthuis BK, Majoie CB, Albrecht KW, Rinkel GJ. Yield of short-term follow-up CT/MR angiography for small aneurysms detected at screening. *Stroke.* 2006;37:414-418.
4. Matsubara S, Hadeishi H, Suzuki A, Yasui N, Nishimura H. Incidence and risk factors for the growth of unruptured cerebral aneurysms: observation using serial computerized tomography angiography. *J Neurosurg.* 2004;101:908-914.
5. Adams WM, Laitt RD, Jackson A. The role of MR angiography in the pretreatment assessment of in intracranial aneurysms: a comparative study. *AJNR Am J Neuroradiol.* 2000;21:1618-1628.

Microsurgical management of incompletely coiled and recurrent aneurysms: trends, techniques, and observations on coil extrusion

Waldron JS, Halbach VV, Lawton MT (Univ of California, San Francisco)

Neurosurgery 64:ons301-ons317, 2009

Objective.—With the growing volume of aneurysms treated with endovascular methods and the unavoidable risks of incomplete coiling or recurrence, the volume of coiled aneurysms requiring surgical management is growing. We present a consecutive surgical experience with previously coiled aneurysms to examine clinical trends, the phenomenon of coil extrusion, microsurgical techniques, and morphological features affecting clippability.

Methods.—During a 10-year period, 43 patients underwent surgical management of an incompletely coiled or recurrent aneurysm (Gurian group B). Most patients (88%) presented initially with subarachnoid hemorrhage, most commonly (28%) located in the anterior communicating artery, and 42% of aneurysms were large or giant sized.

Results.—Twenty-one patients had incompletely coiled aneurysms and 22 patients had recurrent aneurysms, with a mean time to recurrence of 28 months. Coil extrusion was observed in 1 of the incompletely coiled (5%) and 12 of the recurrent aneurysms (55%). Overall, 33 aneurysms were clipped directly, 7 unclippable aneurysms were bypassed, and 3 were wrapped. Three patients died (surgical mortality, 7%), 1 patient (2%) experienced permanent neurological morbidity, and the remaining 39 patients (91%) had good outcomes (mean follow-up, 4.3 years).

Conclusion.—This study demonstrated a sharp increase in the incidence of coiled aneurysms requiring surgery, reflecting the increasing numbers of patients opting for endovascular therapy initially. Coil extrusion occurs more often than expected, is often misdiagnosed on angiography as simply compaction, and seems to be a time-dependent process not seen acutely. Direct clipping is the preferred microsurgical treatment of coiled aneurysms and may be predicted by the relationship between coil width and compaction height ($C/H < 2.5$, or a wedge angle < 90 degrees). We recommend a bypass strategy for unclippable coiled aneurysms because it can be executed methodically; has predictable ischemia times; and is associated with more favorable results than thrombectomy, coil extraction, and clip reconstruction.

▶ This article is a retrospective review of previously coiled aneurysms that were subsequently treated with open surgery. During a 10-year period, 43 patients underwent this surgery at a high-volume cerebrovascular center. It is notable that 88% of these patients presented initially with subarachnoid hemorrhage, and the outcomes obtained after open surgery were excellent in 91% of the cases.

The illustrations and operative photographs are excellent, and the discussion includes valuable and thoughtful commentary on the phenomenon of recurrent or incompletely treated aneurysms that were initially treated endovascularly.

Because a larger proportion of aneurysms is likely to be treated endovascularly in the future, this phenomenon is of increasing relevance in the practice of neurosurgery.

A. S. Arthur, MD, MPH

16 Functional

A Multicenter, Prospective Pilot Study of Gamma Knife Radiosurgery for Mesial Temporal Lobe Epilepsy: Seizure Response, Adverse Events, and Verbal Memory

Barbaro NM, Quigg M, Broshek DK, et al (Univ of California at San Francisco; Univ of Virginia, Charlottesville; et al)

Ann Neurol 65:167-175, 2009

Objective.—The safety, efficacy, and morbidity of radiosurgery (RS) must be established before it can be offered as an alternative to open surgery for unilateral mesial temporal lobe epilepsy. We report the 3-year outcomes of a multicenter, prospective pilot study of RS.

Methods.—RS was randomized to 20 or 24Gy targeting the amygdala, hippocampus, and parahippocampal gyrus. Seizure diaries evaluated the final seizure remission between months 24 and 36, Verbal memory was evaluated at baseline and 24m with the Wechsler Memory Scale–Revised (WMS-R) and California Verbal Learning Test (CVLT). Patients were classified as having "significant improvement," "no change," and "significant impairment" based on relative change indices.

Results.—Thirteen high-dose and 17 low-dose patients were treated. Both groups showed significant reductions in seizures by 1 year after treatment. At the 36-month follow-up evaluation, 67% of patients were free of seizures for the prior 12 months (high dose: 10/13, 76.9%; low dose: 10/17, 58.8%). Use of steroids, headaches, and visual field defects did not differ by dose or seizure remission. The prevalence of verbal memory impairment was 15% (4/26 patients); none declined on more than one measure. The prevalence of significant verbal memory improvements was 12% (3/26).

Interpretation.—RS for unilateral mesial temporal lobe epilepsy offers seizure remission rates comparable with those reported previously for open surgery. There were no major safety concerns with high-dose RS compared with low-dose RS. Additional research is required to determine whether RS may be a treatment option for some patients with mesial temporal lobe epilepsy.

▶ This multicenter trial, sponsored by the National Institutes of Health with assistance from Elekta, was designed to provide safety and efficacy data regarding the use of radiosurgery to treat mesial temporal lobe epilepsy. These data are intended to serve as the foundation for a planned phase 3 trial of radiosurgery for this condition.

Although no medical therapy or surgical resection groups were used for direct comparison with the radiosurgery treatment, this was an extremely well-designed and well-executed trial by a group of the most experienced investigators in the United States. The trial used rigorous methodology to build on single-center observations of radiosurgical therapy. Strengths of the trial design worth noting include clinically applicable inclusion criteria, centrally reviewed radiosurgery treatment plans, and an independent National Institute of Neurological Disorders and Stroke safety monitoring board. In addition to seizure outcomes, verbal memory was prospectively tracked.

Sixty-seven percent of patients treated with either 20-Gy or 24-Gy dosing were free from seizures between 2 and 3 years after therapy. Patients who received the higher radiation dose experienced a higher seizure-free rate. Although these results compare well with those achieved with standard surgical resection, patients did experience an interval of continued seizures while the radiation effects took place. Verbal memory impairment was seen in 25% of dominant hemisphere cases. Interestingly, the occurrence of auras was transiently increased after therapy.

Overall, this prospective study documents very favorable responses to radiosurgery in patients suffering from mesial temporal lobe epilepsy. Larger trials will be required to arrive at optimal dosing and direct outcome comparisons with traditional temporal lobe resections.

P. A. House, MD

Efficacy of Steroid and Nonsteroid Caudal Epidural Injections for Low Back Pain and Sciatica: A Prospective, Randomized, Double-Blind Clinical Trial

Sayegh FE, Kenanidis EI, Papavasiliou KA, et al (Aristotle Univ of Thessaloniki Med School, Greece)

Spine 34:1441-1447, 2009

Study Design.—Prospective, double-blind, randomized, case-control study.

Objective.—To evaluate the efficacy of caudal epidural injections (CEI) containing steroid *versus* nonsteroid preparations when treating patients suffering from low back pain (LBP) and sciatica.

Summary of Background Data.—Literature seems to be deprived of well-designed randomized, controlled studies that evaluate the effectiveness of CEI in the treatment of chronic LBP; hence the value of CEI remains still the subject of controversy.

Methods.—Patients suffering from severe chronic LBP and sciatica were randomly allocated into 2 groups. Steroid-group's patients (n = 93) underwent CEI containing 12 mL of xylocaine 2% and 1 mL of betamethasone dipropionate and betamethasone phosphate (2 + 5) mg/dL. Water for Injection (WFI)-group's patients (n = 90) underwent CEI containing 12 mL of xylocaine 2% and 8 mL of WFI. Both groups were statistically comparable as far as their demographic data and the cause and duration of symptoms were concerned. Patients answered the Oswestry Disability

Index questionnaire and underwent physical examination, before and at 1 week, 1 month, 6 months, and 1 year following the CEI.

Results.—Symptoms improved in 132 patients (72.1%) following CEI. The mean Oswestry Disability Index questionnaire score of steroid-group's patients was statistically significant lower than that of the WFI-group at all postinjection re-evaluations. Patients receiving steroid CEI experienced faster relief during the first postinjection week. The Straight Leg Rising test improved in both groups following CEI; this improvement was faster among steroidgroup's patients. Fifty-one patients (27.8%), noticed no improvement 1 week post-CEI and underwent a second CEI (with the same preparation) 7 to 14 days later. Nineteen of them reported improvement; 32 (steroid-group:13, WFI-group: 19) did not respond well and underwent operative decompression (n = 15) or spinal fusion (n = 17).

Conclusion.—CEI containing local anesthetic and steroids or WFI seems to be effective when treating patients with LBP and sciatica. CEI containing steroid preparations demonstrated better and faster efficacy.

▶ Despite widespread use of caudal epidural steroid injections to treat low back pain, data supporting their benefits are limited primarily to short-term studies. The mechanism of pain relief and nearly every technical detail of the procedure (including indications, fluoroscopic guidance, volume of injection, and drugs used) have been debated. The study by Sayegh et al is a rigorous investigation into the use of epidural injections for low back and radicular pain. The study was performed in a double-blind, prospective manner, with patients randomized to receive either sterile water with xylocaine or xylocaine mixed with betamethasone injected into the caudal epidural space. One hundred fifty-one (of 183 patients treated) patients were followed for 1 year. Both groups of patients experienced significant improvement in their scores on disability rating scales, with those receiving steroids having a much faster, more significant, and sustained overall response. This study strongly supports the use of caudal epidural steroid injections for patients with back and leg pain related to MRI-confirmed disc disease. This study contains some of the most compelling data to date regarding this topic.

P. A. House, MD

Financial impact of spinal cord stimulation on the healthcare budget: a comparative analysis of costs in Canada and the United States

Kumar K, Bishop S (Univ of Saskatchewan, Canada)

J Neurosurg Spine 10:564-573, 2009

Object.—Many institutions with spinal cord stimulation (SCS) programs fail to realize that besides the initial implantation cost, budgetary allocation must be made to address annual maintenance costs as well as complications as they arise. Complications remain the major contributing factor to the overall expense of SCS. The authors present a formula that, when applied, provides a realistic representation of the actual costs necessary to implant and maintain SCS systems in Canada and the US.

Methods.—The authors performed a retrospective analysis of 197 cases involving SCS (161 implanted and 36 failed trial stimulations) between 1995 and 2006. The cost of patient workup, initial implantation, annual maintenance, and resources necessary to resolve complications were assessed for each case and a unit cost applied. The total cost allocated for each case was determined by summing across healthcare resource headings. Using the same parameters, the unit cost was calculated in both Canadian (CAD) and US dollars (USD) at 2007 prices.

Results.—The cost of implanting a SCS system in Canada is $21,595 (CAD), in US Medicare $32,882 (USD), and in US Blue Cross Blue Shield (BCBS) $57,896 (USD). The annual maintenance cost of an uncomplicated case in Canada is $3539 (CAD), in US Medicare $5071 (USD), and in BCBS $7277 (USD). The mean cost of a complication was $5191 in Canada (range $136–18,837 [CAD]). In comparison, in the US the figures were $9649 (range $381–28,495) for Medicare and $21,390 (range $573–54,547) for BCBS (both USD). Using these calculations a formula was derived as follows: the annual maintenance cost (a) was added to the average annual cost per complication per patient implanted (b); the sum was then divided by the implantation cost (c); and the result was multiplied by 100 to obtain a percentage ($a + b \div c \times 100$). To make this budgetary cap universally applicable, the results from the application of the formula were averaged, resulting in an 18% premium.

Conclusions.—For budgeting purposes the institution should first calculate the initial implantation costs that then can be "grossed up" by 18% per annum. This amount of 18% should be in addition to the implantation costs for the individual institution for new patients, as well as for each actively managed patient. This resulting amount will cover the costs associated with annual maintenance and complications for every actively managed patient. As the initial cost of implantation in any country reflects their current economics, the formula provided will be applicable to all implanters and policy makers alike.

▶ Contentious debates filled the headlines and airwaves this year regarding the possibility of health care reform in the United States. While functional neurosurgery remains a small component of neurosurgery in general—both in terms of the number of procedures performed and in total costs—innovative procedures, such as deep brain stimulation and spinal cord stimulation require implantable devices that are very costly. The significant profits associated with these devices have even become a target of windfall corporate taxes.

Although the costs of the implanted devices are easy to identify, the total costs associated with providing therapy through such devices are more difficult to calculate. The article by Kumar et al provides an in-depth analysis of all costs associated with providing spinal cord stimulation therapy. The records of nearly 200 patients who were evaluated for, and most of whom were subsequently treated with, spinal cord stimulation were reviewed. The authors provide detailed cost breakdowns and illustrate costs in the Canadian health care system, the United States Medicare system, and the United States Blue Cross/Blue Shield payment system.

The primary conclusion, surprising in amount, is that complications associated with device implantation are actually one of the most expensive aspects of care. It becomes necessary to increase the cost of device implantation by nearly 20% to cover the costs associated with complications. The detailed data tabulated regarding each component of patient care provide a snapshot of current health care expenses and serve to illustrate sharp contrasts in private versus nationalized payment schedules. Recognizing the significant cost of surgical complications should help focus attention to modifiable surgical technique details and device design details that could help curtail health care expenditures in a rational fashion.

P. A. House, MD

High-Frequency Electroencephalographic Oscillations Correlate With Outcome of Epilepsy Surgery

Jacobs J, Zijlmans M, Zelmann R, et al (McGill Univ, Montreal, Quebec, Canada)

Ann Neurol 67:209-220, 2010

Objective.—High-frequency oscillations (HFOs) in the intracerebral electroencephalogram (EEG) have been linked to the seizure onset zone (SOZ). We investigated whether HFOs can delineate epileptogenic areas even outside the SOZ by correlating the resection of HFO-generating areas with surgical outcome.

Methods.—Twenty patients who underwent a surgical resection for medically intractable epilepsy were studied. All had presurgical intracerebral EEG (500Hz filter and 2,000Hz sampling rate), at least 12-month postsurgical follow-up, and a postsurgical magnetic resonance imaging (MRI). HFOs (ripples, 80–250Hz; fast ripples, >250Hz) were identified visually during 5 to 10 minutes of slow-wave sleep. Rates and extent of HFOs and interictal spikes in resected versus nonresected areas, assessed on postsurgical MRIs, were compared with surgical outcome (Engel's classification). We also evaluated the predictive value of removing the SOZ in terms of surgical outcome.

Results.—The mean duration of follow-up was 22.7 months. Eight patients had good (Engel classes 1 and 2) and 12 poor (classes 3 and 4) surgical outcomes. Patients with a good outcome had a significantly larger proportion of HFO-generating areas removed than patients with a poor outcome. No such difference was seen for spike-generating regions or the SOZ.

Interpretation.—The correlation between removal of HFO-generating areas and good surgical outcome indicates that HFOs could be used as a marker of epileptogenicity and may be more accurate than

spike-generating areas or the SOZ. In patients in whom the majority of HFO-generating tissue remained, a poor surgical outcome occurred.

▶ Obtaining seizure freedom through surgical resection is particularly challenging in cases of neocortical and especially nonlesional epilepsy. A wide variety of imaging and noninvasive electrophysiological markers have been used to refine surgical planning, but intracranial electroencephalography (iEEG) remains necessary in a large number of patients despite its well-described risks. Frustratingly, even when localized seizure onset can be demonstrated through iEEG, surgical resection results in seizure-freedom rates of approximately 50%. iEEG patterns that are indicative of probable surgical success have been widely sought and many variations described. Two new contributions to this literature focus on iEEG frequencies higher than those often used in clinical analysis.

In the study by Wetjen et al,[1] the surgical outcomes of patients without lesions that could be demonstrated on optimized magnetic resonance imaging were reviewed and compared with iEEG patterns in those patients. The most notable finding is that focal high-frequency (> 20 Hz) activity at the seizure-onset zone correlated with seizure-free outcomes. Importantly, broadband digitized recordings were used—allowing for frequency analysis up to ~100 Hz. Perhaps just as importantly, patterns of diffuse high-frequency activity or only increased delta activity at the defined seizure-onset zone did not correlate with any seizure-free outcomes.

Jacobs et al evaluated much higher frequency activity (> 250 Hz) that had been recorded through stereotactically implanted depth electrodes. Five-minute intervals of interictal activity during slow-wave sleep were intensively analyzed retrospectively. The analysis was undertaken without knowledge of the determined seizure-onset zone. Several types of interictal activity at different frequency bands (ripples, fast-ripples, and spikes) were analyzed, and a wide variety of exploratory comparisons (such as relative ratios of activity type to percentage of electrodes and relative ratio of activity types at resection sites) were conducted. The somewhat surprising finding is that seizure-free outcome correlated more strongly with the percentage of tissue removed containing frequent high-frequency (> 80 Hz) activity than with the percentage of tissue removed from the defined seizure-onset zone.

In each study, small numbers of patients were evaluated and thus definitive conclusions cannot be drawn; however, each of these studies offer new insights into possible classification criteria of iEEG information with potential clinical implications. The iEEG evaluations performed are complex and time consuming and require validation. Clearly, large repositories of digitized iEEG information sampled at high frequencies and automated algorithms for pattern detection are needed to truly extend either set of findings. It is likely that such undertakings would be well rewarded, however, as enhancing even the ability to predict poor outcomes from surgical resections would significantly advance the field.

P. A. House, MD

Reference

1. Bell ML, Rao S, So EL, et al. Epilepsy surgery outcomes in temporal lobe epilepsy with a normal MRI. *Epilepsia*. 2009;50:2053-2060.

Intracranial electroencephalography seizure onset patterns and surgical outcomes in nonlesional extratemporal epilepsy

Wetjen NM, Marsh WR, Meyer FB, et al (Mayo Clinic, Rochester, MN)

J Neurosurg 110:1147-1152, 2009

Object.—Patients with normal MR imaging (nonlesional) findings and medically refractory extratemporal epilepsy make up a disproportionate number of nonexcellent outcomes after epilepsy surgery. In this paper, the authors investigated the usefulness of intracranial electroencephalography (iEEG) in the identification of surgical candidates.

Methods.—Between 1992 and 2002, 51 consecutive patients with normal MR imaging findings and extratemporal epilepsy underwent intracranial electrode monitoring. The implantation of intracranial electrodes was determined by seizure semiology, interictal and ictal scalp EEG, SPECT, and in some patients PET studies. The demographics of patients at the time of surgery, lobar localization of electrode implantation, duration of follow-up, and Engel outcome score were abstracted from the Mayo Rochester Epilepsy Surgery Database. A blinded independent review of the iEEG records was conducted for this study.

Results.—Thirty-one (61%) of the 51 patients who underwent iEEG ultimately underwent resection for their epilepsy. For 28 (90.3%) of the 31 patients who had epilepsy surgery, adequate information regarding follow-up (> 1 year), seizure frequency, and iEEG recordings was available. Twenty-six (92.9%) of 28 patients had frontal lobe resections, and 2 had parietal lobe resections. The most common iEEG pattern at seizure onset in the surgically treated group was a focal high-frequency discharge (in 15 [53.6%] of 28 patients). Ten (35.7%) of the 28 surgically treated patients were seizure free. Fourteen (50%) had Engel Class I outcomes, and overall, 17 (60.7%) had significant improvement (Engel Class I and IIAB with ≥ 80% seizure reduction). Focal high-frequency oscillation at seizure onset was associated with Engel Class I surgical outcome (12 [85.7%] of 14 patients, $p = 0.02$), and it was uncommon in the nonexcellent outcome group (3 [21.4%] of 14 patients).

Conclusions.—A focal high-frequency oscillation (> 20 Hz) at seizure onset on iEEG may identify patients with nonlesional extratemporal epilepsy who are likely to have an Engel Class I outcome after epilepsy surgery. The prospect of excellent outcome in nonlesional extratemporal lobe epilepsy prior to intracranial monitoring is poor (14 [27.5%] of 51

patients). However, iEEG can further stratify patients and help identify those with a greater likelihood of Engel Class I outcome after surgery.

▶ Obtaining seizure freedom through surgical resection is particularly challenging in cases of neocortical and, especially, nonlesional epilepsy. A wide variety of imaging and noninvasive electrophysiological markers have been used to refine surgical planning, but intracranial electroencephalography (iEEG) remains necessary in a large number of patients despite its well-described risks. Frustratingly, even when localized seizure onset can be demonstrated through iEEG, surgical resection results in seizure-freedom rates of approximately 50%. iEEG patterns that are indicative of probable surgical success have been widely sought and many variations described. Two new contributions to this literature focus on iEEG frequencies higher than those often used in clinical analysis.

In the study by Wetjen et al, the surgical outcomes of patients without lesions that could be demonstrated on optimized magnetic resonance imaging were reviewed and compared with iEEG patterns in those patients. The most notable finding is that focal high-frequency (> 20 Hz) activity at the seizure-onset zone correlated with seizure-free outcomes. Importantly, broadband digitized recordings were used—allowing for frequency analysis up to ~100 Hz. Perhaps just as importantly, patterns of diffuse high-frequency activity or only increased delta activity at the defined seizure-onset zone did not correlate with any seizure-free outcomes.

Jacobs et al[1] evaluated much higher frequency activity (> 250 Hz) that had been recorded through stereotactically implanted depth electrodes. Five-minute intervals of interictal activity during slow-wave sleep were intensively analyzed retrospectively. The analysis was undertaken without knowledge of the determined seizure-onset zone. Several types of interictal activity at different frequency bands (ripples, fast-ripples, and spikes) were analyzed, and a wide variety of exploratory comparisons (such as relative ratios of activity type to percentage of electrodes and relative ratio of activity types at resection sites) were conducted. The somewhat surprising finding is that seizure-free outcome correlated more strongly with the percentage of tissue removed containing frequent high-frequency (> 80 Hz) activity than with the percentage of tissue removed from the defined seizure-onset zone.

In each study, small numbers of patients were evaluated and thus definitive conclusions cannot be drawn; however, each of these studies offer new insights into possible classification criteria of iEEG information with potential clinical implications. The iEEG evaluations performed are complex and time consuming and require validation. Clearly, large repositories of digitized iEEG information sampled at high frequencies and automated algorithms for pattern detection are needed to truly extend either set of findings. It is likely that such undertakings would be well rewarded, however, as enhancing even the ability to predict poor outcomes from surgical resections would significantly advance the field.

P. A. House, MD

Reference

1. Jacobs J, Zijlmans M, Zelmann R, et al. High-frequency electroencephalographic oscillations correlate with outcome of epilepsy surgery. *Ann Neurol.* 2010;67: 209-220.

Long-term outcome of gamma knife radiosurgery for treatment of typical trigeminal neuralgia

Han JH, Kim DG, Chung H-T, et al (Seoul Natl Univ College of Medicine, Korea)

Int J Radiat Oncol Biol Phys 75:822-827, 2009

Purpose.—To analyze the long-term outcomes of patients with typical trigeminal neuralgia treated with gamma knife radiosurgery (GKRS).

Patients and Methods.—A total of 62 consecutive patients with typical trigeminal neuralgia were treated with GKRS between 1998 and 2004. Of the 62 patients, 2 were lost to follow-up; the remaining 60 patients were followed for >12 months. The mean prescribed maximal dose was 79.7 Gy (range, 75–80), using a 4-mm shot.

Results.—Of the 60 patients, 48 were followed for >4 years. An additional 3 patients, followed for <4 years, experienced recurrent pain after a favorable initial response and were incorporated into the long-term response analysis. Of these 51 patients (mean age, 61 ± 11 years; 37 women [72.5%]; and mean follow-up duration, 58 ± 14 months), 46 (90.2%) responded to GKRS, as demonstrated by an improvement in their Barrow Neurological Institute pain intensity score. Of the 46 patients, 24 (52.2%) had pain recurrence. The actuarial recurrence-free survival rate was 84.8%, 76.1%, 69.6%, 63.0%, and 45.8% at 1, 2, 3, 4, and 5 years after radiosurgery, respectively. Patient age >70 years correlated with a favorable outcome in terms of pain recurrence after radiosurgery (hazard ratio, 0.125; 95% confidence interval, 0.016–0.975; $p = .047$) on multivariate analysis.

Conclusion.—GKRS seems to be an effective treatment modality for patients with typical trigeminal neuralgia considering the initial response rate; however, fewer than one-half of patients might continue to benefit from GKRS after long-term follow-up. Elderly patients might be good candidates for radiosurgery considering the long-term durability of efficacy.

► Radiosurgery is likely the most frequently used surgical intervention for medically refractory trigeminal neuralgia. Radiosurgery has become widely used primarily because of its safety profile and known short-term efficacy, as long-term efficacy has not been well described. The studies by Dhople et al,[1] from the University of Maryland, and Han et al, from Seoul National University, add significantly to our understanding of the long-term outcomes of radiosurgical therapy for trigeminal neuralgia. The University of Maryland group performed Gamma Knife radiosurgery with 75 Gy average dosing, while the

Seoul National University group used an average of 79.7 Gy. As expected, each group had very few complications, and their initial response rates were in agreement with those in previous publications (̃80% of patients had improvement in pain within 6 months of treatment). Notably, Han et al found a much better response rate in patients over 70 years of age and Dhople et al found a better response rate in patients who had not undergone previous invasive procedures.

The most significant contribution of each group is detailed in actuarial plots of cumulative freedom from severe pain. By 4.5 years, half of the patients had experienced recurrence of their trigeminal neuralgia pain that could not be adequately controlled by medications in the study by Han et al. The work by Dhople et al, which documents longer follow-up in a larger group of patients, reveals that half of the patients experienced recurrence within 2 years of therapy. Combined, these important articles give the most detailed analysis to date on long-term pain outcomes. Proponents and detractors of radiosurgery alike will find much to consider.

P. A. House, MD

Reference

1. Dhople AA, Adams JR, Maggio WW, Naqvi SA, Regine WF, Kwok Y. Long-term outcomes of Gamma Knife radiosurgery for classic trigeminal neuralgia: implications of treatment and critical review of the literature. Clinical article. *J Neurosurg*. 2009;111:351-358.

Long-term outcomes of Gamma Knife radiosurgery for classic trigeminal neuralgia: implications of treatment and critical review of the literature

Dhople AA, Adams JR, Maggio WW, et al (Univ of Maryland School of Medicine, Baltimore)

J Neurosurg 111:351-358, 2009

Object.—Few long-term studies of Gamma Knife surgery (GKS) for trigeminal neuralgia (TN) exist. The authors report their long-term experience with the use of GKS in a previously reported cohort of patients with TN that has now been followed since 1996.

Methods.—One hundred twelve patients with TN were treated with GKS at the University of Maryland between June 1996 and July 2001. Of these, 67% had no invasive operations for TN prior to GKS, 13% had 1, 4% had 2, and 16% had ≥ 3. The right side was affected in 56% of cases, predominantly involving V2 (26%), V3 (24%), or a combination of both (18%) branches. The median age at diagnosis was 56 years, and median age at GKS was 64 years. The median prescription dose of 75 Gy (range 70–80 Gy) was delivered to the involved trigeminal nerve root entry zone. The authors assessed the degree of pain before and after GKS by using the Barrow Neurological Institute (BNI) pain scale.

Results.—In total, 102 patients took the survey at least once, for a response rate of 91%. Although not found to alter the conclusions of this study, 7 cases of atypical TN were found and these patients were removed, for a total of 95 cases herein analyzed. The median follow-up was 5.6 years (range 13–115 months). Before GKS, 88% of patients categorized their pain as BNI IV or V (inadequate control or severe pain on medication), whereas the remainder described their pain as BNI III (some pain, but controlled on medication). After GKS, 64% reported a BNI score of I (no pain, no medications), 5% had BNI II (no pain, still on medication), 12% had BNI III, and 19% reported a BNI score of IV or V. The median time to response was 2 weeks (range 0–12 weeks) and the median response duration was 32 months (range 0–112 months). Eighty-one percent reported initial pain relief, and actuarial rates of freedom from treatment failure at 1, 3, 5, and 7 years were 60, 41, 34, and 22%, respectively. Response duration was significantly better for those who had no prior invasive treatment versus those in whom a previous surgical intervention had failed (32 vs 21 months, $p < 0.02$). New bothersome facial numbness was reported in 6% of cases.

Conclusions.—This study represents one of the longest reported median follow-up periods and actuarial results for a cohort of patients with classic TN treated with GKS. Although GKS achieves excellent rates of initial pain relief, these results suggest a steady rate of late failure, particularly among patients who had undergone prior invasive surgical treatment. Despite a higher than expected recurrence rate, GKS remains a viable treatment option, particularly for patients who have had no prior invasive procedures. Patients with recurrences can still be offered salvage therapy with either repeat GKS, microvascular decompression, or rhizotomy.

▶ Radiosurgery is likely the most frequently used surgical intervention for medically refractory trigeminal neuralgia. Radiosurgery has become widely used primarily because of its safety profile and known short-term efficacy, as long-term efficacy has not been well described. The studies by Dhople et al, from the University of Maryland, and Han et al,[1] from Seoul National University, add significantly to our understanding of the long-term outcomes of radiosurgical therapy for trigeminal neuralgia. The University of Maryland group performed Gamma Knife radiosurgery with 75 Gy average dosing, while the Seoul National University group used an average of 79.7 Gy. As expected, each group had very few complications, and their initial response rates were in agreement with those in previous publications (~80% of patients had improvement in pain within 6 months of treatment). Notably, Han et al found a much better response rate in patients over 70 years of age, and Dhople et al found a better response rate in patients who had not undergone previous invasive procedures.

The most significant contribution of each group is detailed in actuarial plots of cumulative freedom from severe pain. By 4.5 years, half of the patients had experienced recurrence of their trigeminal neuralgia pain that could not be adequately controlled by medications in the study by Han et al. The work by Dhople et al, which documents longer follow-up in a larger group of patients, reveals that half of the patients experienced recurrence within 2 years of therapy. Combined, these important articles give the most detailed analysis to date on long-term pain outcomes. Proponents and detractors of radiosurgery alike will find much to consider.

P. A. House, MD

Reference

1. Han JH, Kim DG, Chung HT, et al. Long-term outcome of gamma knife radiosurgery for treatment of typical trigeminal neuralgia. *Int J Radiat Oncol Biol Phys.* 2009;75:822-827. Epub 2009 Jun 8.

Medically intractable epilepsy in Sturge-Weber syndrome is associated with cortical malformation: Implications for surgical therapy

Maton B, Kršek P, Jayakar P, et al (Miami Children's Hosp, FL; Charles Univ, Prague, Czech Republic; et al)

Epilepsia 51:257-267, 2010

Purpose.—Anecdotal reports have described cortical malformations in epileptic patients with Sturge-Weber syndrome (SWS). No data are available regarding the prevalence and significance of this association.

Methods.—We reviewed retrospectively the clinical profile, preoperative magnetic resonance imaging (MRI) studies, and pathology reports of all patients with SWS and medically intractable epilepsy evaluated in our epilepsy surgery program between 1979 and 2006.

Results.—Twelve patients (male/female = 7/5) were identified. Mean age at seizure onset was 11.1 ± 16.7 months. Seizures occurred daily in seven patients and weekly in five patients. A facial port-wine stain was noted in 10 cases. Eleven patients evidenced developmental delay and eight were hemiparetic. Eight patients underwent excisional surgery for epilepsy (mean age 10.3 ± 6.5 year), including hemispherectomy (n = 4) and focal cortical resection (n = 4). Tissue was available for neuropathology in six operated cases and revealed polymicrogyria (n = 3) and cortical dysplasia (n = 4). Polymicrogyria was associated with cortical dysplasia in one child. Brain MRIs were reviewed in 10 of 12 patients and were consistent with cortical malformations in all cases.

Conclusions.—We conclude that cortical malformations are frequent in patients with medically intractable epilepsy and Sturge-Weber-syndrome and may be the primary cause of epilepsy.

► Epilepsy associated with Sturge-Weber syndrome that presents during the first year of life is often catastrophic and difficult to control. Seizures are typically assumed to occur as a result of cortical alterations secondary to chronic ischemia. If localized seizure onset can be electrophysiologically demonstrated, a cortical area associated with a vascular malformation is generally sought to explain the physiology.

The study by Maton et al presents an analysis of the histological findings regarding 12 patients sequentially evaluated for surgery to treat medically refractory seizures. Eight of the 12 underwent surgical resections. Their primary finding is that polymicrogyria and cortical dysplasia were noted in all 6 histological specimens that were available for review. When magnetic resonance imaging studies were re-examined (available for 10 of the 12 patients), findings consistent with cortical dysplasia were identified. The authors postulate that cortical dysplasia plays a significant pathological role in the epilepsy that affects approximately 80% of patients with Sturge-Weber syndrome. If confirmed, these results suggest that a wide range of histological abnormalities might lead to seizures in these patients and that identification and resection of areas containing cortical dysplasia might lead to improvements in seizure control.

P. A. House, MD

Motor Homunculus: Passive Mapping in Healthy Volunteers by Using Functional MR Imaging—Initial Results

Kocak M, Ulmer JL, Sahin Ugurel M, et al (Med College of Wisconsin, Milwaukee)

Radiology 251:485-492, 2009

Purpose.—To determine the concurrence of activation in the primary motor cortex, induced by paradigms of active and passive movement of extremities, by using blood oxygen level–dependent functional magnetic resonance (MR) imaging.

Materials and Methods.—The HIPAA-compliant study was approved by the institutional review board, and written informed consent was obtained from the participating volunteers. Functional MR imaging data were collected from 11 healthy volunteers (four women, seven men; age range, 24–42 years) during active and passive movements of hand, elbow, shoulder, ankle, knee, and hip. These data were then mapped onto three-dimensional anatomic images. Volumes of activation were determined by using cross-correlation analysis at a coefficient threshold of 0.4 ($P < .01$). Regions of interest were drawn in pre- and postcentral gyri based on anatomic criteria. The mean number of activated voxels in the pre- and postcentral gyri induced by active and passive movements was compared by using Wilcoxon analysis. Concurrence ratios and proportional ratios of activation between active and passive movements were calculated for each somatotopic location.

Results.—Primary motor cortex activation tended to increase with active compared with passive movements, although in the precentral gyrus, hand, elbow, and shoulder movements showed no statistically significant difference in mean number of activated voxels. In the postcentral gyrus, only the shoulder revealed a significant difference ($P < .05$). Concurrence ratios (activation volume overlap of two tasks/combined activation area of both tasks) ranged from 0.44 to 0.57. Proportional ratios (activation volume overlap of passive task with active task/total activation volume of passive task) ranged from 0.64 to 0.82.

Conclusion.—Passive movement paradigms may be an alternative to or complement to active movement tasks in patient populations.

▶ In this quite interesting study, the authors used functional MRI (fMRI) to demonstrate that motor cortex activation may occur to a significant degree by the utilization of passive movements. The study used several joints in the hand, elbow, shoulder, ankle, and knees in 11 volunteers, whereby the differences between active and passive motion of these joints were measured using blood oxygen level-dependent (BOLD) measurements in the precentral and postcentral gyri at various anatomic landmarks. A statistical analysis was then applied comparing these landmarks in the active versus the passive states. As expected, there was somewhat greater activation overall in the active versus the passive state with most movements; however, surprisingly, there were no significant differences specifically for the ankle, knee, and hip in the precentral gyri between active versus passive states. The authors point out an anatomic basis for this activation based on previous research describing how afferent inputs may modulate efferent outputs from the primary motor cortex. These results may significantly further the abilities of fMRI research by enabling passive studies of the primary motor homunculus in the precentral gyrus. One of the greatest potential utilities in this author's opinion is in early pediatric patients and in developmental delay, although this has yet to be proven facile and validated in the sedated population. Research in animals or in patients with dementia, Parkinson, or other neurologic conditions preventing voluntary motor control, or possibly even intraoperatively, are other possibilities that come immediately to mind. Hence, this preliminary study points to a significant alternative method of evaluating motor cortex activation via passive movement paradigms, which will require further studies in various populations to determine the reproducibility of these results.

A. M. McKinney IV, MD

Spinal cord stimulation for failed back surgery syndrome: Outcomes in a workers' compensation setting

Turner JA, Hollingworth W, Comstock BA, et al (Univ of Washington, Seattle; Univ of Bristol, UK; et al)
Pain 148:14-25, 2010

Questions remain concerning effectiveness and risks of spinal cord stimulation (SCS) for chronic back and leg pain after spine surgery ("failed back surgery syndrome" [FBSS]). This prospective, population-based controlled cohort study evaluated outcomes of workers' compensation recipients with FBSS who received at least a trial of SCS (SCS group, $n = 51$) versus those who (1) were evaluated at a multidisciplinary pain clinic and did not receive SCS (Pain Clinic, $n = 39$) or (2) received neither SCS nor pain clinic evaluation (Usual Care, $n = 68$). Patients completed measures of pain, function, medication use, and work status at baseline and 6, 12, and 24 months later. We also examined work time loss compensation over 24 months. Few (<10%) patients in any group achieved success at any follow-up on the composite primary outcome encompassing less than daily opioid use and improvement in leg pain and function. At 6 months, the SCS group showed modestly greater improvement in leg pain and function, but with higher rates of daily opioid use. These differences disappeared by 12 months. Patients who received a permanent spinal cord stimulator did not differ from patients who received some pain clinic treatment on the primary outcome at any follow-up (<10% successful in each group at each follow-up) and 19% had them removed within 18 months. Both trial and permanent SCS were associated with adverse events. In sum, we found no evidence for greater effectiveness of SCS versus alternative treatments in this patient population after 6 months.

▶ Previous randomized controlled trials have shown favorable results when spinal cord stimulation (SCS) was used to treat failed back syndrome. Stimulation proved superior to continued medical therapy alone, and it also proved more favorable than repeat lumbar operations. As with many controlled trials, important limitations, such as a lack of workers' compensation patients in the study population and sponsorship by the device manufacturer, have restricted the conclusions that can be drawn from these studies.

Turner et al proposed to evaluate SCS in more typical clinical settings and focused on patients with workers' compensation claims in the state of Washington. Patients were treated with usual care (not referred to specialty clinics), referral to a multidisciplinary pain clinic, or referral to a pain clinic that also incorporated SCS. A composite outcome index (incorporating measures of pain, function, and opioid medication use) was chosen as the primary outcome. The researchers found no statistically significant difference among the groups at 6, 12, or 24 months. Very few patients (<10%) achieved success on the composite index with any therapy. At 6 months, SCS patients did show modestly improved leg pain and functional status and consumed more opioid medications than the other treatment groups. These improvements were not sustained at 12 or 24 months.

This study failed to show superiority of SCS to other forms of therapy for patients with failed back syndrome and workers' compensation claims. These results suggest that a high level of scrutiny should be applied to the decision-making process regarding the use of SCS to treat this population.

P. A. House, MD

Trigeminal neuralgia and pain related to multiple sclerosis

Cruccu G, Biasiotta A, Di Rezze S, et al (Università La Sapienza, Roma, Italy; et al)

Pain 143:186-191, 2009

Although many patients with multiple sclerosis (MS) complain of trigeminal neuralgia (TN), its cause and mechanisms are still debatable.

In a multicentre controlled study, we collected 130 patients with MS: 50 patients with TN, 30 patients with trigeminal sensory disturbances other than TN (ongoing pain, dysaesthesia, or hypoesthesia), and 50 control patients. All patients underwent pain assessment, trigeminal reflex testing, and dedicated MRI scans. The MRI scans were imported and normalised into a voxel-based, 3D brainstem model that allows spatial statistical analysis. The onset ages of MS and trigeminal symptoms were significantly older in the TN group. The frequency histogram of onset age for the TN group showed that many patients fell in the age range of classic TN. Most patients in TN and non-TN groups had abnormal trigeminal reflexes. In the TN group, 3D brainstem analysis showed an area of strong probability of lesion ($P < 0.0001$) centred on the intrapontine trigeminal primary afferents. In the non-TN group, brainstem lesions were more scattered, with the highest probability for lesions ($P < 0.001$) in a region involving the subnucleus oralis of the spinal trigeminal complex. We conclude that the most likely cause of MS-related TN is a pontine plaque damaging the primary afferents. Nevertheless, in some patients a neurovascular contact may act as a concurring mechanism. The other sensory disturbances, including ongoing pain and dysaesthesia, may arise from damage to the second-order neurons in the spinal trigeminal complex.

▶ The medical and surgical treatment of trigeminal neuralgia symptoms associated with multiple sclerosis (MS) remains challenging. It is well known that surgical interventions are less likely to have durable success in the setting of MS; however, the underlying pathophysiology of the pain is not fully characterized. The authors of this article performed the largest analysis to date of MRI findings in patients with trigeminal neuralgia. Most significantly, patients with typical trigeminal neuralgia symptoms were found to harbor lesions in the ventrolateral pons between the trigeminal root entry zone and the trigeminal nucleus. Patients with other forms of facial sensory disturbance displayed lesions in the lower pons in the region of the trigeminal nucleus. The results of this study suggest that typical trigeminal neuralgia symptoms are most likely due to injury to afferents of first-order neurons within the pons. The authors were not able to address how often a dual mechanism, such as neurovascular compression, is also present.

P. A. House, MD

17 Miscellaneous

A Comparison of 3% Hypertonic Saline and Mannitol for Brain Relaxation During Elective Supratentorial Brain Tumor Surgery

Wu C-T, Chen L-C, Kuo C-P, et al (Tri-Service General Hosp, Taipei, Taiwan; Kaohsiung Armed Forces General Hosp, Taiwan; et al)

Anesth Analg 110:903-907, 2010

Background.—In this study, we compared the effects of 3% hypertonic saline (HTS) and 20% mannitol on brain relaxation during supratentorial brain tumor surgery, intensive care unit (ICU) stays, and hospital days.

Methods.—This prospective, randomized, and double-blind study included patients who were selected for elective craniotomy for supratentorial brain tumors. Patients received either 160 mL of 3% HTS (HTS group, $n = 122$) or 150 mL of 20% mannitol infusion (M group, $n = 116$) for 5 minutes at the start of scalp incision. The Pco_2 in arterial blood was maintained within 35 to 40 mm Hg, arterial blood pressure was controlled within baseline values ±20%, and positive fluid balance was maintained intraoperatively at a rate of 2 mL/kg/h. Outcome measures included fluid input, urine output, arterial blood gases, serum sodium concentration, ICU stays, and hospital days. Surgeons assessed the condition of the brain as "tight," "adequate," or "soft" immediately after opening the dura.

Results.—Brain relaxation conditions in the HTS group (soft/adequate/tight, $n = 58/43/21$) were better than those observed in the M group (soft/adequate/tight, $n = 39/42/35$; $P = 0.02$). The levels of serum sodium were higher in the HTS group compared with the M group over time ($P < 0.001$). The average urine output in the M group (707 mL) was higher than it was in the HTS group (596 mL) ($P < 0.001$). There were no significant differences in fluid input, ICU stays, and hospital days between the 2 groups.

Conclusions.—Our results suggest that HTS provided better brain relaxation than did mannitol during elective supratentorial brain tumor surgery, whereas it did not affect ICU stays or hospital days.

▶ This is a very well-designed, double-blind, prospective randomized study evaluating the effects of 3% hypertonic saline (HTS) and 20% mannitol on intraoperative brain relaxation during supratentorial surgery. At the time of scalp incision, the patient was administered either 160 cc of 3% or 150 cc of 20% mannitol. Other variables were controlled such as the Pco_2. The surgeon, who was also blind to the drug administered, was asked to judge the brain after opening the

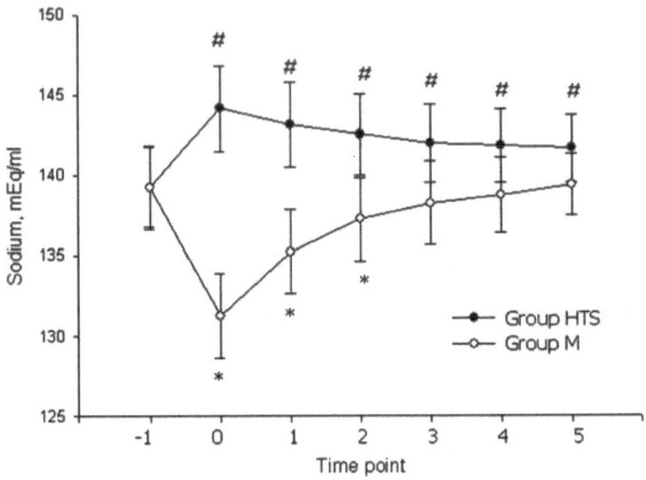

FIGURE 1.—Sodium (Na) concentration in arterial blood. Hypertonic saline (HTS) administration caused an increase in serum Na concentration at points 0, 1, 2, 3, 4, and 5 compared with the baseline (point −1) and mannitol (#$P < 0.001$). In the presence of mannitol, Na concentration decreased at points 0, 1, and 2 compared with point −1 (∗$P < 0.001$). Point −1 indicates the onset of hyperosmotic solution infusion; point 0 indicates the time of dural opening; point 1 indicates 1 hour after the end of the infusion; points 2, 3, and 4 indicate 2, 3, and 4 hours after the end of the infusion; and point 5 indicates the end of surgery. M = mannitol. (Reprinted from Wu C-T, Chen L-C, Kuo C-P, et al. A comparison of 3% hypertonic saline and mannitol for brain relaxation during elective supratentorial brain tumor surgery. *Anesth Analg*. 2010;110:903-907.)

dura as either tight, adequate, or soft. HTS clearly provided more satisfactory brain relaxation. The authors also found that HTS was able to increase the serum Na and thus the serum osmolarity, compared with mannitol (Fig 1). Mannitol, on the other hand, induced a greater diuretic and natriuretic effect. Both of these agents work by improving blood rheology with shrinkage of erythrocytes, decrease cerebrospinal fluid (CSF) production, but Na is completely impermeable to an intact blood-brain-barrier (reflection coefficient = 1), while mannitol is slightly permeable (reflection coefficient = 0.9). Therefore, a lower solute leakage from the intravascular space to the brain interstitial space may evoke a greater increase in serum osmolality and a higher transendothelial osmotic gradient in the vascular compartment which will then lead to increased brain water extraction into the intravascular space.

This article adds to the growing literature favoring the use of HTS over mannitol for the management of traumatic and nontraumatic cerebral edema.

P. Klimo, Jr, MD, MPH

Efficacy of intravenous patient-controlled analgesia after supratentorial intracranial surgery: a prospective randomized controlled trial

Morad AH, Winters BD, Yaster M (Hopkins Med Insts, Baltimore, MD)

J Neurosurg 111:343-350, 2009

Object.—Opioid administration following major intracranial surgery is often limited by a presumed lack of need and a concern that opioids will adversely affect postoperative outcome and interfere with the neurological examination. Nevertheless, evidence is accumulating that these patients suffer moderate to severe postoperative pain and that this pain is often undertreated. The authors hypothesized that intravenous patient-controlled analgesia (PCA) would safely and more effectively treat postoperative supratentorial craniotomy pain than conventional as needed (PRN) therapy.

Methods.—Following a standardized course of general anesthesia, adult patients who underwent elective supratentorial intracranial surgery were randomized in the neurosciences intensive care unit to receive either PRN intravenous fentanyl 25–50 μg every 30 minutes or PCA intravenous fentanyl 0.5 μg/kg every 15 minutes (maximum 4 doses/hour). The authors measured pain (self-reported scale score [0–10]), sedation (Ramsay Sedation Scale score), Glasgow Coma Scale score, fentanyl use, and major adverse events (excessive sedation, respiratory depression, pruritus, nausea, or vomiting) hourly.

Results.—Sixty-four patients with a mean age of 48 years (range 22–77 years) were randomized to intravenous PCA (29 patients) or PRN fentanyl (35 patients) groups. There were no statistically significant demographic differences between the 2 groups. Patients receiving intravenous PCA had significantly lower pain scores than those receiving intravenous PRN fentanyl (2.53 ± 1.96 vs 3.62 ± 2.11 [$p = 0.039$]) and received significantly more fentanyl than the PRN group (44.1 ± 34.5 vs 23.6 ± 23.7 μg/hour [$p = 0.007$]). There were no differences between the 2 groups regarding the number of patients with adverse events.

Conclusions.—Intravenous PCA more effectively treats the pain of supratentorial intracranial surgery than PRN fentanyl, and patients in the former group did not experience any untoward events related to the self-administration of opioids.

▶ Morad et al present the first randomized controlled trial directly comparing standard intravenous PCA fentanyl with PRN therapy for postcraniotomy patients. Not surprisingly, intravenous PCA was superior to PRN opioid administration in terms of pain relief. Patients were routinely assessed during their entire stay in the neurocritical care unit. Both groups also received regularly scheduled acetaminophen. Concordantly, patients in the PCA group received significantly more fentanyl than the PRN group. Respiratory depression and excessive sedation did not occur in the PCA group, although there was a trend toward greater nausea and vomiting.

This is a very clean study with no design flaws. Dissemination of this work will hopefully lead to improved postcraniotomy pain management.

P. Klimo, Jr, MD, MPH

Emergency transorbital ventricular puncture: refinement of external landmarks

Tubbs RS, Loukas M, Shoja MM, et al (Children's Hosp, Birmingham, AL; St George's Univ, Grenada, West Indies; Indiana Univ, Indianapolis)

J Neurosurg 111:1191-1192, 2009

Object.—Emergency access to the ventricular system is sometimes necessary for the treatment of raised intracranial pressure with ensuing herniation. One procedure described in the literature is a transorbital approach performed using a spinal needle. Because past publications have been case reports with minimal definition of external landmarks, the present study was performed.

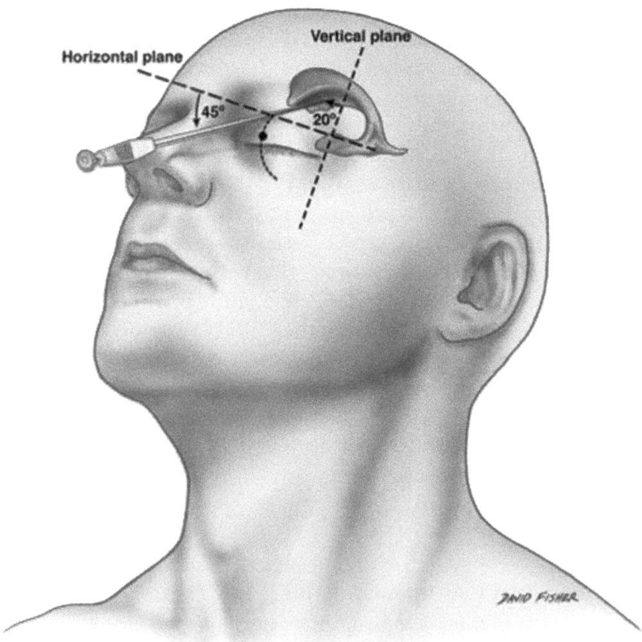

FIGURE 1.—Schematic drawing illustrating the refined landmarks found in the present study. Note that the needle tip is placed under the upper lid and punctures into the orbital roof just medial to the midpupillary line. The trajectory for entering the frontal horn of the lateral ventricle was on average 45° inferior to a horizontal line and 15–20° medial to a vertical line. Entrance into the frontal horn and to a point just superior to the foramen of Monro was on average 8 cm. (Reprinted from Tubbs RS, Loukas M, Shoja MM, et al. Emergency transorbital ventricular puncture: refinement of external landmarks. *J Neurosurg*. 2009;111:1191-1192.)

Methods.—Five adult cadavers (10 sides) underwent transorbital puncture of the lateral ventricles. This approach was performed following an axial section through the cranium that exposed the lateral ventricular system. Landmarks for the ideal placement of catheters into the ventricular system were then evaluated.

Results.—The authors found that the lateral ventricular system was consistently entered just superior to the level of the foramen of Monro by puncturing the roof of the orbit just medial to a midpupillary line, with the trajectory of the perforation aimed 45° from a horizontal line and 15–20° medial to a vertical line.

Conclusions.—Although it is uncommon, transorbital ventriculostomy may be used in emergency cases of raised intracranial pressure. Such refined landmarks as described in the present study may be of use to the neurosurgeon.

▶ I have only heard or read about the transorbital ventricular puncture, never performing it myself or seeing it done, but I read this article with fascination. Although it would be uncommon to need to do such a procedure, it is useful to know the landmarks, as described by the authors, in order to perform an emergent decompression of the ventricles in a situation where one has a high suspicion of hydrocephalus and no external ventricular access kits are available. The procedure can be done in a matter of seconds using an 18-gauge spinal needle that needs to be at least 9 cm long since the mean distance to ventricle was 8 cm (Fig 1). It should be noted that the needle tip is placed under the upper lid and punctures the orbital roof just medial to the midpupillary line.

P. Klimo, Jr, MD, MPH

Hospital Costs Associated With Shunt Infections in Patients Receiving Antibiotic-Impregnated Shunt Catheters Versus Standard Shunt Catheters

Attenello FJ, Garces-Ambrossi GL, Zaidi HA, et al (Johns Hopkins Univ School of Medicine, Baltimore, MD)

Neurosurgery 66:284-289, 2010

Background.—The average hospital cost for shunt infection treatment is $50 000, making it the most financially costly implant-related infection in the United States. We set out to determine whether introduction of antibiotic-impregnated shunts (AISs) in our practice has decreased the incidence of shunt infection or decreased infection-related hospital costs at our institution.

Methods.—Clinical and hospital billing records of pediatric patients undergoing cerebrospinal fluid (CSF) shunt insertion at a single institution from April 2001 to December 2006 were retrospectively reviewed. Eighteen months before October 2002, all CSF shunts included standard, non-AIS catheters. During the 4 years after October 2002, all CSF shunts included AIS catheters. Patients were followed at least 18 months after surgery.

Results.—A total of 406 pediatric patients underwent 608 shunt placement procedures (400 AISs, 208 non-AISs). Of patients with non-AIS catheters, 25 (12%) experienced shunt infection, whereas only 13 patients (3.2%) with AIS catheters experienced shunt infection during follow-up ($P < .001$). The total hospital cost to treat 25 non-AIS shunt infections over the first 18 months was $1,234,928. The total hospital cost to treat 13 AIS shunt infections over the past 4 years was $606,328. The mean hospital cost per shunt infection was similar for infected AIS and non-AIS catheters ($46 640 vs. $49 397). However, the infection-related hospital cost per 100 patients shunted was markedly lower in the AIS cohort than in the non-AIS cohort ($151 582 vs. $593 715).

Discussion.—The introduction of AIS catheters in our institutional practice reduced the incidence of shunt infection and resulted in significant hospital cost savings. AIS systems are efficient and cost-effective instruments to prevent perioperative colonization of CSF shunt components.

▶ This is yet another article that demonstrates a lowering in shunt infection rates when an institution switches from a standard silicone shunt system to an antibiotic impregnated system (AIS). At the authors' institution (Johns Hopkins University), the infection rate dropped from 12% to 3.2%. The cost analysis in this article is striking: the mean cost to treat a shunt infection was $48 454 (with no significant difference between those with a regular shunt and AIS), and thus the difference in cost between the treatment of 25 non-AIS shunt infections and 13 AIS infections was $628 600. Infection-related cost savings per 100 AIS patients was $442 133. When factoring the additional cost of the AIS ($400), it decreased the savings by only $40 000 per 100 shunt operations.

Another interesting finding of this study is the difference in the cost of a typical shunt infection in the United States (this study) compared with Germany.[1] Eymann et al performed a similar cost-analysis study that was actually reviewed last year. At their institution, the average costs of a single shunt infection were $17 300 and $13 000 in children and adults, respectively. This large difference in costs further strengthens the argument that in the United States, where health care cost containment is of immense concern, all shunt surgeries should be done with AIS.

P. Klimo, Jr, MD, MPH

Reference

1. Eymann R, Chehab S, Strowitzki M, et al. Clinical and economic consequences of antibiotic-impregnated cerebrospinal fluid shunt catheters. *J Neurosurg Pediatrics.* 2008;1:444-450.

Legacy and current understanding of the often-misunderstood Foix-Alajouanine syndrome

Ferrell AS, Tubbs RS, Acakpo-Satchivi L, et al (Univ of Alabama at Birmingham)

J Neurosurg 111:902-906, 2009

Foix-Alajouanine syndrome has become a well-known entity since its initial report in 1926. The traditional understanding of this clinical syndrome is as a progressive spinal cord venous thrombosis related to a spinal vascular lesion, resulting in necrotic myelopathy. However, spinal venous thrombosis is extremely rare and not a feature of any common spinal vascular syndrome. A translation and review of the original 42-page French report revealed 2 young men who had presented with progressive and unrelenting myelopathy ultimately leading to their deaths. Pathological analysis demonstrated endomesovasculitis of unknown origin, including vessel wall thickening without evidence of luminal narrowing, obliteration of cord vessels, or thrombosis. Foix and Alajouanine also excluded the presence of intramedullary arteriovenous malformations. At the time, dural arteriovenous fistulas (dAVFs) had not been described, and therefore this type of lesion was not specifically sought. In retrospect, it seems possible that both patients had progressive myelopathy due to Type I dAVFs. In the decades since that original report, numerous authors have included spinal cord venous thrombosis as a central feature of Foix-Alajouanine syndrome. The inclusion of thrombosis in the clinical picture of this syndrome is not only incorrect but may leave one with the impression of therapeutic futility, thus possibly preventing successful surgical or endovascular therapy.

► Foix-Alajouanine syndrome is a rare syndrome that is classically attributed to patients with progressive myelopathy and a type I spinal arteriovenous fistula (AVF). Apparently, this syndrome has been traditionally defined as a subacute myelopathy produced by a thrombotic disorder of the spinal cord. The article by Ferrell et al is an interesting trip back in history. They review the origin of this syndrome by translating from French the pertinent findings in the 2 cases described by Foix and Alajouanine in the 42-page article in 1926. Although the patients have many features typical of type I spinal AVF, there are some features that raise some doubt. Although we will never know what the real diagnosis was in their patients, the important findings described by these 2 French neurologists were the presence of endomesovasculitis with hypertrophy of the tunica media, myelitis, and spinal cord necrosis. No thrombosis was found. It is now generally accepted that patients with type I AVF have a progressive myelopathy due to venous hypertension that is potentially reversible with interruption of the fistula, whereas venous thrombosis would probably cause an irreversible spinal cord injury. Although Alajouanine lived 90 years before dying in 1980, Foix, arguably the first stroke neurologist, died at the young age of 43 in 1927, shortly after developing fever and abdominal pain. He died very soon after surgery.

P. Klimo, Jr, MD, MPH

Perioperative management of neurosurgical patients with methicillin-resistant *Staphylococcus aureus*

Akins PT, Belko J, Banerjee A, et al (Kaiser Permanente, Sacramento, CA)

J Neurosurg 112:354-361, 2010

Object.—The emergence of methicillin-resistant *Staphylococcus aureus* (MRSA) has posed a challenge in the treatment of neurosurgical patients. The authors investigated the impact of MRSA colonization and infection in the neurosurgical population at a community-based, tertiary care referral center.

Methods.—Hospitalized patients under the care of the Kaiser Permanente inpatient neurosurgery service were prospectively entered into a database. In Phase I of the study, 492 consecutive patients were followed. Per hospital policy, the 260 patients from this group who were admitted to the intensive care unit (ICU) underwent screening for MRSA based on nasal swab cultures and a review of their medical history for prior MRSA infections. These patients were designated as either MRSA positive (17 patients, 6.5% of screened patients) or MRSA negative (243 patients). The 232 patients admitted to non-ICU nursing units did not undergo MRSA screening and were designated as unscreened. In Phase II of the study, the authors reviewed 1005 neurosurgical admissions and completed a detailed chart review in 62 MRSA-positive patients (6.2%). Eleven patients received nonoperative treatment. Five patients presented with community-acquired neurosurgical infections, and the causative organism was MRSA in 3 cases. Forty-six patients underwent 55 procedures, and the authors reviewed their perioperative management.

Results.—In Phase I of the study, the authors found that for the MRSA-positive, MRSA-negative, and unscreened groups, the rates of postoperative neurosurgical wound infections caused by all pathogens were 23.5, 4.1, and 1.3%, respectively. For MRSA wound infections, the rates were 23.5, 0.8, and 0%, respectively. In Phase II, patients with MRSA were noted to have the following clinical features: male sex in 63%, a malignancy in 39.1%, diabetes in 34.8%, prior MRSA infection in 21.7%, immunosuppressed state in 17.4%, and a traumatic injury in 15.2%. The rate of postoperative neurosurgical wound infection in patients who received MRSA-specific prophylactic antibiotic therapy (usually vancomycin) was 7.4% (27 procedures) compared with 32.1% (28 procedures) in patients who received the standard treatment (usually cefazolin) ($p = 0.04$). Wound care for ICU patients was standardized for postoperative Days 0–7 with chlorhexidine cleaning at bandage changes at 3-day intervals. Wound cultures from neurosurgical site infections in patients with prior MRSA colonization or infection grew MRSA in 7 of 11 patients.

Conclusions.—Neurosurgical patients identified with MRSA colonization or a prior history of MRSA infections benefit from specific perioperative care, including prophylactic antibiotics active against MRSA (such as vancomycin) and postoperative wound care with coverings and chlorhexidine antisepsis to reduce MRSA wound colonization.

▶ As resistant organisms become more and more common in surgical practice, identifying factors to help minimize postoperative infections will be critical. This is a very well-conducted study evaluating the impact of methicillin-resistant *Staphylococcus aureus* (MRSA) on neurosurgical patients. The authors identify patients with MRSA prior to any surgical intervention and then follow these patients through their surgical procedures. Positive MRSA status was profoundly associated with any postoperative complication. Not surprisingly, the infection rate was significantly higher in the MRSA-positive group. Importantly, preoperative identification of MRSA-positive patients with subsequent MRSA-specific antibiotic prophylaxis significantly reduced the postoperative infection rate.

G. Rao, MD

Relationships between essential cortical language sites and subcortical pathways

Ellmore TM, Beauchamp MS, O'Neill TJ, et al (The Univ of Texas Med School at Houston)

J Neurosurg 111:755-766, 2009

Object.—Maps produced using either electrical stimulation or functional imaging have demonstrated a distributed network of cortical regions involved in expressive and receptive language tasks. The pattern of connectivity among components of this network has begun to be explored with diffusion tensor (DT) imaging, but has yet to be completely characterized. In this study the authors used DT imaging–based tractography to examine the interrelationship between cortical areas found to be essential for language by intraoperative electrical stimulation.

Methods.—The authors localized the arcuate fasciculus (AF), a white matter fiber system connecting frontal and parietotemporal areas in 10 patients, 9 of whom subsequently underwent left hemispheric language mapping.

Results.—The authors found that 81 (79%) of 102 essential language sites (ELSs) were closely related to the AF. Of all ELSs, 59% were located within 7.5 mm of AF fiber pathway terminations, and another 20% contained pathways terminating closer to the AF than would be expected by chance ($p < 0.05$). Additionally, direct subcortical stimulation of the AF following focal cerebral resections produced transient language deficits. The close spatial relationship found between ELSs and the AF suggests that tractography data alone may be used for localization of ELSs.

Conclusions.—The deficits evoked by subcortical stimulation validate and demonstrate the utility of this AF localization technique, and provide further evidence that the AF is an important pathway for fluent language. Taken together, these results demonstrate that DT imaging of the AF may be used to predict the location of brain areas that will be eloquent by the standards of stimulation mapping.

▶ The arcuate fasciculus (AF), which is considered part of the superior longitudinal fasciculus, is thought to connect the frontal speech areas (Broca's) with posterior temporal and parietal cortical areas (Wernicke's). The authors of this study were able to map out the AF preoperatively using diffusion tensor imaging (DTI). Intraoperatively, they localized essential language sites using cortical stimulation mapping and then mapped these to the preoperative AF projections to determine how well the DTI tractography predicted the locations of the essential language sites. Fifty-nine percent of the essential language sites had a direct relationship with the AF fiber pathway terminations, defined as being within 7.5 mm of the AF fiber end points (Fig 4 in the original article). Twenty percent of the language sites had an indirect relationship with the AF projections, defined as being beyond 7.5 mm from the AF end points but still closer to the AF than would be expected by chance (< 5%) alone (Fig 5 in the original article). Although parts of this article are difficult to follow, such as the Methods section in which the authors detail their statistical methods and modeling, and the authors do not explain how they came to use 7.5 mm in their assumptions, this article suggests that preoperative analysis of AF end points based on DTI can be used to guide cortical stimulation mapping, which is considered the gold-standard test in finding cortical language centers. The importance of the AF was also demonstrated by subcortical stimulation.

P. Klimo, Jr, MD, MPH

Spontaneous intracranial hypotension syndrome: a novel speculative physiopathological hypothesis and a novel patch method in a series of 28 consecutive patients

Franzini A, Messina G, Nazzi V, et al (Istituto Nazionale Neurologico "Carlo Besta," Milan, Italy)

J Neurosurg 112:300-306, 2010

Object.—Spontaneous intracranial hypotension (SIH) is a potentially serious pathological syndrome consisting of specific symptoms and neuroradiological signs that can sometimes be used to assess the efficacy of the treatment. In this paper the authors report a series of 28 patients with this syndrome who were all treated with an epidural blood patch at the authors' institution. The authors propose a novel physiopathological theory of SIH based on some anatomical considerations about the spinal venous drainage system.

Methods.—Between January 1993 and January 2007, the authors treated 28 patients in whom SIH had been diagnosed. Twenty-seven of the 28 patients presented with the typical findings of SIH on brain MR imaging (dural enhancement and thickening subdural collections, caudal displacement of cerebellar tonsils, and reduction in height of suprachiasmatic cisterns). The sites of the patients' neuroradiologically suspected CSF leakage were different, but the blood patch procedure was performed at the lumbar level in all patients. The patients were then assessed at 3-month and 1- and 3-year follow-up visits. At the last visit (although only available for 11 patients) 83.3% of patients were completely free from clinical symptoms and 8.3% complained of sporadic orthostatic headache.

Results.—The authors think that in the so-called SIH syndrome, the dural leak, even in those cases in which it can be clearly identified on neuroradiological examinations, is not the cause of the disease but the effect of the epidural hypotension maintained by the inferior cava vein outflow to the heart. The goal of their blood patch procedure (a sort of epidural block obtained using autologous blood and fibrin glue at the L1–2 level) is not to seal CSF leaks, but instead to help in reversing the CSF-blood gradient within the epidural space along the entire cord.

Conclusions.—The authors' procedure seems to lead to good and long-lasting clinical results.

▶ The authors present an intriguing theory on the development of spontaneous intracranial hypotension (SIH). They postulate that the inferior vena cava is a negative sump that preferentially drains the venous blood from the epidural spinal vein network via large lumbar collectors through 1-way valves (Fig 1 in the original article). This creates a gradient for cerebrospinal fluid (CSF) to aspirate from the subarachnoid into the epidural space and then into the venous system (inferior vena cava system).

Their theory would explain the SIH syndrome even in those patients without an obvious CSF leak—the aspiration mechanism may act diffusely on the dural surface and at the origin of spinal roots with a considerable outflow of CSF from the subarachnoid compartment to the radicular veins. The treatment should therefore focus on blocking the flow of venous blood from the epidural space by creating a block formed by a lumbar epidural blood patch.

However, their theory seems physiologic, meaning that the flow of venous blood preferentially to the lower pressure inferior vena cava system probably occurs in all individuals and not just those with SIH. The authors state that the development of SIH would require an additional process—constitutional weakness of dura or multiple subarachnoidal microdiverticula. The authors found that the sites of suspected CSF leakage, based on evidence of irregularity or cystic appearance of the sleeves of the radicular roots, were noted in 20 out of 28 patients. The next logical study would be to compare spinal imaging (MRIs and myelograms) in those patients with SIH versus those without to see whether there is a difference in the incidence of these radicular root irregularities (case-control study). The practical application of this article is that it would argue against surgical treatment of an identified cerebrospinal fluid (CSF) leak site, as the leak "...is not the cause of the disease but the effect of the epidural hypotension maintained by the inferior vena cava outflow to the heart."

P. Klimo, Jr, MD, MPH

Surface landmarks for the junction between the transverse and sigmoid sinuses: application of the "strategic" burr hole for suboccipital craniotomy

Tubbs RS, Loukas M, Shoja MM, et al (Children's Hosp, Birmingham, AL; St George's Univ, Grenada, West Indies; Indiana Univ, Indianapolis)

Neurosurgery 65:ons37-ons41, 2009

Objective.—Localization of internal cranial anatomy based on superficial landmarks is paramount in identifying and avoiding various important structures and, thus, decreasing surgical morbidity. We have studied external skull bony landmarks to facilitate the placement of the initial "strategic" burr hole just inferior and medial to the junction of transverse-sigmoid venous sinuses during standard retrosigmoid craniotomy.

Methods.—One hundred adult skulls (200 sides) underwent intracranial drilling of a small hole from the inside surface of the cranium, 5 mm inferior and medial to the border of the transverse sigmoid sinus junction (defined as the ideal location for the center of the strategic burr hole). Localization of this hole from the external surface of the skull was made based on easily identifiable superficial landmarks, including the mastoid process and zygomatic arch. A horizontal line was established parallel to the superior border of the zygomatic arch ("zygomatic line"), and a vertical line was fashioned by connecting the mastoid notch superiorly to the squamosal suture ("mastoid line").

Results.—For left sides, 81% of the strategic burr holes were inferior to the zygomatic line and 86% were medial to the mastoid line. For right sides, 91% of the strategic burr holes were inferior to the zygomatic line and 97% were medial to the mastoid line. For left and right sides, the mean distance for the center of the burr holes from the zygomatic line was 4.5 and 7.7 mm, respectively. For left and right sides, the mean distance from the mastoid line was 9.1 and 9.8 mm, respectively.

Conclusion.—Because landmark data in the literature for externally identifying the transverse sigmoid sinus junction is variable, we have attempted to refine this location with the largest sample size to date. These data can assist surgeons to localize the external cranial projection of the area just inferior and medial to the junction between the transverse and sigmoid sinuses when image guidance devices are not available. This localization is important in creation of appropriate size for craniotomy/craniectomy during the posterolateral approaches to the cranial base (Fig 1).

▶ The asterion, which is the confluence of the lambdoid, parietomastoid, and occipitomastoid sutures, has classically been cited as the junction of the transverse-sigmoid junction. This is an important landmark when planning the initial burr hole for lateral suboccipital approaches. Incorrect placement of the burr hole can lead to sinovenous injury. However, several anatomic studies have demonstrated that the location of the asterion can be quite variable in its relation to these venous structures. Furthermore, it is often difficult to palpate.

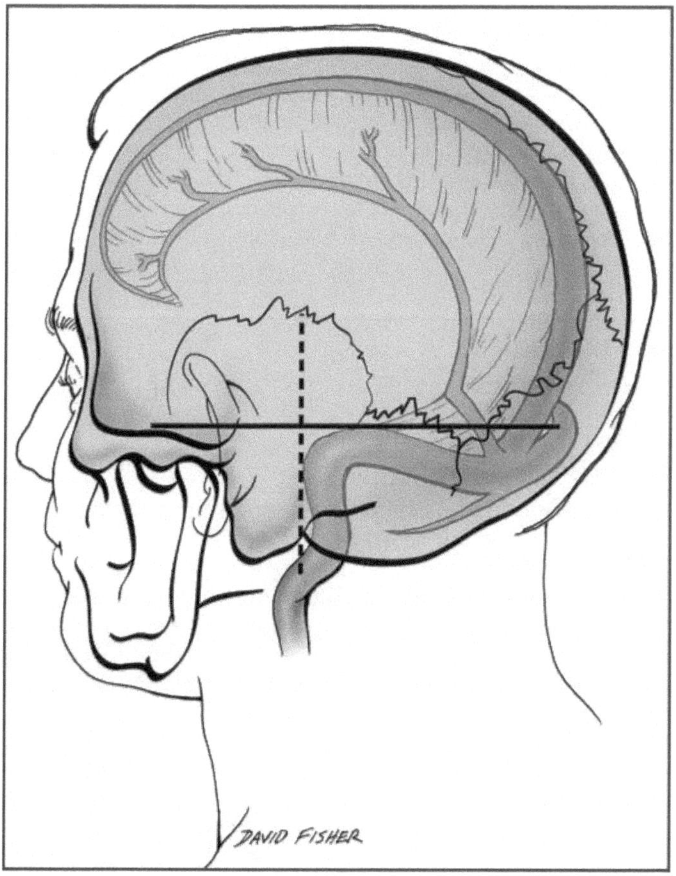

FIGURE 1.—Schematic drawing illustrating the intracranial transversesigmoid sinus junction and extracranial landmarks used in the present study. Note a horizontal line from the superior aspect of the zygomatic arch ("zygomatic line") and a vertical line from the mastoid notch ("mastoid line"). (Reprinted from Tubbs RS, Loukas M, Shoja MM, et al. Surface landmarks for the junction between the transverse and sigmoid sinuses: application of the "strategic" burr hole for suboccipital craniotomy. *Neurosurgery*. 2009;65:ons37-ons41.)

The authors of this cadaveric study identified the location of the ideal burr hole, that being 5 mm inferior to the transverse and 5 mm medial to the sigmoid sinus. The burr hole, which was drilled from the inside of the skull, was then referenced to 2 external surface landmarks as described above—the horizontal line was the superior border of the zygomatic arch and the vertical line was in line with the mastoid notch (Fig 1). This simple article has clinical relevance, as many neurosurgeons continue to use external landmarks to approximate the location of the transverse-sigmoid sinus junction. Although average distances from the lines for left- and right-sided specimens are provided in the abstract, what is important to note is that there is a wide range. For example, for left-sided specimens, the average distance of the drill hole from the zygomatic line was 4.5 mm, but this ranged from −16 mm to +15 mm (− signifies superior to the line, + signifies inferior to the line). A similar wide range from the zygomatic line was observed on the right side: −10 mm to +20 mm. For the mastoid line, most of the variability was located medial to the mastoid notch. In conclusion, 1 cm inferior to the zygomatic line and 1 cm medial to the mastoid notch line is a safe starting point in most patients, but the anatomy is variable enough in patients that one should try to confirm the position of the burr hole by analyzing the preoperative contrast-enhanced MRI or CT images or simply use intraoperative stereotaxy. In this day and age of intraoperative technology, I see no reason why neuronavigation should not be used routinely even for the purpose of placing burr holes accurately.

P. Klimo, Jr, MD, MPH

Syndrome of the trephined

Joseph V, Reilly P (Christian Med College Hosp, Tamil Nadu, India; Royal Adelaide Hosp, North Terrace, Adelaide, Australia)

J Neurosurg 111:650-652, 2009

"Syndrome of the trephined" or "sinking skin flap syndrome" is an unusual syndrome in which neurological deterioration occurs following removal of a large skull bone flap. The neurological status of the patient can occasionally be strongly related to posture. A 77-year-old male patient with an acute subdural hematoma was treated using a hemicraniectomy and evacuation of the hematoma. On the 9th postoperative day there was deterioration in sensorium associated with a sunken scalp flap and worsening midline shift on CT. A significant improvement in sensorium and a filling up of the scalp flap occurred after maintaining the patient's head in a dependent position. The patient subsequently made an excellent recovery following replacement of the bone flap. The pathophysiology of "syndrome of the trephined" or "sinking skin flap syndrome" is reviewed.

▶ The authors present a case of an elderly gentleman who required a decompressive craniectomy for an acute intracranial hemorrhage and several days later had a decline neurologically with midline shift and depression of the scalp flap. This was attributed to the infamous "syndrome of the trephined."

It has also been described as the "syndrome of the sinking skin flap" or the "posttraumatic syndrome." The patient made a rapid recovery after his head was placed just below the horizontal plane and then had his bone flap replaced the next day. The key feature of this syndrome is its rapid reversibility with either lowering the head to fill-up the brain or replacing the bone flap. There are a number of theories that have been put forth to explain this syndrome as reviewed by the authors, from changes in blood flow to disruption of cerebrospinal fluid dynamics. What is more intriguing is why this is such a rare complication after a decompressive craniectomy. In all patients, their brain is now subjected to atmospheric pressure, but yet this syndrome is rarely observed. This may be in part due to the vague definition of this syndrome. Some define it as the onset of neurologic symptoms and others define it vaguely as a constellation of subjective symptoms such as fatigability, feeling of apprehension, and discomfort at the craniectomy site. Nonetheless, in my personal experience while deployed to Afghanistan treating many patients with decompressive craniectomy, I cannot recall 1 patient who I thought developed this syndrome.

P. Klimo, Jr, MD, MPH

Treatment for Blunt Cerebrovascular Injuries: Equivalence of Anticoagulation and Antiplatelet Agents

Cothren CC, Biffl WL, Moore EE, et al (Univ of Colorado School of Medicine, Denver)

Arch Surg 144:685-690, 2009

Hypothesis.—We hypothesize that the 2 antithrombotic treatment regimens, systemic heparin sodium vs antiplatelet agents, are equivalent for the treatment of blunt cerebrovascular injuries (BCVIs) to prevent devastating injury-related strokes.

Design.—Retrospective review of a prospective database.

Setting.—Level I trauma center.

Patients.—Patients with BCVIs from January 1, 1997, to January 1, 2007.

Main Outcome Measures.—Incidence of cerebrovascular accident (CVA), stratified by treatment.

Results.—During the study period, 422 BCVIs were identified in 301 patients (64.8% men; mean [SEM] age, 37.0 [0.8] years; mean [SEM] injury severity score, 27.0 [0.9]). A total of 22 patients presented with neurologic ischemia, and 5 patients sustained CVAs after embolization and/or stenting of an injury. Treatment was initiated for 282 asymptomatic BCVIs (heparin, 192; aspirin, 67; aspirin and/or clopidogrel, 23); 1 patient had a CVA (0.5%). Of 107 patients with untreated, asymptomatic BCVIs, 23 (21.5%) had a CVA. For untreated patients sustaining BCVI-related CVAs, the mean (SEM) time to diagnosis was 58(10) hours. For those who did not exhibit symptoms within 2 hours of injury, mean time to diagnosis of CVA was 75(11) hours. Injury healing rates (heparin, 39%;

aspirin, 43%; aspirin/clopidogrel, 46%) and injury progression rates (12%; 10%; 15%) were equivalent between therapeutic regimens.

Conclusions.—With an overall CVA risk of 21% and a documented latent period, comprehensive screening, early diagnosis, and institution of antithrombotic therapy for BCVI are clearly warranted. The type of treatment, heparin vs antiplatelet agents, does not appear to affect either stroke risk or injury healing rates.

▶ Trauma patients with unrecognized, untreated blunt cerebrovascular injuries (BCVI) carry a stroke rate between 20% to 50%.[1] Stroke from BCVI often presents 2 to 3 days after trauma, giving clinicians a diagnostic window to act.[2] The Denver Health Medical Center has been at the forefront of the diagnosis and treatment of BCVI for the past 12 years. Over this time, 18 431 trauma admits showed 422 BCVIs in 301 patients (1.6%). In this study, the stroke rate of asymptomatic BCVI patients that were treated and not treated was 0.3% (1/282) and 21.5% (23/107), respectively. Of treated patients, 8 patients had bleeding complications (4 patients requiring blood transfusions for falling hematocrits, 3 craniotomies for intracranial bleeds, and 1 nasal packing for epistaxis). Although best treatment regime is still in question (ie, heparin drip only, aspirin only, aspirin, and/or clopidogrel), the reduction in stroke rate is clear. This data add to what other authors have reported—detect trauma-associated blunt cerebrovascular injuries early and discuss treatment in a multidisciplinary fashion taking into account all injuries involved.

B. T. Ragel, MD

References

1. Biffl WL, Ray CE Jr, Moore EE, et al. Treatment-related outcomes from blunt cerebrovascular injuries: importance of routine follow-up arteriography. *Ann Surg.* 2002;235:699-706.
2. Davis JW, Holbrook TL, Hoyt DB, Mackersie RC, Field TO Jr, Shackford SR. Blunt carotid artery dissection: incidence, associated injuries, screening, and treatment. *J Trauma.* 1990;30:1514-1517.

18 Pediatric Neurosurgery

Decompression of Chiari malformation with and without duraplasty: morbidity versus recurrence

Mutchnick IS, Janjua RM, Moeller K, et al (Univ of Louisville, KY; Univ of South Florida, Tampa; Kosair Children's Hosp, Norton Neuroscience Inst, Louisville, KY)

J Neurosurg Pediatr 5:474-478, 2010

Object.—The optimal surgical management of Chiari malformation (CM) is evolving. Evidence continues to accrue that supports decompression without duraplasty as an effective treatment to achieve symptomatic relief and anatomical decompression. The risks and benefits of this less invasive operation need to be weighed against decompression with duraplasty.

Methods.—The authors performed a retrospective review of all CM decompressions from 2003 to 2007. All operations were performed by a single surgeon at a single institution. Data were analyzed for outcome, postoperative morbidity, and recurrence.

Results.—Of 121 unique patients, 56 underwent posterior fossa decompressions without duraplasty (PFD) and 64 patients underwent posterior fossa decompressions with duraplasty (PFDD). Of the 56 PFD patients, 7 (12.5%) needed a subsequent PFDD for symptomatic recurrence. Of the 64 patients who underwent a PFDD, 2 (3.1%) needed a repeated PFDD for symptomatic recurrence. Patients treated with PFDD had an average operative time of 201 minutes in contrast to 127 minutes for those who underwent PFD ($p = 0.0001$). Patients treated with PFDD had average hospital stays of 4.0 days, whereas that for patients treated with PFD was 2.7 days ($p = 0.0001$). While in the hospital, patients treated with PFDD used low-grade narcotics, intravenous narcotics, muscle relaxants, and antiemetic medications at statistically significant differing rates.

Conclusions.—While PFD was associated with a higher rate of recurrent symptoms requiring repeated decompression, this may be justified by the significantly lower morbidity rate. Clearer delineation of the trade-off

between morbidity and recurrence may be used to help patients and their families make decisions regarding care.

▶ This article raises more questions than it answers. The authors state that all patients with a syrinx were treated with decompression and duraplasty, whereas those without a syrinx were preferentially treated with a bony decompression only, unless "...intraoperative observations led the surgeon to believe that a duraplasty was required for adequate decompression. Specifically, the surgeon looked for intradural pulsatility and the reestablishment of a subarachnoid space; if these were not unquestionably present after a full [decompression], then a [decompression and duraplasty] were performed." There are several issues with this statement. The authors briefly give a description of their surgical technique. Although they state that the suboccipital craniectomy was wide, how wide was it? Was the surgical technique the same among the surgeons? The critical part of this article, in my mind, is how the authors determined intraoperatively which patients would get a duraplasty and which would not. Was the assessment of pulsatility and subarachnoid space made with any objective measurements? Was a radiologist involved in the decision making (ie, who interpreted what I presume was the intraoperative ultrasound)? What specifically did the authors look for to make them satisfied that the subarachnoid space was re-established and that pulsatility was present?

As for the results, it comes to no surprise that hospital stay, narcotic and antiemetic usage, intraoperative OR time, and overall cost were more in the duraplasty group than in the nonduraplasty group. However, I submit that none of these differences would be important enough to convince a surgeon or the family to choose one over the other. The main factors that go into this decision are the risk of recurrence and the incidence of significant postoperative complications. Only 2 out of 64 patients who underwent duraplasty had a pseudomeningocele (3%). The authors make no mention whether these 2 patients required any further treatment for their pseudomeningocele, but I presume not. The recurrence rate was 4 times higher (12.5% vs 3.1%) in the duraplasty group, and I would argue that this is a big difference, not slightly higher as concluded by the authors. A subgroup analysis comparing only those patients without a syrinx (duraplasty vs nonduraplasty) would have been preferred. One could argue that patients with a syrinx could have a more aggressive or different spectrum of pathology than those without a syrinx, and thus comparing them with a group (the nonduraplasty patients) in which none of the patients had a syrinx raises some questions as to the validity of this comparison. What is the difference in recurrence rate between those patients who did not have syrinx? This would have provided more clinically applicable information.

Although the authors present some interesting albeit predictable data, this article brings us no closer to "...better patient understanding and decision making."

P. Klimo, Jr, MD, MPH

Endoscopic biopsy of brain tumors in children: diagnostic success and utility in guiding treatment strategies

Ahn ES, Goumnerova L (Johns Hopkins Univ School of Medicine, Baltimore, MD; Children's Hosp Boston, MA)

J Neursurg Pediatr 5:255-262, 2010

Object.—Endoscopic biopsy is an important minimally invasive method of diagnosis in the initial management of lesions in children with intraventricular and periventricular tumors. The procedure can be performed in conjunction with CSF-diverting procedures for obstructive hydrocephalus. The authors present their single-institution experience in a predominantly pediatric series with respect to diagnostic efficacy, utility in guiding treatment plans, and safety.

Methods.—A retrospective review was conducted in a consecutive series of patients who underwent endoscopic biopsy of brain tumors during a 13-year period.

Results.—There were 33 endoscopic biopsies in 31 patients (16 males and 15 females). The average age of the patients was 11.3 years, with a mean follow-up duration of 2.4 years. The majority of biopsies were performed in conjunction with CSF-diverting procedures, such as endoscopic third ventriculostomy or fenestration of the septum pellucidum. Overall, 23 (70%) of 33 biopsies were diagnostic, with results that directed subsequent treatment. When stratified by tumor location, biopsy samples obtained in the lateral ventricle or pineal region were more favorable toward a successful diagnosis than those in the thalamus or tectal region. In 4 cases, elevated CSF tumor marker levels led to modification of the diagnosis and appropriate adjustment of treatment. The endoscopic third ventriculostomy success rate was 82.4%. There were 2 major complications (6.1%), which resulted in neurological deficits. There were no procedure-related deaths.

Conclusions.—Endoscopic biopsy is an effective means of diagnosis of brain tumors in children. The diagnostic power may be more favorable with tumors in the lateral ventricle or pineal region. Collection of CSF during the procedure for tumor marker analysis is an integral component of diagnosis.

► The results of this article demonstrate the use of endoscopy in the management of children with intraventricular tumors. Endoscopy can potentially achieve 3 goals: (1) obtain CSF for the analysis of germ cell tumor markers (α-fetoprotein and β-human chorionic gonadotropin); (2) treat the hydrocephalus by an endoscopic third ventriculocisternostomy (ETV) or septostomy; and (3) perform biopsy of the tumor for diagnosis.

Although not all patients were candidates for an ETV after a biopsy was performed (2 patients had imaging evidence of disseminated CSF seeding with tumor, and thus it was thought that they had communicating hydrocephalus), the ETV success rate was 82.4%. The biopsy success rate was 70% and was a function of tumor location, type of endoscope used, and surgical technique.

Tumors located in the lateral ventricle (100%) and pineal region (62.5%) had higher biopsy success rates than those in the anterior third ventricle/suprasellar (57.1%) and thalamic or tectal region (25%). The larger rigid endoscope, since it is able to obtain a larger sample size, had a higher success rate (81%) than the flexible endoscope (45.5%). Finally, procedures that were performed by the senior author in the second half of this series had a higher diagnostic success (87.5%) rate than the first half (52.9%). Traditionally, the major fear about endoscopic biopsies is the limited ability to control bleeding. This is a valid concern. Not only are you limited in what you can use and do to control bleeding, but also even a small amount of blood can have a serious impact on visualization through the endoscope. The authors state that in their experience, most bleeding can be easily controlled with irrigation and the application of cautery through the endoscope.

P. Klimo, Jr, MD, MPH

Hemispherotomy: efficacy and analysis of seizure recurrence

Limbrick DD Jr, Narayan P, Powers AK, et al (Washington Univ School of Medicine, St Louis, MO; Princeton Brain and Spine Care, NJ; et al)

J Neurosurg Pediatr 4:323-332, 2009

Object.—Hemispherotomy generally is performed in hemiparetic patients with severe, intractable epilepsy arising from one cerebral hemisphere. In this study, the authors evaluate the efficacy of hemispherotomy and present an analysis of the factors influencing seizure recurrence following the operation.

Methods.—The authors performed a retrospective review of 49 patients (ages 0.2–20.5 years) who underwent functional hemispherotomy at their institution. The first 14 cases were traditional functional hemispherotomies, and included temporal lobectomy, while the latter 35 were performed using a modified periinsular technique that the authors adopted in 2003.

Results.—Thirty-eight of the 49 patients (77.6%) were seizure free at the termination of the study (mean follow-up 28.6 months). Of the 11 patients who were not seizure free, all had significant improvement in seizure frequency, with 6 patients (12.2%) achieving Engel Class II outcome and 5 patients (10.2%) achieving Engel Class III. There were no cases of Engel Class IV outcome. The effect of hemispherotomy was durable over time with no significant change in Engel class over the postoperative follow-up period. There was no statistical difference in outcome between surgery types. Analysis of factors contributing to seizure recurrence after hemispherotomy revealed no statistically significant predictors of treatment failure, although bilateral electrographic abnormalities on the preoperative electroencephalogram demonstrated a trend toward a worse outcome.

Conclusions.—In the present study, hemispherotomy resulted in freedom from seizures in nearly 78% of patients; worthwhile

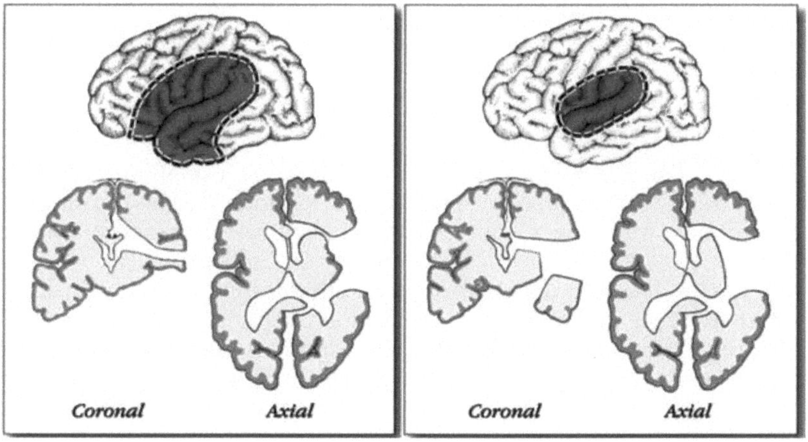

FIGURE 1.—Schematic representations of the 2 hemispherotomy techniques used in the current study. *Left:* A surface rendering showing the area resected in FH. Below are coronal and axial views showing the areas transected for the disconnection. Note that the anterior temporal lobe has been resected and the insular cortex remains intact (although this was resected in 4 of 14 cases). *Right:* The surface rendering the limited area of frontal and temporal opercula removed to permit the hemispheric disconnection in PIH. Coronal and axial views illustrate the disconnection. For the PIH, the corpus callosotomy is performed by subpial aspiration following the anterior cerebral arteries. A selective amygdalohippocampectomy is performed rather than a temporal lobectomy. (Reprinted from Limbrick DD Jr, Narayan P, Powers AK, et al. Hemispherotomy: efficacy and analysis of seizure recurrence. *J Neurosurg Pediatr.* 2009;4:323-332.)

improvement was demonstrated in all patients. The seizure reduction observed after hemispherotomy was durable over time, with only rare late failure. Bilateral electrographic abnormalities may be predictive of posthemispherotomy recurrent seizures.

▶ The authors present excellent seizure outcomes in 49 patients who underwent one of 2 hemispherotomy techniques: functional hemispherotomy or peri-insular hemispherotomy (Fig 1). Almost 90% of their patients had Engel class I (seizure free) or class II (rare seizures) seizure outcome. There were only 5 patients who had class III outcome (worthwhile improvement in seizure frequency) and no patients with class IV outcome. Because of the small sample size, no factors were identified that predicted seizure outcomes, including surgical technique, although the peri-insular hemispherotomy typically took longer to perform. Seven patients had surgical complications, 6 of them being related to the development of hydrocephalus (4 de novo shunts, 1 shunt revision, and 1 de novo subduroperitoneal shunt). Patients with malformation of cortical development—cortical dysplasia, polymicrogyria, and hemimegalencephaly—seemed to be at higher risk of postoperative seizure recurrence. Three out of 9 patients with hemimegalencephaly and 2 out of 7 patients with cortical dysplasia had class III outcomes.

P. Klimo, Jr, MD, MPH

Linear vein–based arteriovenous malformations in children

Maher CO, Scott RM (Univ of Michigan, Ann Arbor; Children's Hosp Boston, and Harvard Med School, MA)

J Neurosurg Pediatr 4:12-16, 2009

Object.—The authors reviewed the experience of a single surgeon in the surgical treatment of arteriovenous malformations (AVMs) in children, with specific attention to the angioarchitectural appearance of these lesions.

Methods.—The authors performed a retrospective review of pediatric cases of AVM treated at a single institution over a 15-year period. Inclusion criteria consisted of pediatric age at time of treatment and resection of a pial AVM. The AVMs were considered linear-based if they had a single, centrally located, dominant vein with a linear configuration rather than the typical central nidus.

Results.—Sixty-seven patients, ranging in age from 6 months to 17 years, underwent surgical treatment of an AVM between January 1, 1990, and December 30, 2005. In these patients, 31 AVMs (46%) had a distinct linear configuration that was centered on a dominant draining vein ("vein-based"). These AVMs presented with hemorrhage (61%), incidental findings on imaging (16%), or seizures (13%). In 4 cases, AVM recurrence was noted on angiographic follow-up after postoperative angiography showed no residual lesion. Recurrence was seen at 1 year in 2 cases, and at 3 and 11 years in 1 case each.

Conclusions.—A linear vein–based morphological pattern is common in pediatric AVMs and may recapitulate the embryological origins of the cerebral circulation. Surgical treatment in these cases can also be vein-based, through a narrow surgical corridor, which leads to minimal cortical disruption.

▶ Maher and Scott have described a rather unique arteriovenous malformation (AVM) in their pediatric series. These AVMs were termed linear vein-based if they had a single, centrally located, dominant vein and had a linear configuration rather than a typical globoid nidus with the central vein usually being oriented perpendicularly to the cortical surface. Of the 67 children who underwent surgery for AVMs over a 15-year-period, this linear vein-based configuration was found in a surprisingly high percentage (31 patients, 46%). All were successfully treated with surgery except one patient that had a transient postoperative neurologic deficit as a result of a small infarct. The authors state that patients with these AVM types were less likely to experience postoperative complications compared with patients with other AVM types.

There are several issues with this article. More detailed analysis of these patients would have been preferable. For example, there is no mention of the classic Spetzler-Martin grading of these patients, no mention of size or location, and postoperative data were limited. There is no mention of the follow-up period. If these vein-based malformations are so common, why have they not been described by other authors? The authors rely heavily on a 13-year-old article by Mullan et al[1] to support their findings and provide an embryological explanation for these lesions.

One patient with a linear vein-based malformation did have a delayed recurrence, reinforcing the fact that pediatric patients with AVM are at much higher risk of delayed recurrence than adults, but the authors do not provide any further details such as when this recurrence was discovered and how it was treated.

The authors also make no mention of any preoperative or alternative treatment modalities for these lesions, such as embolization or radiosurgery.

In conclusion, this article describes what could be a unique morphological AVM in children. I hope that other centers will add to this data.

P. Klimo, Jr, MD, MPH

Reference

1. Mullan S, Mojrahedi S, Johnson DL, MacDonald RL. Embryological basis of some aspects of cerebral vascular fistulas and malformations. *J Neurosurg.* 1996;85:1-8.

Long-term results of a second endoscopic third ventriculostomy in children: retrospective analysis of 40 cases

Peretta P, Cinalli G, Spennato P, et al (Regina Margherita Children's Hosp, Turin, Italy; Santobono-Pausilipon Children's Hosp, Naples, Italy)

Neurosurgery 65:539-547, 2009

Objective.—To evaluate retrospectively the operative findings and long-term results of a repeat endoscopic third ventriculostomy (ETV) in pediatric hydrocephalic patients readmitted after the first procedure with symptoms and/or signs of intracranial hypertension and/or radiological evidence of increased ventricular dilation and/or occluded stoma on follow-up radiological examinations.

Methods.—We analyzed a series of 482 ETVs in pediatric patients from 2 Italian departments of pediatric neurosurgery. The clinical charts of 40 patients undergoing a second ETV were selected and reviewed retrospectively. The pre- and postoperative radiological findings and operative films were analyzed retrospectively.

Results.—Forty patients underwent a total of 82 ETVs. Thirty-eight patients were operated on twice and 2 were operated on 3 times. During the second procedure, the stoma was found to be closed in 28 patients without underlying adhesions, to be open but with significant arachnoid adhesions in the prepontine cistern in 8 patients, to be open without adhesions in 2 patients, to have a pinhole orifice in 1 patient, and to be closed with underlying adhesions in 1 patient. The second procedure allowed reopening of the stoma or lysis of the arachnoid adhesions in 35 patients and was abandoned in 3 patients because of extensive arachnoid adhesions or because the stoma was found to be wide open (2 patients). In 30 patients (75%), the second ETV was effective, and the 2 patients who underwent a third ETV remained shunt free. In 10 patients (25%), a ventriculoperitoneal shunt was eventually placed. Age younger than 2 years at the time of the first procedure and arachnoid adhesions in the subarachnoid cisterns observed during the second procedure are the main negative prognostic factors for the success of a second ETV.

Conclusion.—A second ETV can be performed with a reasonable chance of restoring patency of the stoma and avoiding placement of an extrathecal shunt. Every effort should be made to detect subarachnoid adhesions in the cistern on preoperative imaging study to select potential candidates and avoid unnecessary procedures.

▶ Endoscopic third ventriculocisternostomy (ETV) is viewed by many neurosurgeons—pediatric and adult—as a preferred treatment of certain forms of obstructive hydrocephalus. An ETV may fail due to either progressive scarring of the orifice at the level of the floor of the third ventricle (tuber cinereum) or by the formation of arachnoid adhesions in the interpeduncular/prepontine cisterns or both.

This article by Peretta et al looks at children who had an initial ETV and then developed recurrent symptoms and underwent a repeat ETV. Forty of their 482 patients underwent a second ETV and of these 28 (70%) patients remained asymptomatic and symptom free. Two additional patients who had recurrent symptoms underwent a third ETV attempt and remained shunt free. This is how the authors came up with their 75% success rate (30/40 patients).

This study shows that those patients who were deemed a candidate for their initial ETV should be considered a candidate for a repeat ETV if needed. The authors of this study found that a repeat ETV was most effective in patients older than 2 years and with no arachnoid membranes seen at the time of reoperation. A larger study is required to hopefully elucidate more prognostic factors for success or failure of an ETV. In such higher-risk patients, it may be prudent to leave a permanent ventricular catheter with reservoir.

P. Klimo, Jr, MD, MPH

Modified orbitozygomatic craniotomy for craniopharyngioma resection in children

Golshani KJ, Lalwani K, Delashaw JB Jr, et al (Oregon Health and Science Univ, Portland)

J Neurosurg Pediatr 4:345-352, 2009

Object.—In this study, the authors evaluated the efficacy and safety of modified orbitozygomatic craniotomy for resection of craniopharyngioma in children.

Methods.—A prospective, institutional review board–approved database was retrospectively reviewed for pediatric patients undergoing craniopharyngioma resection performed by a single surgeon.

Results.—Ten patients underwent craniopharyngioma resection surgery between July 2000 and January 2006 (4 girls and 6 boys, ages 1.5–17 years). Nine patients presented to the authors' institution, and 1 patient was referred after surgery and radiation therapy were administered elsewhere. Nine patients presented with visual field deficits (2 with unilateral or bilateral light perception only) and 5 with endocrine dysfunction. Eight patients had large tumors that significantly displaced the optic chiasm and hypothalamus. All patients underwent a modified frontotemporal orbitozygomatic osteotomy in a single piece. The lamina terminalis was opened in 4 patients with third ventricular extension. One patient required a staged transsphenoidal operation to remove residual tumor in the sella turcica, and 1 patient underwent a contralateral subtemporal approach to resect a daughter lesion in the prepontine cistern. Complete radiographic resection was achieved in all patients. Follow-up averaged 55 months (range 12–95 months). Vision was improved in 8 patients and remained stable in 2. All patients had postoperative endocrine dysfunction. One patient experienced transient cranial nerve IV palsy and 1 suffered a small caudate stroke 5 months after surgery without sequelae. Two patients experienced polyphagia and weight gain without other symptoms of hypothalamic dysfunction. There were no other new neurological deficits.

Conclusions.—Modified orbitozygomatic craniotomy provides excellent exposure of the suprasellar region with minimal brain retraction, allowing complete resection of craniopharyngiomas with good visual and neurological results.

▶ This article describes the modified orbitozygomatic craniotomy for the resection of craniopharyngiomas (Fig 1 in the original article). The approach really is a standard frontotemporal (pterional) craniotomy with an orbital extension (orbital rim and room osteotomy); the zygoma is kept intact. There are traditionally 3 main approaches for craniopharyngiomas: a more lateral or anterolateral trajectory with the pterional, an anterior trajectory using the subfrontal approach, or a combination of both. Some authors feel that the lower starting profile—anterior-inferior approach as described by the authors—achieved by removing the orbital rim and roof allows easier subfrontal retraction and greater visualization of the posterior and superior aspects of the tumor. In my opinion, the added orbital osteotomies are rarely needed. Exposure via a combined approach allows access to multiple surgical corridors, which is usually adequate for tumor removal. Craniopharyngiomas are often cystic, and with aspiration of the cyst, the superior aspects of the tumor will fall away and can be dissected into the surgical field.

The authors used a lumbar drain intraoperatively to facilitate brain relaxation. I have not found this to be necessary, as cerebrospinal fluid can be aspirated with dissection of the basal arachnoid cisterns, and osmotic agents can be given shortly after intubation. The authors use angled fiberoptic endoscopes to better visualize areas that are somewhat blind, such as the sella and behind the clivus. I have tried angled mirrors, but I think the endoscope would be far superior. Finally, the authors state that there are 3 factors that influence the ability to perform a total tumor resection: size, anatomical complexity of the mass, and history of cyst leakage. I think the third item is very important and one that can have the greatest impact on surgical extirpation. It is important to look for this when taking a history from the patient and family. I would have liked the authors to be more specific with the term "anatomical complexity of the mass"—are they referring to proximity to surrounding neurovascular structures, or are they referring to extension to areas beyond the sellar/suprasellar region?

P. Klimo, Jr, MD, MPH

Multiple-suture nonsyndromic craniosynostosis: early and effective management using endoscopic techniques

Jimenez DF, Barone CM (The Univ of Texas Health Science Ctr at San Antonio)

J Neurosurg Pediatr 5:223-231, 2010

Object.—The authors present the results of treating infants with multiple-suture nonsyndromic craniosynostosis in whom the authors used minimally invasive endoscopy-assisted techniques and postoperative cranial molding over an 11-year period.

Methods.—A total of 21 patients who presented with multiple-suture (nonsyndromic) craniosynostosis were treated using minimally invasive endoscopy-assisted craniectomies. Surgery was followed by treatment with custom-made cranial orthoses for up to 12 months. A total of 48 sutures were treated. The most common was the coronal suture (38 cases) and this was followed by the sagittal (11 cases), metopic (6 cases), and lambdoid (3 cases) sutures. There were 13 male and 8 female pediatric patients. Their ages ranged between 3 weeks and 9 months (mean 3.2 months, median 2.5 months). The sagittal suture was treated with a wide vertex craniotomy via 2 incisions located behind the anterior fontanel and in front of the lambda. The metopic suture underwent a suturectomy as did the coronal and lambdoid sutures.

Results.—The mean follow-up duration was 61 months (range 3–135 months). There were no deaths. In patients with bicoronal synostosis, brachycephaly was corrected. Patients presenting with vertical dystopia or nasal deviation had these deformities corrected as well. The mean blood loss was 42 ml (range 10–120 ml). The mean hospital length of stay was 1 day. The intraoperative transfusion rate was 0%. The results indicate that nonsyndromic multiple-suture synostosis can be safely and effectively treated using endoscopic techniques.

Conclusions.—Early treatment of complex multiple-suture synostosis with endoscopic techniques provides an excellent surgical alternative. The results of the present study indicate marked correction of skull base and craniofacial deformities. Endoscopy provides a safe and effective way to treat these patients.

▶ The debate on whether craniosynostosis repair should be done in the classic open approach or the newer endoscopic approach continues. The lead author

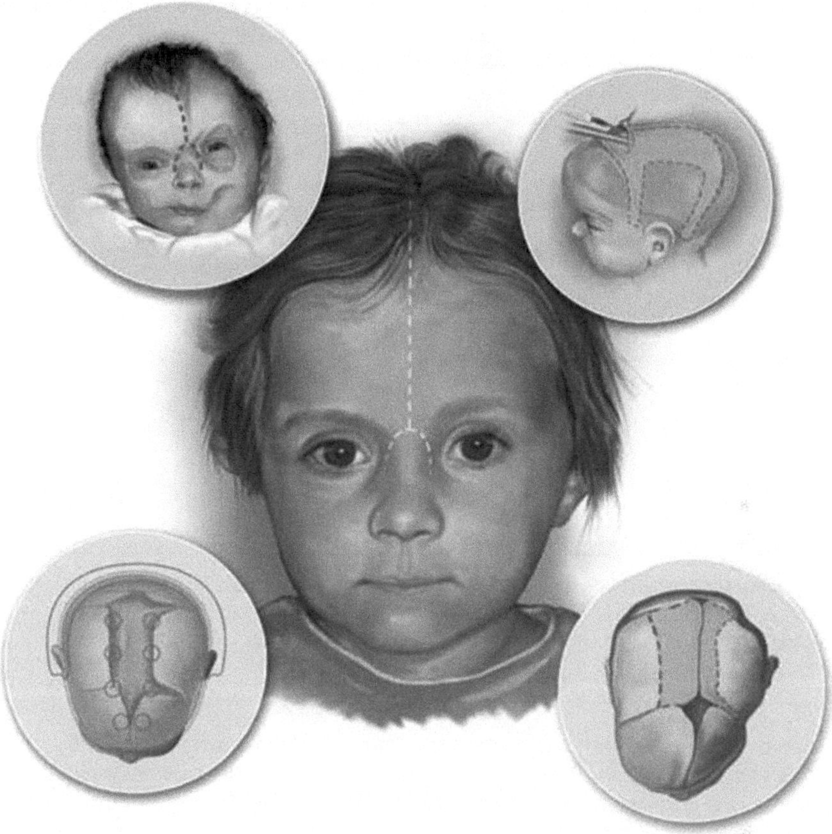

FIGURE 2.—Case 1. Artist's rendition of the treatment and outcome in the patient with coronal, sagittal, and lambdoid craniosynostosis. The *upper left inset* shows preoperative dystopia and other compensatory changes. The *upper right inset* shows the extent of osseous resection and the endoscopic approach. The *lower right inset* shows aerial view of the patient's head preoperatively and the amount of bone removed during surgery. The *lower left inset* demonstrates cranial expansion and normalization while the helmet is still worn. The *center* image shows almost complete normalization of the craniofacial skeleton at 1 year of age. (Reprinted from Jimenez DF, Barone CM. Multiple-suture nonsyndromic craniosynostosis: early and effective management using endoscopic techniques. *J Neurosurg Pediatr.* 2010;5:223-231.)

in this article, arguably the father of endoscopic synostosis repair, reports his 11-year experience treating children with multisuture nonsyndromic synostosis. His argument for intervening early (usually within the first 3-6 months of life) is to halt the progression of complex deformities involving the calvarial, orbital facial, and skull base skeleton (Fig 2). At this age, the minimally invasive endoscopic technique is the only one that can be performed. The classic open approach needs to be done at an age when the child can tolerate such a larger surgery (typically 6-12 months of age), and such delay allows these deformities to worsen.

There were 21 patients with 48 sutures involved, the most common being the coronal. The authors provide a good description of the surgical procedure for each suture involved, including patient positioning, placement of the burr hole, and extent of the strip craniectomy performed. On the fourth postoperative day, the patient undergoes a scan so that the physician may obtain anthropometric measurements for a helmet that is typically worn for the next 10 to 12 months or until the child is 18 months of age, whichever comes first. This aspect of endoscopic synostosis surgery—prolonged helmet therapy—is often cited by proponents of open surgery as a significant disadvantage.

The most striking finding of this article is that the authors were able to halt the progression of the various deformities, and most, if not all, of the deformities were reversed. The authors provide fascinating chronologic pictures of cases in which one can see the severity of the deformity preoperatively and how it corrects with time. Based on the results of this long-term follow-up study, the authors make a strong case that endoscopic repair should be considered the primary means of treating children with multisuture nonsyndromic craniosynostosis.

P. Klimo, Jr, MD, MPH

Neurosurgical management of intracranial epidermoid tumors in children

Ahmed I, Auguste KI, Vachhrajani S, et al (The Univ of Toronto, Ontario, Canada)

J Neurosurg Pediatr 4:91-96, 2009

Object.—Epidermoid tumors are benign lesions representing 1% of all intracranial tumors. There have been few pediatric series of intracranial epidermoid tumors reported previously. The authors present their experience in the management of these lesions.

Methods.—The neurosurgical database at the Hospital for Sick Children was searched for children with surgically managed intracranial epidermoid tumors. The patients' charts were reviewed for demographic data, details of clinical presentation, surgical therapy, and follow-up. Ethics board approval was obtained for this study.

Results.—Seven children, all girls, were identified who met the inclusion criteria between 1980 and 2007. The average age at surgery was 11.2 years (range 8–15 years), and the mean maximal tumor diameter was 2.1 cm. Headache was the most common presenting symptom, and 1 tumor was found incidentally. Most patients had normal neurological examinations, but meningism was found in 2 cases. There were 3 cerebellopontine angle lesions, 1 pontomedullary lesion, and 3 supratentorial tumors. Hydrocephalus developed in 1 patient after aseptic meningitis, and she underwent shunt placement. There were no operative deaths. Complete resection could be performed in 2 patients. One patient experienced a small recurrence that did not require a repeated operation, while 1 subtotally resected lesion recurred and the patient underwent a second operation.

Conclusions.—Intracranial epidermoid tumors are rare in the pediatric population. Total resection is desirable to minimize the risk of postoperative aseptic meningitis, hydrocephalus, and tumor recurrence. Aggressive neurosurgical resection may be associated with cranial nerve or ischemic deficits, however. In these cases, neurosurgical judgment at the time of surgery is warranted to ensure maximum resection while minimizing postoperative neurological deficits.

▶ Intracranial epidermoid lesions are benign tumors arising from ectodermal cellular remnants due to incomplete cleavage of the neural ectoderm from the cutaneous ectoderm. These tumors grow very slowly through progressive accumulation of normally dividing epidermal cells (termed linear growth) and typically insinuate through the subarachnoid space. Although most tumors present in adulthood, Ahmed et al present the first series of exclusively pediatric patients. Seven children with ages ranging from 8 to 15 years presented with 3 supratentorial and 4 infratentorial tumors. This well written article discusses all of the major issues in working up and treating these patients and is summarized here:

1. Imaging: These lesions are considered extra-axial as they almost always grow from within the subarachnoid space. As such, they will often appear as an arachnoid cyst on CT and on most sequences on MRI, but the increased signal intensity on diffusion weighted imaging (DWI) is what differentiates them.
2. Presentation: This is primarily dependent on location. Headache was the most common presenting symptom and cranial nerve involvement and cerebellar dysfunction was the most common presentation of posterior fossa tumors. Two of their patients presented with signs and symptoms of meningitis presumably due to spillage of the tumor contents into the cerebrospinal fluid (CSF).
3. Surgical treatment: The aim of treatment should be total resection without harm to surrounding structures, but this is often difficult to do. A gross total resection could be achieved in only 2 of their patients. These tumors can infiltrate into brain parenchyma and be very adherent to surround neurovascular structures. Herein lies the source of most postoperative complications. Cranial nerve (CN) palsies developed in 5 patients with 2 of them having permanent deficits. One patient went blind as a result of central retinal artery occlusion and the anterior choroidal artery was sacrificed in another, leading to a visual field defect.
4. Chemical meningitis: This may occur preoperatively or postoperatively as a result of spillage of the cyst contents into the subarachnoid space. This may lead to communicating hydrocephalus, which occurred in 1 patient. The authors advocate irrigating the surgical site with hydrocortisone and administering perioperative systemic steroids.

5. Follow-up: Tumors that are incompletely resected should be followed with serial imaging. Only one patient required repeat resection for progressive increase in tumor size.

P. Klimo, Jr, MD, MPH

Neurosurgical management of intractable rolandic epilepsy in children: role of resection in eloquent cortex

Benifla M, Sala F, Jane J Jr, et al (The Univ of Toronto, Ontario, Canada; Univ of Virginia Health System, Charlottesville)

J Neurosurg Pediatr 4:199-216, 2009

Object.—The authors undertook this study to review their experience with cortical resections in the rolandic region in children with intractable epilepsy.

Methods.—The authors retrospectively reviewed the medical records obtained in 22 children with intractable epilepsy arising from the rolandic region. All patients underwent preoperative electroencephalography (EEG), MR imaging, prolonged video-EEG recordings, functional MR imaging, magnetoencephalography, and in some instances PET/SPECT studies. In 21 patients invasive subdural grid and depth electrode monitoring was performed. Resection of the epileptogenic zones in the rolandic region was undertaken in all cases. Seizure outcome was graded according to the Engel classification. Functional outcome was determined using validated outcome scores.

Results.—There were 10 girls and 12 boys, whose mean age at seizure onset was 3.2 years. The mean age at surgery was 10 years. Seizure duration prior to surgery was a mean of 7.4 years. Nine patients had preoperative hemiparesis. Neuropsychological testing revealed impairment in some domains in 19 patients in whom evaluation was possible. Magnetic resonance imaging abnormalities were identified in 19 patients. Magnetoencephalography was performed in all patients and showed perirolandic spike clusters on the affected side in 20 patients. The mean duration of invasive monitoring was 4.2 days. The mean number of seizures during the period of invasive monitoring was 17. All patients underwent resection that involved primary motor and/or sensory cortex. The most common pathological entity encountered was cortical dysplasia, in 13 children. Immediately postoperatively, 20 patients had differing degrees of hemiparesis, from mild to severe. The hemiparesis improved in all affected patients by 3–6 months postoperatively. With a mean follow-up of 4.1 years (minimum 2 years), seizure outcome in 14 children (64%) was Engel Class I and seizure outcome in 4 (18%) was Engel Class II. In this series, seizure outcome following perirolandic resection was intimately related to the child's age at the time of surgery. By univariate logistic regression analysis, age at surgery was a statistically significant factor predicting seizure outcome ($p < 0.024$).

Conclusions.—Resection of rolandic cortex for intractable epilepsy is possible with expected morbidity. Accurate mapping of regions of functional cortex and epileptogenic zones may lead to improved seizure outcome in children with intractable rolandic epilepsy. It is important to counsel patients and families preoperatively to prepare them for possible worsened functional outcome involving motor, sensory and/or language pathways.

▶ This article discusses the surgical management and outcomes in children who have medically intractable epilepsy arising from the rolandic region that is defined as the region (primary motor and primary sensory cortex) surrounding the central sulcus. Specifically, the authors discuss their results with cortical resections in this area. The group started performing cortical resections because of a high relapse rate in their patients who had undergone multiple subpial transections. There are several important points made in this article.

Children with this kind of epilepsy are typically young at the time of seizure onset, have a long history of seizures prior to surgery, and have failed multiple drugs. Indeed, the mean number of seizures per day for the group was 21, the mean number of seizure types was 2.5/patient, the mean number of anticonvulsants tried before surgery per patient was 6, and the mean number of anticonvulsants at the time of surgery was 3 per patient.

All patients underwent a magnetoencephalography that localized abnormal rolandic spiking in 20 of 22 patients, and using somatosensory evoked fields, the somatosensory cortex was mapped and then fused with intraoperative neuronavigational systems. MR imaging demonstrate dabnormalities in 19 of 22 patients, but all patients had a neuropathologic diagnosis, with cortical dysplasia being the most common. A good seizure outcome (Engle class I or II) was achieved in 81% of patients, and favorable seizure outcome was associated with older children.

Not surprisingly, the risk of postoperative deficits is very high in these patients. Twenty of 22 patients exhibited an immediate postoperative deficit. This included patients whose primary motor cortex was spared any resection, suggesting that the postcentral cortex also contributes fibers to the corticospinal tract. However, most of these patients who had sparing of the motor cortex exhibited improvement of their weakness within the first week and nearly complete by 6-week to 3-month follow-up. The authors speculate that in cases where there was a postoperative hemiparesis and the primary motor cortex was spared, this may not represent a true weakness but rather a profound sensory neglect or proprioceptive disturbance. Likewise, dysphasia in patients in which the resection spared the language centers may be due to a neuropraxia from impairment of unilateral face and tongue motor pathways. The authors correctly state that the most difficult decision to make is whether motor hand or leg cortex should be included in any nonlesional resection to control epilepsy arising from the rolandic region.

P. Klimo, Jr, MD, MPH

Occipitocervical instrumentation in the pediatric population using a custom loop construct: initial results and long-term follow-up experience

Couture D, Avery N, Brockmeyer DL (Univ of Utah, Salt Lake City; Flagstaff Med Ctr, AZ)

J Neurosurg Pediatr 5:285-291, 2010

Object.—Rigid occipitocervical instrumentation for craniovertebral instability is gaining widespread acceptance for use in pediatric patients; however, most of the instrumentation has been modified from adult-sized hardware. The Wasatch loop system (formerly the Avery-Brockmeyer-Thiokol loop system) is a rigid occipitocervical fixation device designed specifically for use in children. It affixes to the occiput and incorporates either C1–2 transarticular screws or C-2 pars screws. It is preformed and is available in a variety of sizes. The authors describe their clinical experience and long-term follow-up experience with the first 22 patients.

Methods.—An institutional review board-approved retrospective review of medical records and radiographs was performed for patients who underwent occipitocervical fusion with the Wasatch loop. The mean patient age was 4.9 years (1.2–13 years), and the overall mean follow-up was 4 years (1.5–6.5 years). Six patients had posttraumatic instability, and 16 patients had congenital instability.

Results.—Twelve patients underwent placement of bilateral C1–2 transarticular screws, 6 patients had placement of a combination of C1–2 transarticular and C-2 pars screws, and 4 patients had placement of bilateral C-2 pars screws. One patient required a halo orthosis; the others were treated postoperatively with a hard cervical collar. All patients had radiographic evidence of solid occipitocervical arthrodesis on last follow-up examination.

Conclusions.—The Wasatch loop system is a novel internal fixation device for children who have posttraumatic or congenital occipitocervical instability. Successful arthrodesis was achieved in all patients with minimal use of halo orthoses (Fig 3).

► The Wasatch plate, designed by Dr Brockmeyer and others at the University of Utah, is the first occipitocervical instrumentation device specifically designed and sized for pediatric patients. It is a preformed 3-mm thick titanium U-shaped loop that is contoured to lie against the occiput and the posterior aspect of C-2. It is fixated against the occiput with three 4-mm screws and held against C-2 by either 3.5-mm C1-2 transarticular screws or C-2 pars screws (Fig 3). The authors report their results using this system in 22 patients requiring occipitocervical stabilization for various etiologies over a 6-year period. All patients went on to fuse in an average of 4.3 months. Only 1 child was placed in a halo postoperatively; otherwise a hard collar was used for 2 to 3 months. Three children had hardware complications that required reoperations.

Although the authors state in the Methods section that the plate is coupled to C-2 pars or transarticular screws, in the Discussion section they also add C-2

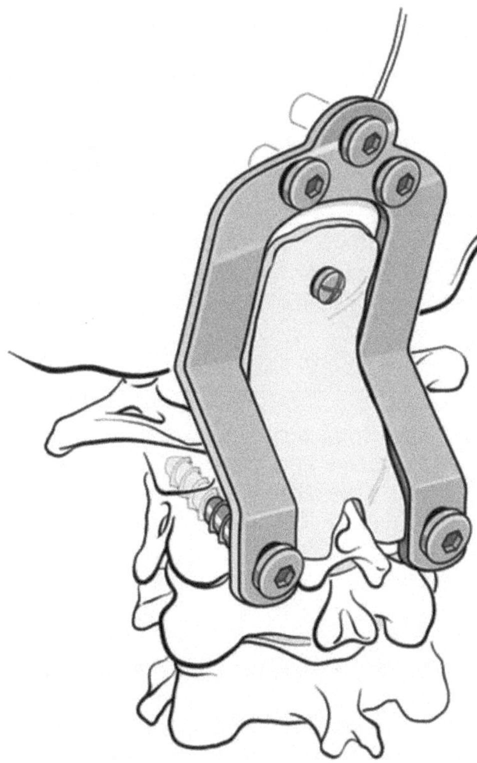

FIGURE 3.—Drawing depicting the final appearance of the Wasatch plate spanning the suboccipital region to C-2. Note the placement of the iliac crest bone graft between the arms of the plate with a small screw placed through the graft and into the suboccipital bone. For purposes of clarity, the retention cable holding the graft in place has been omitted. (Reprinted from Couture D, Avery N, Brockmeyer DL. Occipitocervical instrumentation in the pediatric population using a custom loop construct: initial results and long-term follow-up experience. *J Neurosurg Pediatr.* 2010;5:285-291.)

laminar screws. However, to accommodate the latter would seem to require a significant change in the design of the plate. The screw heads for the C-2 laminar screws are resting higher and more medial than the C-2 pars/transarticular screw heads and oriented in a completely different direction. It would have been helpful for the authors to provide more details on this, as translaminar screws have become increasingly more popular in occipitocervical fusions.

The authors also state that at 3 to 4 months after surgery, they obtain a thin-cut CT to evaluate for fusion. If fusion has not yet matured, they recommend repeating the CT in 2- to 3-month intervals. This to me seems like too much radiation for a child. I'm not sure whether they were obtaining more frequent CT scans because they were using a new device. However, I would argue that if plain films cannot show a fusion (which I think they could in the majority of cases), then a single CT scan at 6 months should be sufficient to show fusion mass.

Finally, the authors used rib or posterior iliac crest autograft in their patients. I think the next study would be to evaluate other fusion materials in an effort to spare the patient a second surgical site and potential morbidity of graft harvest. For example, the use of synthetic onlay graft material with or without the use of BMP could be an alternative.

P. Klimo, Jr, MD, MPH

Postoperative cerebellar mutism syndrome following treatment of medulloblastoma: neuroradiographic features and origin

Wells EM, Khademian ZP, Walsh KS, et al (George Washington Univ School of Medicine and Health Sciences, DC)

J Neurosurg Pediatr 5:329-334, 2010

Object.—The origin and long-term outcome of cerebellar mutism syndrome (CMS), a postoperative syndrome of diminished speech, hypotonia, and ataxia that affects approximately 25% of patients with medulloblastoma, is poorly elucidated. The current study was undertaken to determine factors associated with development of CMS, a means to determine its severity or cause, and outcomes of patients with this syndrome.

Methods.—The study included 28 children with medulloblastoma who either underwent an operation or were referred to the authors' institution soon after surgery. Eleven (39%) of these children had CMS. The preoperative, immediate postoperative, and 1-year postoperative MR images were reviewed by a neuroradiologist blinded to diagnosis of CMS. The severity of mutism and neurological and neurocognitive outcomes were examined.

Results.—Preoperative MR images showed no differences in tumor size, hydrocephalus, or peritumoral edema in patients with and without CMS. An association with brainstem invasion was significant ($p < 0.05$), and there was a trend toward an association with involvement of the cerebellomedullary angle ($p = 0.08$). Images obtained immediately postoperatively showed cerebellar edema in 92% of all patients; there were trends for more middle and superior cerebellar peduncle edema in patients with CMS ($p = 0.05$ and 0.07, respectively). At 1 year postoperatively, patients with CMS showed more moderate to severe atrophy/gliosis of total cerebellum ($p < 0.01$), vermis ($p < 0.01$), and brainstem ($p < 0.05$). Mean IQ was 16 points lower in patients with CMS ($IQ = 84.2 \pm 15.8$) compared with those without CMS ($IQ = 100.4 \pm 17.4$), with a trend toward significance ($p = 0.07$).

Conclusions.—This study demonstrates that CMS is associated with postoperative damage to the cerebellum and brainstem, damage not predicted by immediate postoperative MR imaging, and with poorer associated functional outcome.

▶ Cerebellar mutism syndrome (CMS) consists of diminished speech, hypotonia, ataxia, and emotional lability following resection of a posterior fossa tumor. Tumors in a vermal location, particularly medulloblastomas, have the highest rates of CMS. No studies have demonstrated any specific demographic, clinical, or radiographic predictive factors, and it is not localizable to a specific neuroanatomic region but thought to be due to the disruption of the dentato-thalamocortical outflow tracts.

This article was undertaken to determine the factors associated with CMS. What is unique is that the authors evaluated CMS symptoms and MRI findings 1 year postoperatively. Over a 15-year period, CMS was found in 11 (39%) of 28 patients with medulloblastoma. The authors found that patients with CMS had more brainstem tumor invasion preoperatively. There was no difference in the amount of postoperative edema between those who did and did not get CMS. MR imaging at 1 year revealed significantly more atrophy of total cerebellum and vermis as well as more brainstem atrophy in patients with CMS (Fig 1 in the original article). It appears that only those patients who have mild initial CMS deficits will have a full recovery. At 1 year, all patients in this study who had either moderate or severe symptoms continued to have speech deficits, and 83% of patients had persistent ataxia.

Unfortunately, CMS will continue to be a risk for patients undergoing posterior fossa tumor resection and at this time, there is little that can be done to avoid it. Although the authors suggest that the use of brain and cranial neurophysiologic monitoring, less aggressive retraction, and avoidance of the CUSA have improved the risk, this is speculative at best. In my opinion, I agree with minimizing the retractor use and that using perioperative steroids, avoiding the extension of resection into the cerebellar peduncles or brainstem, and limiting the degree of vermis splitting can hopefully decrease the development of CMS.

P. Klimo, Jr, MD, MPH

The natural history of pineal cysts in children and young adults

Al-Holou WN, Maher CO, Muraszko KM, et al (Univ of Michigan, Ann Arbor)

J Neursurg Pediatr 5:162-166, 2010

Object.—The authors reviewed their experience with pediatric pineal cysts to define the natural history and clinical relevance of this common intracranial finding.

Methods.—The authors identified all patients with pineal cysts who had been clinically evaluated at their institution over an 11.5-year interval and were < 25 years of age at the time of diagnosis. All inclusion criteria were met in 106 patients, and included repeated MR imaging as well as repeated clinical evaluation over at least a 6-month interval.

Results.—The mean age at diagnosis was 11.7 ± 7.2 years. Forty-two patients were male and 64 were female. On follow-up MR imaging evaluation at a mean interval of 3.0 years from the initial study, 98 pineal cysts had no increase in size and no change in imaging appearance. Six pineal cysts increased in size and 2 others had a change in imaging characteristics without associated growth. Younger age was associated with cyst change or growth on follow-up imaging ($p = 0.02$). The mean age of patients with cysts that changed or grew was 5.5 years, and the mean age of patients with stable pineal cysts was 12.2 years. Initial cyst size and appearance on MR imaging were not significant predictors of growth or change in imaging appearance at follow-up. Similarly, the patient's sex was not a significant predictor of growth or change in imaging characteristics.

Conclusions.—Follow-up imaging and neurosurgical evaluation may be considered optional in older children with pineal cysts.

▶ Pineal cysts are a common incidental finding on MRI. Patients often end up being evaluated by neurosurgeons. This article follows a number of patients with pineal cysts (> 5 mm), with at least 6 months of clinical and radiographic follow-up. Of 106 patients, only 8 patients showed either a growth or change in MRI appearance with follow-up. Only 1 patient underwent a resection for what was subsequently diagnosed as a pineocytoma.

The authors found that young age was a predictor of cyst growth or change in imaging characteristics; however, with only 8 patients who had these outcomes, it is hard to justify performing statistical analysis. Furthermore, with such small numbers, a subgroup analysis (older patients vs younger patients) is also limited but would have been helpful. How many patients were there in each group? What was the follow-up for each group? Did limited follow-up in the older patients explain the perceived difference in risk of pineal cysts changing with time?

The use of this article is to show just how few patients with pineal cysts eventually require surgical intervention (< 1%). However, the authors do not have enough patients with outcomes (change in cyst imaging characteristics and growth of cyst) to make any meaningful conclusions about these changes. With this study, one needs to question the need for repeat imaging on any patient, especially those who are asymptomatic. Although the authors state in their final sentence that their practice is to offer these patients a "...neurosurgical evaluation," I would argue that pediatricians should be made aware of the results of this study and hopefully prevent unnecessary and costly consultations, much in the way that should be done for other nonsurgical entities such as positional plagiocephaly.

P. Klimo, Jr, MD, MPH

The outcome of tethered cord release in secondary and multiple repeat tethered cord syndrome

Al-Holou WN, Muraszko KM, Garton HJ, et al (Univ of Michigan, Ann Arbor)

J Neurosurg Pediatr 4:28-36, 2009

Object.—After primary repair of a myelomeningocele or a lipomyelomeningocele, patients can present with symptoms of secondary tethered cord syndrome (TCS). After surgical untethering, a small percentage of these patients can present with multiple repeat TCS. In patients presenting with secondary or multiple repeat TCS, the role as well the expected outcomes of surgical untethering are not well defined.

Methods.—Eighty-four patients who underwent spinal cord untethering after at least 1 primary repair were retrospectively evaluated using scaled and subjective outcome measures at short-term and long-term follow-up visits. Outcomes were analyzed for predictive measures using multivariate logistic regression.

Results.—Surgical untethering was performed in 66 patients with myelomeningoceles and 18 patients with lipomyelomeningoceles. Fourteen patients underwent multiple repeat spinal cord untethering. Patients were followed up for an average of 6.2 years. Most patients had stability of function postoperatively. Motor function and weakness improved in 7 and 16% of patients at 6 months, respectively, and 6 and 19% of patients at long-term follow-up evaluation, respectively. Of the patients who presented with back pain, 75% had improvement in symptoms at 6 months postoperatively. Younger age at untethering was significantly associated with worse long-term neurological outcomes. The number of previous untethering procedures, original diagnosis, sex, anatomical level, and degree of untethering had no effect on surgical outcomes.

Conclusions.—Patients presenting with secondary or multiple repeat TCS may benefit from surgical untethering.

▶ Al-Holou et al provide an excellent review of patients from their institution (University of Michigan) undergoing 1 or more spinal cord untethering surgeries after the index untethering (defined as 'secondary' and 'multiple' tethering) over a 25-year interval. There were 84 patients with 66 of them having a tethered cord due to myelomeningocele and 18 for a lipomyelomeningocele. Of these patients, 50 had repeat surgery because of progressive symptoms, whereas 34 had prophylactic surgery in the setting of a spinal fusion and deformity correction.

The authors used scales for measurement of various dimensions of clinical function, including motor, ambulation, bladder, bowel, and sensory function. This raises a question. The oldest data in this study predate the existence and use of many of these scales by a significant time period. How were they able to categorize all of their patients in a retrospective manner? Because this is not a prospective study, how did the authors manage data that were not present in the charts? Did they call the patients' parents? The authors do not mention whether their surgical technique or use of technology changed over the 25-year period.

Nonetheless, this study yielded some interesting results. In the short and intermediate (6 months) follow-up, >80% of symptomatic patients were stable with respect to the functional parameters studied, and of the remainder roughly half improved and half deteriorated. However, at long-term follow-up, a substantial percentage exhibited functional deterioration:

In patients with preoperative score >1, which indicates some degree of function:

- motor function (Necker-Enfants Malades [NEM] scale): 57% deteriorated

- ambulation (modified Hoffer ambulatory scale): 52% deteriorated
- bowel and bladder function (NEM Bladder and Bowel Scales): 20/31% deteriorated
- sensory function (NEM sensory scale): 21% deteriorated

These numbers indicate that in a substantial percentage of patients, this is a progressive disease that will worsen despite surgery. It is unclear whether the deterioration of function in these patients would have been worse if no surgery was performed. We presume so because the vast majority of patients did exhibit improvement in the short and intermediate follow-up. Pain generally responded well to surgery.

The authors also found that outcomes of patients were not different in:

- patients with myelomeningocele versus patients with lipomyelomeningocele
- multiple versus secondary untethering
- complete versus incomplete circumferential untethering

The only factor that correlated with worse long-term neurological outcome was younger age at untethering.

This study demonstrates that, analogous to patients with shunted hydrocephalus, there is a subgroup of patients with tethered cord whose disease will not be halted with the index surgery and will continue to have a progressive decline in neurologic function despite surgery. These patients need to be identified and followed closely. The authors should be commended on their study and they should now pursue a prospective study using the same or similar outcome measures while standardizing their operative technique.

P. Klimo, Jr, MD, MPH

The transsphenoidal resection of pediatric craniopharyngiomas: a case series

Jane JA Jr, Prevedello DM, Alden TD, et al (Univ of Virginia Health System, Charlottesville; Univ of Pittsburgh Med Ctr, PA; Northwestern Univ, Chicago, IL; et al)

J Neursurg Pediatr 5:49-60, 2010

Object.—The majority of pediatric craniopharyngiomas are treated using a transcranial approach. Although there is an increasing acceptance of transsphenoidal resection in adults, there are few reports describing this approach in the pediatric population. The purpose of this study is to report the outcomes after transsphenoidal surgery in a consecutive series of pediatric patients with craniopharyngiomas treated at a single institution with the goal of gross-total resection (GTR).

Methods.—Twenty-three patients with pathologically proven craniopharyngiomas were identified who were 18 years of age or less at the time of surgery. The medical records and imaging studies of the patients were retrospectively reviewed. One patient who was lost to follow-up after surgery was excluded.

Results.—Among the 22 patients included in the study, 11 underwent transsphenoidal surgery as the primary procedure and 11 underwent transsphenoidal surgery as a secondary procedure after a previous procedure. All patients had at least some sellar component to their tumor and all had either anterior or posterior pituitary dysfunction at presentation. In the entire cohort, a GTR was achieved in 15 (68%) of 22 patients, a radical subtotal resection in 4 (18%) of 22 patients, a subtotal resection in 1 patient, and a partial resection in 2 patients. The degree of resection was higher in the primary transsphenoidal group. After a mean follow-up of 82 months, 4 patients (18%) experienced recurrence. Recurrence occurred in 13% after GTR compared with 28.5% after all other degrees of resection. Tumor recurred in 9% of the primary transsphenoidal group and in 30% of patients who had undergone other therapies prior to the transsphenoidal operation. No patient who had panhypopituitarism experienced a gain of function postoperatively, 67% developed new panhypopituitarism, and 56% experienced new diabetes insipidus. Vision improved or normalized in 9 (64%) of 14 patients presenting with visual loss. Complications included 1 death 3 weeks postoperatively, 2 CSF leaks, and new obesity in 37%.

Conclusions.—Transsphenoidal resection of pediatric craniopharyngiomas results in a high rate of both visual improvement and GTR with a low associated risk of recurrence. The transsphenoidal approach should be considered in selected pediatric patients with craniopharyngioma, especially those with infradiaphragmatic origin.

▶ The transsphenoidal approach in children with sellar or sellar/suprasellar craniopharyngiomas is very underutilized, primarily due to a lack of experienced pediatric pituitary surgeons. This report, with the senior author being arguably one of the most experienced pituitary surgeons in the world, represents the largest series of children treated with a transsphenoidal operation. There were a total of 22 patients—11 with de novo tumors and 11 with recurrent tumors. All patients had suprasellar extension except for 1 patient with a purely sellar tumor. Ten patients had a total of 14 prior craniotomies.

Overall, 13 of 16 patients with intrasellar or intrasellar/suprasellar extension experienced a gross total resection compared with only 33% of the 6 patients with tumors extending into the third ventricle, retroclival region, or anterior cranial fossa. The authors reported an 18% recurrence rate at an average of 22 months postoperatively. Thirty-five percent of patients had major or minor complications; the most frequent is new obesity due to hypothalamic injury. New obesity did not seem to correlate with tumor size, location, or extent of resection.

Because of the unique anatomy in children with respect to transsphenoidal surgery (aeration of sinuses, configuration of sinuses, and small nasal aperture), only 6 patients could have an endonasal approach and the rest underwent a sublabial approach. The sphenoid sinus was poorly pneumatized in 6 patients, and the bone had to be resected with curettes or drilled to expose the cortical bone of the sella. The authors make the point that for these cases, frameless stereotaxy and intraoperative videofluoroscopy are invaluable and necessary, especially the latter.

The authors present a very detailed analysis of preoperative and postoperative data, including endocrinopathies, visual impairment, imaging data, and complications. With time, hopefully more pediatric neurosurgeons will gain experience with this surgery or elicit the assistance of their adult colleagues, but for now and the immediate future, craniotomy will be the treatment of choice for the vast majority of children with craniopharyngiomas.

P. Klimo, Jr, MD, MPH

19 Peripheral Nerve Surgery

Carpal tunnel release in patients with negative neurophysiological examinations: clinical and surgical findings

Lama M (Santa Maria di Loreto Hosp, Naples, Italy)

Neurosurgery 65:A171-A173, 2009

Objective.—In 16% to 34% of patients with classic symptoms of carpal tunnel syndrome (CTS), neurophysiology is negative. Few studies have concentrated on patients with symptoms compatible with CTS with normal examinations. The purpose of our study was to examine the clinical and surgical characteristics of this subtype of CTS in order to clarify a correct approach toward these patients.

Methods.—We studied a subpopulation of 25 patients (31 hands) with typical CTS symptoms despite normal neurophysiological examinations. All of the patients were initially treated with conservative therapy, and patients with work-related symptoms were advised to change their duties. In patients with persistent symptoms, wrist ultrasound and radiographic and blood examinations with rheumatic screenings were performed. Cervical magnetic resonance imaging was performed in some cases to exclude cervical radiculopathy. Other pathologies were found in 5 cases. Nine patients improved with nonsurgical therapy. Six months later, electric examinations were repeated and 3 patients with a confirmed median nerve injury underwent surgery. Eight patients with negative examinations underwent surgery (10 hands). All patients were advised of the possibility of incomplete pain remission after surgery.

Results.—All patients improved after surgery. Median nerve injury was confirmed by operative findings according to Tuncali grading.

Conclusion.—A combination of clinical findings and instrumental procedures is required when selecting patients for successful surgery.

▶ Carpal tunnel syndrome (CTS) is the most common compressive peripheral neuropathy and is typically diagnosed with a combination of history (such as hand shaking, nocturnal symptoms, exacerbation with hand activity), examination (sensory loss in the median nerve distribution), and nerve conduction studies (NCS). This article looked at the surgical results of patients with CTS by history and examination but with a negative NCS. In this situation, it is important to perform a careful workup and in some cases, make the diagnosis of CTS one of exclusion. This includes, as suggested by the author, ancillary studies as magnetic resonance neurography or wrist ultrasound to look for evidence of entrapment such as a thickened transverse carpal ligament, blood work to evaluate for rheumatoid arthritis, radiographs of the wrist and cervical spine, and MRI of the cervical spine. These should be performed when the clinician has any doubt as to the diagnosis. The author failed to mention the use of provocative maneuvers such as Tinel's test, Phalen's test, and compression of the carpal tunnel. Positive, provocative tests like these, in my opinion, would be a very important finding in a patient with classic symptoms and history but negative neurophysiologic testing. The authors also did not mention the use of steroid injections in the carpal tunnel that would be both diagnostic and therapeutic. Out of 25 patients, eventually only 8 patients underwent surgery (10 hands), and all had improvement in their symptoms.

Like the author, I too continue to confirm my clinical findings with electrophysiologic testing for CTS, but this article shows to me, as I have found repeatedly in my clinic, the limited usefulness of neurophysiologic testing in evaluating peripheral neuropathy (and radiculopathy too). A thorough history, examination, and a host of other less invasive tests will provide enough data for diagnosis in virtually all patients. But I, like most surgeons, continue to order electrophysiologic tests to satisfy both the patient and ourselves that, in an objective manner, a diagnosis of CTS has been made. We do this despite the fact that the only useful result for NCS is a positive one. As this study shows, a negative NCS is of limited benefit to the clinician because of the possibility that it represents a false-negative result.

P. Klimo, Jr, MD, MPH

Evidence of improvement in distal conduction of ulnar nerve sensory fibers after carpal tunnel release

Mondelli M, Ginanneschi F, Rossi A (EMG Service, Siena, Italy; Univ of Siena, Italy)

Neurosurgery 65:696-701, 2009

Objective.—The aim of this study was to verify any effect of carpal tunnel release (CTR) on distal ulnar nerve conduction findings, using the database of a previous study performed to establish a protocol for CTR outcome.

Methods.—The motor and sensory ulnar distal conduction findings of 251 consecutive hands belonging to 217 patients (175 women and 42 men; mean age, 55.6 years) with idiopathic carpal tunnel syndrome (CTS) were reanalyzed before and 1 and 6 months after CTR.

Results.—Before surgery, 115 hands (45.8%) showed reduction of ulnar nerve sensory action potential (SAP) amplitude; this number was reduced significantly to 85 (33.9%) after CTR. The SAP amplitude and sensory conduction velocity values of the ulnar nerve showed significant improvement 1 month after CTR; SAP amplitude values showed further significant improvement 6 months after CTR. Patients' ages and occupations were independent predictors of reduced baseline SAP amplitudes of the ulnar nerve in CTS.

Conclusion.—These results demonstrate an improvement in conduction values in sensory ulnar fibers in a percentage of patients with CTS after CTR, providing further support for the conclusion that in CTS ulnar fibers may be subject to compressive forces in the Guyon canal as a consequence of high pressure in the carpal tunnel.

► It is not uncommon to have patients with carpal tunnel syndrome (CTS) present with sensory symptoms outside the typical median nerve territory. The cause for this is not entirely clear, but there is literature to support that mechanical compression of the median nerve in the carpal tunnel is transmitted to Guyon's canal, thus compressing the ulnar nerve. These canals are separated by the pisiform bone, and the transverse carpal ligament forms the roof of the carpal tunnel and the floor of Guyon's canal. The authors of this article show nicely that in patients with idiopathic CTS, the sensory action potential and the sensory conduction velocity values of the ulnar nerve at the wrist were significantly reduced, particularly in younger patients and blue-collar workers, and improved with a standard carpal tunnel release. They excluded patients with medical comorbidities that predispose to neuropathy, as well as patients with concomitant ulnar neuropathy at the elbow.

The implication of this study is that for patients with symptoms involving the ulnar distribution as well as typical CTS symptoms, only the transverse carpal ligament needs to be released. In my experience, I have found that this works well in these patients and there is no need to explore Guyon's canal.

P. Klimo, Jr, MD, MPH

Magnetic resonance neurography for the evaluation of peripheral nerve, brachial plexus, and nerve root disorders

Du R, Auguste KI, Chin CT, et al (Brigham and Women's Hosp, Boston, MA; Univ of California, San Francisco)

J Neurosurg 112:362-371, 2010

Object.—Treatment of spinal and peripheral nerve lesions relies on localization of the pathology by the use of neurological examination, spinal MR imaging and electromyography (EMG)/nerve conduction studies (NCSs). Magnetic resonance neurography (MRN) is a novel imaging technique recently developed for direct imaging of spinal and peripheral nerves. In this study, the authors analyzed the role of MRN in the evaluation of spinal and peripheral nerve lesions.

Methods.—Imaging studies, medical records, and EMG/NCS results were analyzed retrospectively in a consecutive series of 191 patients who underwent MRN for spinal and peripheral nerve disorders at the University of California, San Francisco between March 1999 and February 2005. Ninety-one (47.6%) of these patients also underwent EMG/NCS studies.

Results.—In those who underwent both MRN and EMG/NCS, MRN provided the same or additional diagnostic information 32 and 45% of patients, respectively. Magnetic resonance neurograms were obtained at a median of 12 months after the onset of symptoms. The utility of MRN correlated with the interval between the onset of symptoms to MRN. Twelve patients underwent repeated MRN for serial evaluation. The decrease in abnormal signal detected on subsequent MRN correlated with time from onset of symptoms and the time interval between MRN, but not with resolution of symptoms. Twenty-one patients underwent MRN postoperatively to assess persistent, recurrent, or new symptoms; of these 3 (14.3%) required a subsequent surgery.

Conclusions.—Magnetic resonance neurography is a valuable adjunct to conventional MR imaging and EMG/ NCS in the evaluation and localization of nerve root, brachial plexus, and peripheral nerve lesions. The authors found that MRN is indicated in patients: 1) in whom EMG and traditional MR imaging are inconclusive; 2) who present with brachial plexopathy who have previously received radiation therapy to the brachial plexus region; 3) who present with brachial plexopathy and have systemic tumors; and 4) in patients under consideration for surgery for peripheral nerve lesions or after trauma. Magnetic resonance neurography is limited by the size of the nerve trunk imaged and the timing of the study.

▶ Magnetic resonance neurography (MRN) offers the ability to not only reveal the morphological characteristics of nerves but also provides information on pathological processes, including nerve fibrosis inflammation and edema. It is a coronal and axial short tau inversion recovery sequence obtained through the region of interest. Although it has been more frequently applied in peripheral nerve pathology, it can also be applied to plexopathy and radiculopathy. The authors report their experience with this novel imaging technique in 91 cases at the UCSF. MRN was most useful when the regular MR and electromyography (EMG)/nerve conduction studies (NCSs) were inconclusive. All 91 of their patients underwent both EMG/NCS and MRN, with MRN providing more information than EMG/NCSs in 41 (45%) patients. The authors present several cases with good quality MRN images to show how MRN helped render a diagnosis.

As stated by the authors, MRN is most useful when performed within a year of symptom onset and in the following scenarios:

(1) EMG/NCS and traditional MR imaging are both nondiagnostic;
(2) EMG/NCS is nondiagnostic for suspected peripheral nerve lesion;
(3) traditional MRI is ambiguous or shows multilevel disease, and EMG/NCS is unable to clarify these results;
(4) patient cannot tolerate EMG/NCS;

(5) localization of trauma of the brachial plexus or peripheral nerves;
(6) localization of peripheral nerve lesions; and
(7) in patients with peripheral and spinal nerve tumors.

Based on this report, I would consider obtaining an MRN before an EMG/NCS. I find that the latter very infrequently helps in isolating the problem, often providing a dirty, not clinically useful result. Furthermore, it is a study most patients find uncomfortable. MRN, I suspect, is limited by the available neuroradiological assets at one's place of practice.

P. Klimo, Jr, MD, MPH

The Surgical Management of Symptomatic Peripheral Nerve Sheath Tumors

Levi AD, Ross AL, Cuartas E, et al (Univ of Miami Miller School of Medicine, FL)

Neurosurgery 66:833-840, 2010

Objective.—To determine the clinical presentation and morbidity of the surgical management of peripheral nerve sheath tumors (PNSTs).

Methods.—We performed a retrospective chart review of surgically treated PNSTs at the University of Miami between 1991 and 2008.

Results.—There were a total of 140 cases, including 87 schwannomas, 34 neurofibromas, and 19 malignant peripheral nerve sheath tumors (MPNSTs). The average age of the total study group was 49.0 years; it was significantly lower for patients with neurofibroma. There was a high correlation between neurofibroma tumors and neurofibromatosis-1. Most patients with benign tumors presented with a painful mass, paresthesias, or numbness without significant weakness. Patients who had previously undergone attempted resections and preoperative biopsy had a significantly increased risk (41%) for developing postoperative neurologic deficits when compared with patients who presented with de novo tumors (15%). Intraoperative monitoring appeared to reduce the risk of postoperative motor deficit, particularly in neurofibromas. Most MPNSTs (>80%) were diagnosed at stage IIB or higher and had a combined mortality rate of 31.6% at 78 months. Tumor size was the best predictor of adverse outcome, as all MPNST mortalities occurred in patients with a tumor size of more than 7 cm.

Conclusion.—PNSTs are a heterogeneous group of lesions. Benign tumors respond well to marginal excision, whereas MPNSTs are aggressive sarcomas that require multimodal management. There was a significantly increased risk of postoperative neurologic deficits in patients who

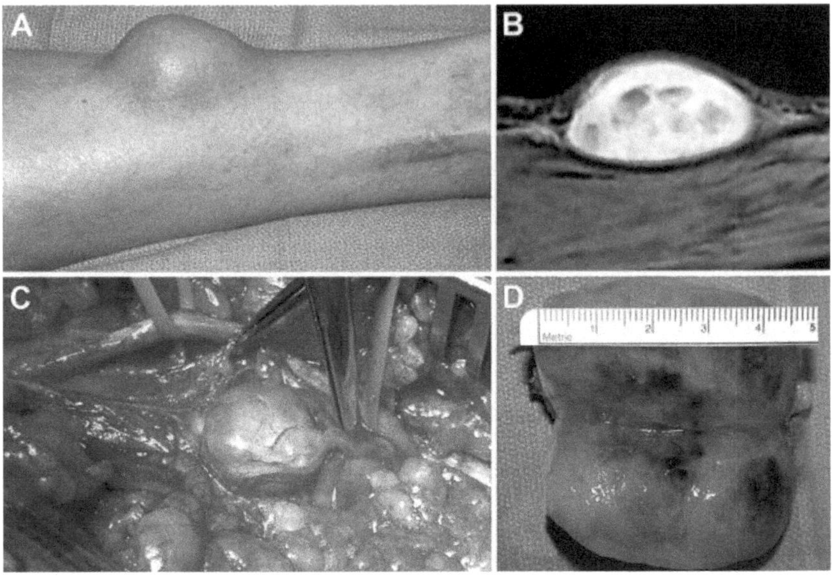

FIGURE 1.—Schwannoma associated with a sural nerve. **A**, photograph showing lobular appearance under the skin. **B**, magnetic resonance imaging (MRI) scan showing evidence of a string sign. **C**, intraoperative photograph from a different case illustrating the ease of dissection of the schwannoma from the associated nerve. **D**, photograph of cross section of a surgical specimen demonstrating a shiny appearance, with areas of hemorrhage and the parent nonfunctioning fascicle leaving and entering the nerve. (Reprinted from Levi AD, Ross AL, Cuartas E, et al. The surgical management of symptomatic peripheral nerve sheath tumors. *Neurosurgery*. 2010;66:833-840.)

had undergone a previous biopsy, and thus tertiary referral without biopsy is recommended when a PNST is suspected (Fig 1).

▶ Peripheral nerve sheath tumors (PNSTs) are a rare entity for neurosurgeons, unless they are at a large tertiary center or at a neurofibromatosis clinic. The authors present an excellent discussion of their experience managing PNSTs, both benign and malignant, over a 17-year period. They provide in-depth preoperative, intraoperative, and postoperative data. They had a total of 132 patients with 140 tumors: 87 schwannomas, 34 neurofibromas, and 19 malignant PNSTs (MPNSTs). Nearly two thirds of the patients with neurofibromas carried a diagnosis of neurofibromatosis type I (NF-1), and 25% of the MPNSTs presented in patients with NF-1.

The authors discuss several important points from their clinical experience. The first is the use of neuromonitoring. They used it relatively infrequently—18.4% of schwannoma cases and 38.2% of neurofibroma cases. The use of neuromonitoring was dependent on the year of surgery and the department performing the surgery (orthopedics vs neurosurgery). The authors found that among neurofibromas there was a decreased risk of developing a neurologic deficit with monitoring, but there was a greater incidence of residual tumor. If electrical stimulation of a nerve fascicle and adjoining tumor produced a motor response at 1 mA, the nerve was not sectioned and a small amount of tumor was left behind. Given the inability to distinguish schwannomas from neurofibromas radiographically or clinically (unless patient has NF-1), I would recommend motor stimulation with EMG on all patients. Neurofibromas, because of their growth pattern, will always be higher risk surgery, but the surrounding nerves may also be injured (although usually temporarily) causing motor or sensory deficits from dissection and manipulation, which can occur with either tumor, and is increased with previous surgery or biopsy at the surgical site—another point stressed by the authors.

Patients with MPNSTs continue to have a poor prognosis. Eighty percent of these patients presented with disease in advanced stage (IIb or higher), and all deaths occurred in patients who had tumors greater than 7 cm. Overall, 36.8% of patients with MPNSTs died at an average of 78 months postoperatively. An important point made by the authors is that if an MPNST is suspected, a biopsy is warranted (needle biopsy in the office). Features that were concerning for malignancy included severe or nocturnal pain, weight loss, itching, and rapid enlargement of the mass.

An interesting finding in this article is the low incidence of nerve sectioning during tumor removal, particularly with the benign tumors: 6.9% of schwannomas and 11.8% of neurofibromas. In my experience, I often find a single fascicle entering a schwannoma that is typically nonfunctional with stimulation and virtually impossible to dissect free from the mass as it enters one end and exits the enter, much in the way the authors show in Fig 1.

P. Klimo, Jr, MD, MPH

20 Spine

2009 ISSLS Prize Winner: Does Discography Cause Accelerated Progression of Degeneration Changes in the Lumbar Disc: A Ten-Year Matched Cohort Study

Carragee EJ, Don AS, Hurwitz EL, et al (Stanford Univ School of Medicine, CA; Univ of Hawaii at Mānoa, Honolulu; et al)

Spine 34:2338-2345, 2009

Study Design.—Prospective, match-cohort study of disc degeneration progression over 10 years with and without baseline discography.

Objectives.—To compare progression of common degenerative findings between lumbar discs injected 10 years earlier with those same disc levels in matched subjects not exposed to discography.

Summary of Background Data.—Experimental disc puncture in animal and in vivo studies have demonstrated accelerated disc degeneration. Whether intradiscal diagnostic or treatment procedures used in clinical practice causes any damage to the punctured discs over time is currently unknown.

Methods.—Seventy-five subjects without serious low back pain illness underwent a protocol MRI and an L3/4, L4/5, and L5/S1 discography examination in 1997. A matched group was enrolled at the same time and underwent the same protocol MRI examination. Subjects were followed for 10 years. At 7 to 10 years after baseline assessment, eligible discography and controlled subjects underwent another protocol MRI examination. MRI graders, blind to group designation, scored both groups for qualitative findings (Pfirrmann grade, herniations, endplate changes, and high intensity zone). Loss of disc height and loss of disc signal were measured by quantitative methods.

Results.—Well matched cohorts, including 50 discography subjects and 52 control subjects, were contacted and met eligibility criteria for follow-up evaluation. In all graded or measured parameters, discs that had been exposed to puncture and injection had greater progression of degenerative findings compared to control (noninjected) discs: progression of disc degeneration, 54 discs (35%) in the discography group compared to 21 (14%) in the control group ($P = 0.03$); 55 new disc herniations in the discography group compared to 22 in the control group ($P = 0.0003$). New disc herniations were disproportionately found on the side of the anular puncture ($P = 0.0006$). The quantitative measures of disc height and disc signal also showed significantly greater loss of disc height

($P = 0.05$) and signal intensity ($P = 0.001$) in the discography disc compared to the control disc.

Conclusion.—Modern discography techniques using small gauge needle and limited pressurization resulted in accelerated disc degeneration, disc herniation, loss of disc height and signal and the development of reactive endplate changes compared to match-controls. Careful consideration of risk and benefit should be used in recommending procedures involving disc injection.

▶ Diskography remains a controversial diagnostic test used by some practitioners to ascertain if a degenerated lumbar disk is a pain generator. In 1997, the authors performed MRI imaging and L3 to S1 diskography in 75 asymptomatic patients. Seventy-five matched patients underwent MRI imaging in 1997 and did not undergo diskography.

Ten years later, 50 patients in the diskography group and 52 patients in the control group underwent repeat MRI imaging. Progression of disk degeneration occurred in 35% of the disks in the diskography group versus 14% in the control group. Greater loss of disk height was also seen in the diskography group compared with the control group. Meanwhile, there was no significant radiographic difference between the 2 groups in the L1-2 and L2-3 levels (these levels were not injected in either group).

This study raises the concern that disk degeneration may occur in some patients as a result of diskography. All physicians that use diskography should read this article and reevaluate the risks and possible benefits of this controversial procedure. For those who continue to use diskography I encourage practitioners to discuss the results of this article with their patients as part of the informed consent process.

R. Riesenburger, MD

A Comparison of Posterolateral Lumbar Fusion Comparing Autograft, Autogenous Laminectomy Bone With Bone Marrow Aspirate, and Calcium Sulphate With Bone Marrow Aspirate: A Prospective Randomized Study

Niu C-C, Tsai T-T, Fu T-S, et al (Chang Gung Univ College of Medicine, Taoyuan, Taiwan)

Spine 34:2715-2719, 2009

Study Design.—A prospective clinical study.

Objective.—To evaluate whether the fusion rate of autogenous laminectomy bone chips and calcium sulfate pellets could be augmented by bone marrow aspirate (BMA) in one-level lumbar posterolateral fusion.

Summary of Background Data.—An *in vivo* animal study has indicated that BMA augments spinal arthrodesis.

Methods.—Forty-three patients undergoing surgery for instrumented one-level fusion with decompression were divided into 2 groups. Autologous iliac crest bone graft (ICBG) was placed in 1 posterolateral gutter (control), while on the other side (test), an equal quantity of laminectomy bone chips mixed with BMA while harvesting the iliac bone graft (group 1) or an equal quantity of calcium sulfate pellets soaked in BMA (group 2) was placed. Radiographic assessment was performed every 3 months (3–12 months) and then annually. The statuses of fusion on either side of the vertebra were compared.

Results.—For the 21 patients in group 1, 18 (85.7%) exhibited bone fusion on the test side, and 19 (90.5%) presented evidence of fusion on the control side. Thus, the test side with laminectomy bone chips and BMA achieved a fusion rate similar to that on the control side ($P > 0.05$). For the 22 patients in group 2, 20 (90.9%) exhibited bone fusion on the control side whereas only 10 (45.5%) demonstrated complete fusion on the test side ($P < 0.05$), where calcium sulfate and BMA was applied.

Conclusion.—ICBG performs as expected with high fusion rates and laminectomy bone with BMA performs equally as well. Osteoset is significantly inferior to ICBG despite the addition of BMA, which is osteoinductive and has improved fusion rates and osteogenesis in other models.

▶ This prospective study compared lumbar intertransverse arthrodesis rates of 3 different techniques: (1) autologous iliac crest bone graft, (2) autologous laminectomy bone chips harvested intraoperatively mixed with iliac crest bone marrow aspirate, and (3) calcium sulfate pellets mixed with iliac crest bone marrow aspirate. These 3 different arthrodesis techniques were used in 43 patients undergoing simultaneous decompression and pedicle screw instrumentation for lumbar stenosis with grade I or II spondylolisthesis.

The authors noted successful arthrodesis rates as follows: just under 91% for autologous iliac crest bone graft, 85.7% for autologous laminectomy bone chips harvested intraoperatively mixed with iliac crest bone marrow aspirate, and 45.5% for calcium sulfate pellets mixed with iliac crest bone marrow aspirate. There was no statistically significant difference when comparing fusion rates between the iliac crest bone graft group and the laminectomy bone chip/iliac crest bone marrow aspirate group.

This small study suggests that rates of arthrodesis for locally harvested vertebral autograft mixed with iliac crest bone marrow aspirate and for iliac crest bone graft (the current gold standard for arthrodesis) are similar. Using locally harvested vertebral autograft mixed with iliac crest bone marrow aspirate that can be aspirated with a Jamshidi needle through a tiny separate incision has 2 major advantages: (1) it avoids the morbidity of iliac crest bone graft harvest, and (2) it avoids the costs of commercially available bone graft substitutes/extenders. This method of arthrodesis warrants more studies to confirm the results of this article.

R. Riesenburger, MD

A Randomized Trial of Vertebroplasty for Painful Osteoporotic Vertebral Fractures

Buchbinder R, Osborne RH, Ebeling PR, et al (Monash Univ, Malvern, Australia; Deakin Univ, Melbourne, Australia; Univ of Melbourne Western Hosp, Footscray, Australia; et al)

N Engl J Med 361:557-568, 2009

Background.—Vertebroplasty has become a common treatment for painful osteoporotic vertebral fractures, but there is limited evidence to support its use.

Methods.—We performed a multicenter, randomized, double-blind, placebo-controlled trial in which participants with one or two painful osteoporotic vertebral fractures that were of less than 12 months' duration and unhealed, as confirmed by magnetic resonance imaging, were randomly assigned to undergo vertebroplasty or a sham procedure. Participants were stratified according to treatment center, sex, and duration of symptoms (<6 weeks or ≥6 weeks). Outcomes were assessed at 1 week and at 1, 3, and 6 months. The primary outcome was overall pain (on a scale of 0 to 10, with 10 being the maximum imaginable pain) at 3 months.

Results.—A total of 78 participants were enrolled, and 71 (35 of 38 in the vertebroplasty group and 36 of 40 in the placebo group) completed the 6-month follow-up (91%). Vertebroplasty did not result in a significant advantage in any measured outcome at any time point. There were significant reductions in overall pain in both study groups at each follow-up assessment. At 3 months, the mean (±SD) reductions in the score for pain in the vertebroplasty and control groups were 2.6±2.9 and 1.9±3.3, respectively (adjusted between-group difference, 0.6; 95% confidence interval, −0.7 to 1.8). Similar improvements were seen in both groups with respect to pain at night and at rest, physical functioning, quality of life, and perceived improvement. Seven incident vertebral fractures (three in the vertebroplasty group and four in the placebo group) occurred during the 6-month follow-up period.

Conclusions.—We found no beneficial effect of vertebroplasty as compared with a sham procedure in patients with painful osteoporotic vertebral fractures, at 1 week or at 1, 3, or 6 months after treatment. (Australian New Zealand Clinical Trials Registry number, ACTRN012605000079640.)

▶ In this multicenter, randomized, double-blind study, vertebroplasty showed no benefit compared with a sham procedure. Seventy-eight patients with painful compression fractures less than 1-year-old were randomized to percutaneous vertebroplasty with a 13-gauge needle or to a sham intervention. The percutaneous vertebroplasty was done via the standard transpedicular route with approximately 3 mL of polymethylmethacrylate injected into the vertebral body. The sham procedure started with infiltration of the skin and periosteum of the posterior lamina and was followed by insertion of a 13-gauge needle that rested on the lamina. To be sure the patient remained blinded, the radiologist gently tapped on the needle and prepared the polymethylmethacrylate so the smell permeated the room.

Seventy-one of the 78 patients completed the 6-month study. Significant pain relief was observed in both groups at 1 week, 1 month, 3 months, and 6 months after treatment. When comparing the 2 groups, there was no significant difference in pain scores, quality of life, or perceived improvement.

This study concludes that vertebroplasty has no benefit over a sham procedure, suggesting a possible placebo effect. Since the publication of this article, I have become more conservative in the management of osteoporotic vertebral body compression fractures. I prefer managing these patients nonoperatively for at least 12 weeks. For patients with debilitating pain who fail to improve after 3 months, I offer vertebroplasty as a treatment option. I then review the findings of this article with the patient as part of the informed consent process.

R. Riesenburger, MD

An Anatomic Study of the S2 Iliac Technique for Lumbopelvic Screw Placement

O'Brien JR, Yu WD, Bhatnagar R, et al (George Washington Univ, DC; et al)

Spine 34:E439-E442, 2009

Study Design.—An anatomic study conducted on cadaveric specimens.

Objectives.—The objectives of the study were (1) to determine course of S2 lumbopelvic screws with reference to the articular cartilage of the sacroiliac joint, (2) to determine the length and trajectory of screws placed using anatomic placement techniques, and (3) to determine vital structures at risk using this technique.

Summary of Background Data.—Multiple techniques exist for fixation distal to S1 including alar screws, iliac post bolts, and transiliac rods. Distal fixation is crucial in adult deformity surgery when fusion to the sacrum is indicated.

Methods.—Five female and 5 male cadaveric specimens were instrumented with S1 promontory screws and S2 iliac lumbopelvic screws. The specimens then underwent computed tomography scanning to determine structures at risk, cortical violations, and characteristics of screws placed. The sacroiliac joints were opened to examine articular cartilage penetration.

Results.—Articular violation occurred in 60% of screws placed. Average length was 84 mm. No vital structures were at risk from screw placement. No intrapelvic cortical violations occurred.

Conclusion.—S2 iliac technique is a potential option for distal fixation in spine surgery. Biomechanical and clinical data are required to fully evaluate the potential of this technique.

▶ This cadaveric article describes the technique used to place an S2 sacroiliac screw. The starting point for this screw is 1 mm inferior and 1 mm lateral to the

S1 dorsal foramen. A drill or gearshift is advanced from this point laterally into the S2 sacral ala until the sacroiliac joint (SI) joint is encountered. Drilling is then continued into the ileum. The average screw length placed into the cadaveric specimens was 84 mm.

I recommend that surgeons doing scoliosis surgery or complex lumbosacral revision surgery should become familiar with this technique. This screw has some possible advantages when compared with traditional iliac screw fixation techniques: (1) Less soft tissue dissection is necessary to place a S2 sacroiliac screw. (2) The screw head is in-line with the S1 pedicle screw head, which makes rod placement easier. (3) The portal of entry is via the sacral ala rather than the iliac crest, and thus does not interfere with iliac crest bone graft harvest.

The authors do admit that this technique needs to be studied further. The biomechanical strength of this screw has not been evaluated. In addition, this screw violates the articular cartilage of the SI joint 60% of the time. While traditional iliac screws do not violate this cartilage, they do cross the sacroiliac articulation. We currently do not know if there is a difference between the 2 techniques on the long-term effects of the SI. This certainly warrants additional study.

R. Riesenburger, MD

Comparison of thoracolumbosacral orthosis and no orthosis for the treatment of thoracolumbar burst fractures: interim analysis of a multicenter randomized clinical equivalence trial

Bailey CS, Dvorak MF, Thomas KC, et al (Univ of Western Ontario, London, Canada; Univ of British Columbia, Vancouver, Canada; Univ of Calgary, Alberta, Canada; et al)

J Neurosurg Spine 11:295-303, 2009

Object.—The authors compared the outcome of patients with thoracolumbar burst fractures treated with and without a thoracolumbosacral orthosis (TLSO).

Methods.—As of June 2002, all consecutive patients satisfying the following inclusion criteria were considered eligible for this study: 1) the presence of an AO Classification Type A3 burst fractures between T-11 and L-3, 2) skeletal maturity and age < 60 years, 3) admission within 72 hours of injury, 4) initial kyphotic deformity <35° , and 5) no neurological deficit. The study was designed as a multicenter prospective randomized clinical equivalence trial. The primary outcome measure was the score based on the Roland-Morris Disability Questionnaire assessed at 3 months postinjury. Secondary outcomes are assessed until 2 years of follow-up have been reached, and these domains included pain, functional outcome and generic health-related quality of life, sagittal alignment, length of hospital stay, and complications. Patients in whom no orthotic was used were encouraged to ambulate immediately following randomization, maintaining "neutral spinal alignment" for 8 weeks. The patients in the TLSO group began being weaned from the brace at 8 weeks over a 2-week period.

Results.—Sixty-nine patients were followed to the primary outcome time point, and 47 were followed for up to 1 year. No significant difference was found between treatment groups for any outcome measure at any stage in the follow-up period. There were 4 failures requiring surgical intervention, 3 in the TLSO group and 1 in the non-TLSO group.

Conclusions.—This interim analysis found equivalence between treatment with a TLSO and no orthosis for thoracolumbar AO Type A3 burst fractures. The influence of a brace on early pain control and function and on long-term 1- and 2-year outcomes remains to be determined. However, the authors contend that a thoracolumbar burst fracture, in exclusion of an associated posterior ligamentous complex injury, is inherently a very stable injury and may not require a brace.

▶ In this study, the authors recruited 72 patients with AO classification type A3 burst fractures. (Type A3 fractures are burst fractures caused by axial loading without injury to the posterior ligaments.) Half of these patients were treated with a thoracolumbosacral orthosis (TLSO). The remaining patients were mobilized without bracing. In this interim analysis, the authors report 1-year outcomes in 47 patients (24 in the TLSO group, 23 in the non-TLSO group). No statistically significant difference in outcomes was noted between the 2 groups. Four patients required early surgery before hospital discharge secondary to severe radicular or mechanical pain that prevented meaningful mobilization (3 in the TLSO group, 1 in the nonTLSO group).

The authors reinforce that this is an interim analysis and that final outcomes have not yet been determined. However, this preliminary analysis certainly suggests that TLSO bracing may be unnecessary for this patient population.

I admittedly place all patients with this type of injury in a TLSO brace for 3 months. Most patients find the brace uncomfortable, especially during hot summer weather. During follow-up visits, they often complain more about the brace than they do about the pain from the original injury. I therefore look forward to the final analysis of this study. If the final outcomes are similar to the interim outcomes, we can save these patients the morbidity of orthosis treatment.

R. Riesenburger, MD

Risedronate decreases bone resorption and improves low back pain in postmenopausal osteoporosis patients without vertebral fractures

Ohtori S, Akazawa T, Murata Y, et al (Chiba Univ, Japan; Chiba East Hosp, Japan; Shimoshizu Natl Hosp, Chiba, Japan; et al)

J Clin Neurosci 17:209-213, 2010

Elderly postmenopausal women who have osteoporosis sometimes experience low back pain, however, the relationship between low back pain and osteoporosis in the absence of vertebral fractures remains unclear. We examined the relationship between bone mineral density (BMD), bone resorption and low back pain in elderly female patients who did not have osteoporotic vertebral fractures. The average BMD was 0.675 g/cm^2 when assessed by dual-energy X-ray absorptiometry (DEXA). Patients were excluded from the study if they had vertebral fractures revealed by radiography, CT scans or MRI. Bisphosphonate (risedronate) was administered for 4 months. The visual analogue scale (VAS) pain score, Roland Morris Disability Questionnaire (RDQ), Short Form-36 (SF-36) questionnaire, BMD and N-terminal telopeptide of type I collagen (NTx; a marker for bone resorption) were examined before and after treatment. DEXA did not increase significantly, but serum and urinary NTx were decreased (−51.4% and −62.0%, respectively) after 4 months of risedronate treatment ($p < 0.01$). The assessment was repeated using the VAS score, RDQ and SF-36, which revealed an improvement after risedronate treatment ($p < 0.01$). A decrease in serum and urinary NTx was associated with improvement of low back pain, suggesting that despite the absence of vertebral fractures, bone resorption due to osteoporosis may cause low back pain.

▶ Low back pain in osteoporotic women without compression fractures is a common condition. Physical therapy and nonsteroidal anti-inflammatory drugs (NSAIDs) are first-line treatment options. If these fail to help, there is not much else currently available to offer these patients.

The authors of this study prospectively treated 27 postmenopausal women with once daily oral risedronate (a bisphosphonate) for 4 months. All patients had osteoporosis and low back pain refractory to NSAID treatment. None of the patients had compression fractures.

After 4 months of treatment, there were statistically significant improvements in visual analogue scale pain scores, Roland Morris Disability Questionnaire scores, and all 8 categories of the Short Form-36 questionnaire.

This study suggests that risedronate treatment may be helpful for back pain in osteoporotic postmenopausal women. The major weakness of this study is the absence of a control group. Therefore, it is difficult to assess how much of a placebo effect occurred with risedronate treatment. Hopefully, the authors will organize a randomized study with a control group to further test the effects of risedronate for back pain in this patient population.

R. Riesenburger, MD

21 Surgical Techniques

"Q-tip" Retractor in Endoscopic Cranial Base Surgery

Prevedello DM, Kassam AB, Gardner P, et al (Univ of Pittsburgh, School of Medicine, PA; Saint John's Health Ctr, Santa Monica, CA; et al)

Neurosurgery 66:363-367, 2010

Objective.—A practical alternative for endonasal retraction is presented.

Technique.—Following 100 endoscopic endonasal procedures at the University of Pittsburgh, a simple alternative for gentle tissue retraction was introduced for endoscopic endonasal procedures: the "Q-tip" cotton swab. Its fine shape allows it to be inserted through one of the nostrils, sharing the space with the other instruments and the endoscope while preserving freedom of movement. Its long dimension allows it to reach deep areas while it is actively held by one of the surgeons, and its stiffness allows more or less force to be applied in any direction. Its soft head permits gentle touch of retraction without causing injury to the noble neurovascular structures of the cranial base.

Conclusion.—During endoscopic endonasal surgery, the instruments are operated through the nostrils, which are restricted passages. Any retractor utilized has to be thin to share the space with the other instruments, long enough to reach the cranial base, and soft to avoid tissue damage. All of these characteristics were encountered in the "Q-tip" cotton swab.

▶ The authors of this article report a simple but useful technique for effective retraction in endoscopic skull base surgery. In performing endoscopic skull base procedures, particularly with a 3-hand or 4-hand bi-nostril technique with 2 surgeons (mainly a neurosurgeon and an otolaryngologist), there is often competition for working space through narrow working passages. The Q-tip allows for gentle touch retraction of critical neurovascular structures with low risk of injury. This is also a very cost-effective tool.

J. K. Liu, MD

Janus flap: Bilateral nasoseptal flaps for anterior skull base reconstruction

Nyquist GG, Anand VK, Singh A, et al (New York Presbyterian Hosp)

Otolaryngol Head Neck Surg 142:327-331, 2010

Objective.—Large dural defects after extended endoscopic endonasal skull base resections require meticulous reconstruction to prevent a cerebrospinal fluid leak postoperatively. The nasoseptal flap is a vascularized tissue graft developed to aid in the multilayer reconstruction of the skull base. The purpose of this study is to describe the first experiences with bilateral nasoseptal flaps for reconstruction of very large skull base defects.

Study Design.—Prospective, observational study.

Setting.—Large tertiary referral center (New York Presbyterian Hospital).

Subjects and Methods.—Five patients underwent a multilayer reconstruction after an extended endoscopic transsphenoidal skull base surgery that included bilateral nasoseptal flaps. Pathologies consisted of two pituitary macroadenomas, one planum sphenoidale meningioma, one craniopharyngioma, and one cavernous sinus hemangioma.

Results.—All five patients underwent successful skull base reconstruction without a cerebrospinal fluid leak, complication at the reconstruction site, or anterior extension of the posterior septal perforation.

Conclusion.—Bilateral nasoseptal flaps are a viable option for large dural defects of the anterior and ventral skull base when one nasoseptal flap may not completely seal the entire defect.

▶ The authors here describe a novel technique for reconstructing large anterior skull base defects after endoscopic cranial base surgery. Usually, 1 nasoseptal flap can cover large skull base defects as long as the flap is maximized anteriorly toward the nostril and also laterally along the floor of the nose. In some instances, however, the surface area of the nasoseptal flap can be compromised by tumor involvement, and additional vascularized tissue may need to be mobilized from another source to reconstruct the skull base defect. Using the remaining contralateral nasoseptal flap allows additional coverage of the remaining defect, the so-called Janus flap technique.

J. K. Liu, MD

Limitations of the transcallosal transchoroidal approach to the third ventricle

Ulm AJ, Russo A, Albanese E, et al (Mercer Univ School of Medicine, Macon, GA; et al)

J Neurosurg 111:600-609, 2009

Object.—The aim of this study was to determine the anatomical limitations of the transcallosal transchoroidal approach to the third ventricle.

Methods.—Twenty-six formalin-fixed specimens were studied. Sagittal dissections were used to determine the anatomical relationships of the foramen of Monro, the angle of approach to landmarks, and placement of a callosotomy. Lateral ventricular dissections were performed to quantitate the forniceal anatomy.

Results.—The foramen of Monro was found 1.07 ± 0.11 cm superior and slightly anterior to the mammillary bodies, 1.48 ± 0.16 cm posterosuperior to the optic recess, and 2.26 ± 0.16 cm anterosuperior to the aqueduct. Relative to the genu, a callosal incision 2.64 ± 0.53 cm long and angled 37 ± 4.3° anterior was needed to access the aqueduct, and an incision 4.92 ± 0.71 cm long and angled 49 ± 7.4° posterior was needed to access the optic recess. The fornix progressively widened within the lateral ventricle, from 1.25 ± 0.63 mm at the foramen of Monro to > 7 mm at 2 cm behind the foramen. Three zones of exposure were identified, requiring unique craniotomies, callosotomies, and angles of approach. The major limiting factors in the approach included the columns of the fornix anteriorly, the width of the fornix posteriorly, and the draining veins of the parietal cortex. The choroidal fissure opening was limited to 1.5 cm posterior to the foramen of Monro; this limited opening created an aperture effect that required an anteriorto-posterior angle, an anterior craniotomy, and an anteriorly placed callosotomy to access the posterior landmarks. In contrast, a posterior-to-anterior angle, posteriorly placed craniotomy, and posteriorly placed callosotomy were required to access anterior landmarks.

Conclusions.—The transcallosal transchoroidal approach was ideally suited to access the foramen of Monro and the middle and posterior thirds of the third ventricle. Exposure of the anterior third ventricle was limited by the columns of the fornix and by the presence of parietal cortical draining veins.

▶ This is an excellent article that reviews in detail the anatomy of the third ventricle and the transcallosal-transchoroidal approach. The major limitations are as follows:

(1) The width of the fornix. The body of the fornix progressively widens posteriorly from the foramen of Monro. According to the measurements provided by the authors, it is about 1.25 mm in width just behind the foramen and greater than 7 mm at 2 cm posterior to the foramen. The wider the fornix, the more it would need to be retracted in order to continue to access the third ventricle, thus placing it at risk for injury. Therefore, the choroidal fissure, in the authors' opinion, should not be opened more than 1.5 cm posterior to the foramen of Monro.

(2) The forniceal columns prevent access to the third ventricle anterior to the foramen of Monro. Therefore, access to the anterior third ventricle in front of the columns of the fornix and beneath the lamina terminalis is not possible without sacrificing the column of the fornix.

(3) The typical site at which the corpus callosum is incised is about 2.5 cm behind the genu. This will provide access to the middle portion of the third ventricle around the foramen of Monro. To gain access to the anterior portion of the third ventricle, the incision through the corpus callosum would need to be made more posteriorly. Conversely, access to the

posterior portion of the third ventricle will require a more anteriorly placed corpus callosum entry. Fig 8 in the original article shows these trajectories. Although the angles vary depending on which part of the third ventricle requires access, they all use the same 1.5-cm choroidal fissure opening as discussed above. The surgeon must keep in mind that the greater the corpus callosum incision, greater is the risk of developing disconnection syndrome postoperatively. This usually does not happen if the incision is kept to less than 22 mm.

P. Klimo, Jr, MD, MPH

Middle Turbinate Flap for Skull Base Reconstruction: Cadaveric Feasibility Study

Prevedello DM, Barges-Coll J, Fernandez-Miranda JC, et al (Univ of Pittsburgh School of Medicine, PA; et al)
Laryngoscope 119:2094-2098, 2009

Objectives/Hypothesis.—Surgical resection of intradural pathology through an endonasal corridor creates defects that communicate the subarachnoid space with the sinonasal tract. Reconstruction of these defects with vascularized tissue is superior to any other method. The purpose of this study is to describe a novel vascularized pedicled flap from the middle turbinate (MT) mucosa and to assess its feasibility using a cadaveric model.

Methods.—Twelve middle turbinate flaps (MTFs) were raised in six fresh cadaveric heads previously injected with colored silicone. Arteries supplying the MT were identified as the turbinate mucoperiosteum was harvested from both its medial and lateral aspects. Length and surface area of the flaps, as well as their ability to cover dural defects of the sella, planum sphenoidale, and fovea ethmoidalis reach were noted.

Results.—All MTFs adequately covered defects of the planum and fovea ethmoidalis; however, two of the twelve MTFs were not suitable to cover a sellar defect. The mean surface area of the MTFs was 5.6 cm^2. As an independent factor surface area did not correlate with the ability of the flap to cover the sellar defects. However, those flaps that were not suitable for sellar repair were less than 4.0 cm in length.

Conclusions.—Harvesting of a vascular pedicle flap from the MT is feasible, albeit technically demanding. It should be considered as an alternative for the reconstruction of small defects of the fovea ethmoidalis, planum, and sella, particularly for patients for whom a reconstruction with vascularized tissue is desirable but the nasoseptal flap is not available.

▶ The authors describe an alternative skull base reconstruction technique after expanded endonasal endoscopic surgery using a vascularized pedicled flap from the middle turbinate. Feasibility was demonstrated anatomically in a cadaver model. This can be a useful technique if the nasoseptal flap is not available due to destruction by the existing tumor or if its vascular pedicle has been compromised. The major limitation of the middle turbinate flap is the size of the flap (mean surface area 5.6 cm^2), which is probably most suitable for smaller skull base defects.

J. K. Liu, MD

Occipital transtentorial approach to the precentral cerebellar fissure and posterior incisural space

Moshel YA, Parker EC, Kelly PJ (New York Univ School of Medicine)
Neurosurgery 65:554-564, 2009

Objective.—To describe the surgical techniques and postoperative clinical outcomes with the occipital transtentorial (OT) approach in patients harboring lesions arising from the precentral cerebellar fissure, posterior incisural space, and adjoining structures.

Methods.—Twenty-two patients underwent microsurgical resection of intra-axial lesions arising within the precentral cerebellar fissure and posterior incisural space between 1997 and 2006. Patient demographics, presenting symptoms, pathology, and neurological outcomes were retrospectively reviewed. Pre- and postoperative magnetic resonance imaging scans were evaluated to determine the anatomic extensions of the lesion and the degree of surgical resection. Patients with lesions primarily confined to the pineal and posterior third ventricle approached by a supracerebellar infratentorial trajectory were excluded from this study.

Results.—Of the 22 patients reported in this series, 17 (77%) had contrast-enhancing lesions, and 5 (23%) had nonenhancing lesions arising from the precentral cerebellar fissure and posterior incisural space. The lesions were oriented dorsomedial to the midbrain and diencephalon in 6 patients (27%), dorsolateral in 14 patients (64%), and lateral in 2 patients (9%). A lateral OT approach directed under the occipitotemporal junction was used in 16 patients (73%), and an interhemispheric OT approach was used in 6 patients (27%). Transient visual field loss occurred in 3 patients (14%); it resolved by the third follow-up month. Gross total resection or near-total resection of the imaging-defined lesion volume was achieved in 19 patients (86%).

Conclusion.—The OT approaches provide excellent exposure for lesions of the precentral cerebellar fissure, posterior incisural space, and adjacent structures. The lateral OT approach directed under the occipitotemporal junction provides an inline view for lesions situated posterolateral to the brainstem. It also provides an inferiorly directed view under the venous system into the precentral cerebellar fissure and fourth ventricular roof. Visual field deficits are minimized by directing the trajectory under the occipitotemporal junction instead of retracting along the interhemispheric corridor. The interhemispheric OT approach was primarily used for lesions extending superiorly, in the midline or near midline, above the tentorium and venous system into the splenium of corpus

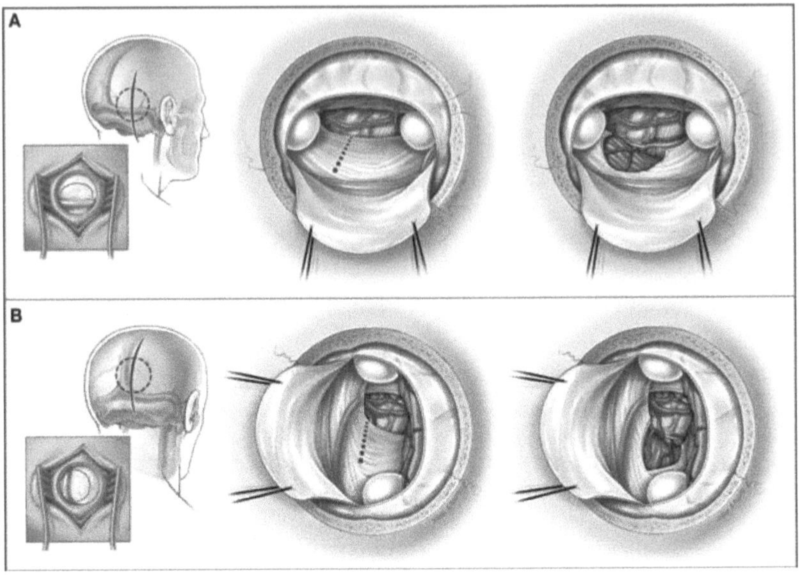

FIGURE 1.—Drawings depicting the lateral (top row) and interhemispheric (bottom row) occipital transtentorial (OT) approach (see Patients and Methods for details). (Courtesy of Moshel YA, Parker EC, Kelly PJ. Occipital transtentorial approach to the precentral cerebellar fissure and posterior incisural space. *Neurosurgery.* 2009;65:554-564.)

callosum, lateral ventricle, and posterior thalamus, where extensive lateral retraction was not required (Fig 1).

▶ The authors describe their experience using 2 occipital transtentorial approaches—the interhemispheric and the lateral—to gain access to the posterior incisural area and the precentral cerebellar fissure, otherwise known as the cerebellomesencephalic fissure, which extends between the cerebellum and the midbrain. Lesions appropriate for these approaches, according to the authors, are those that are located dorsolateral to the brainstem or extend superiorly, above the tentorium and venous system, into the lateral ventricle, posterior thalamus, medial temporal lobe, or splenium of the corpus callosum.

The interhemispheric approach is the one that most surgeons are familiar with and has been classically described for posterior third ventricular or pineal region tumors. The lateral occipital transtentorial approach is less well described. The lateral approach was used for dorsolaterally situated lesions in the midbrain, thalamus, or medial temporal lobe. The lateral approach has the advantage of obtaining exposure by elevating the occipitotemporal junction, thus minimizing the potential visual field deficits compared with the occipital pole retraction required for the interhemispheric approach.

There were several key or unique steps described by the authors (Fig 1). They obtained a preoperative angiogram in all their patients in order to stereotactically plan surgical corridors that would avoid any large cortical veins draining into the tentorial or lateral sinus. This stereotactic guidance allowed the surgeons to make a 50-mm craniotomy for either approach. In my opinion, depending on the lesion configuration, I would not hesitate to make a larger craniotomy, even one that would accommodate both the lateral and interhemispheric trajectories. I don't feel that an angiogram is necessary in all patients. Furthermore, there are few, if any, draining veins into the lateral sinus or posterior superior sagittal sinus. The authors were meticulous in minimizing retraction-induced brain injury. The use of metal retractors was avoided in all cases. Three patients did suffer temporary visual field deficits. The tentorial incision, particularly with the lateral variant, was done only after the trochlear nerve was identified and dissected free from the tentorial edge.

This is a well-written article on surgical techniques for lesions identified by the authors and will introduce many readers to the lateral occipital transtentorial approach.

P. Klimo, Jr, MD, MPH

Supracerebellar Infratentorial Approach to Cavernous Malformations of the Brainstem: Surgical Variants and Clinical Experience With 45 Patients

de Oliveira JG, Lekovic GP, Safavi-Abbasi S, et al (St Joseph's Hosp and Med Ctr, Phoenix, AZ)
Neurosurgery 66:389-399, 2010

Objective.—The supracerebellar infratentorial (SCIT) approach can be performed at the midline (median variant), lateral to the midline (paramedian variant), or at the level of the angle formed by the transverse and sigmoid sinuses (extreme lateral variant). We analyzed our experience with SCIT approaches for the surgical treatment of cavernous malformations of the brainstem (CMBs).

Methods.—Demographic, clinical, radiologic, and surgical data from 45 patients (20 males and 25 females; mean age, 36.2 years) with CMBs surgically removed through SCIT approaches were reviewed retrospectively. Anatomic information was explored using cadaver head dissection.

Results.—Twenty-three lesions were in the midbrain, 3 were at the midbrain and extended to the thalamus, 9 were at the pontomesencephalic junction, and 10 were in the upper pons. All patients presented with hemorrhage. The median variant was used in 13 patients, the paramedian variant in 9, and the extreme lateral variant in 23. Intraoperatively, all CMBs were associated with a developmental venous anomaly. At last follow-up, 88% of the patients were the same or better. After a mean follow-up of 20 months, their mean Glasgow Outcome Scale score was 4.1.

Conclusion.—SCIT approaches provide excellent exposure to CMBs located at the posterior incisural space, not only in the midline but also in the posterolateral surface of the upper pons and midbrain. Careful preoperative planning and neuronavigational assistance are needed to determine the best angle of attack and trajectory for SCIT approaches.

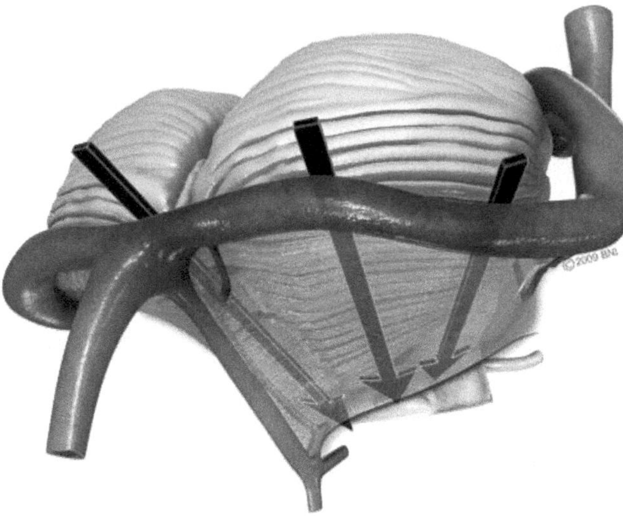

FIGURE 2.—Illustrative drawing showing the trajectories of attack for median (left arrow), paramedian (middle arrow) and extreme lateral (right arrow) variants of SCIT approach. (Used with permission from Barrow Neurological Institute.) (Reprinted from de Oliveira JG, Lekovic GP, Safavi-Abbasi S, et al. Supracerebellar infratentorial approach to cavernous malformations of the brainstem: surgical variants and clinical experience with 45 patients. *Neurosurgery*. 2010;66:389-399.)

Refined microsurgical techniques are paramount to achieve safe surgical removal of CMBs with good outcomes.

▶ This article is one of many excellent surgical approach articles published by the Barrow Neurological Institute group. They report their clinical experience using the 3 variants of the supracerebellar/infratentorial approach to cavernomas located on the posterolateral surface of the upper pons and midbrain: the median, paramedian, and extreme lateral variants (Fig 2). There were 45 patients over a 16-year period, with each patient harboring 1 brainstem cavernoma. A patient was considered for surgical treatment when 1 or more of the following criteria were met: (1) The lesion abutted the pial surface or was exophytic; (2) The lesion produced repeated hemorrhages causing progressive neurologic deficits; (3) Acute hemorrhage extended outside the lesion capsule; and (4) A significant mass effect was produced by a large intralesional hemorrhage. The authors discuss each approach in detail with excellent drawings, cadaveric photos, and MRI images of case examples.

All brainstem cavernomas were associated with developmental venous anomalies that were preserved. Among 45 patients, 20 patients (44%) had new postoperative deficits. Three patients developed hydrocephalus requiring a shunt or had cerebrospinal fluid leaks. Four patients required placement of a midterm tracheostomy and feeding tube. All patients had a gross total resection on the immediate postoperative MRI study, but after a mean follow-up of 37.4 months, 7 patients presented with a recurrence and 4 of these patients required a reoperation.

P. Klimo, Jr, MD, MPH

Article Index

Chapter 1: Alzheimer's Disease and Dementia

Chapter 2: Cerebrovascular Disease

Chapter 3: Epilepsy and Other Seizure Disorders

Chapter 4: Headache

Chapter 5: Infectious Diseases of the Nervous System

Chapter 6: Miscellaneous

Chapter 7: Movement Disorders

Chapter 8: Neoplastic Disease

Chapter 9: Neuromuscular Disease

Chapter 10: Neuro-ophthalmology

Chapter 11: Neuroradiology

Chapter 12: Pediatric Neurology

Chapter 13: Sleep Disorders

Chapter 14: Brain Tumors

Chapter 15: Cerebrovascular

Chapter 16: Functional

Chapter 17: Miscellaneous

Chapter 18: Pediatric Neurosurgery

Chapter 19: Peripheral Nerve Surgery

Chapter 20: Spine

Chapter 21: Surgical Techniques

Author Index

A

B

C

D

E

FSC
www.fsc.org
MIX
Papier | Fördert gute Waldnutzung
FSC® C083411

Kolibri 360 GmbH
Ferdinand-Jühlke-Straße 7
99095 Erfurt, Deutschland
produktsicherheit@kolibri360.de